To

From the:
- Borzi's
- McClay's
- Poitras'
- Thomas'
- Zebrowski's.

Good luck!!!

OTHER MONOGRAPHS IN THE SERIES,
MAJOR PROBLEMS IN PATHOLOGY

Published

Evans and Cruickshank: *Epithelial Tumours of the Salivary Glands*

Mottet: *Histopathologic Spectrum of Regional Enteritis and Ulcerative Colitis*

Whitehead: *Mucosal Biopsy of the Gastrointestinal Tract*

Hughes: *Pathology of Muscle*

Thurlbeck: *Chronic Airflow Obstruction in Lung Disease*

Hughes: *Pathology of the Spinal Cord*

Fox: *Pathology of the Placenta*

Forthcoming

Asbury and Johnson: *Pathology of Peripheral Nerve*

Hartsock: *Diagnostic Histopathology of Lymph Nodes*

Kempson: *Pathology of the Uterine Corpus*

Lee and Ellis: *Bone Marrow Biopsy Pathology*

Mackay: *Soft Tissue Tumors*

Morson et al.: *Polyps and Cancer of the Colon and Rectum*

Newton and Hamoudi: *Histiocytosis*

Sagebiel: *Histopathologic Diagnosis of Melanotic Lesions of Skin*

Smith: *Diagnostic Pathology of the Mouth and Jaws*

GARY E. STRIKER, M.D.
Professor of Pathology
University of Washington School of Medicine
Seattle, Washington

LEONARD J. QUADRACCI, M.D.
Associate Professor of Medicine and Pathology
University of Washington School of Medicine
Seattle, Washington

RALPH E. CUTLER, M.D.
Professor of Medicine
University of Washington School of Medicine
Seattle, Washington

USE AND INTERPRETATION OF RENAL BIOPSY

Volume 8 in the Series
MAJOR PROBLEMS IN PATHOLOGY
JAMES L. BENNINGTON, M.D., *Consulting Editor*
Chairman, Department of Pathology
Children's Hospital of San Francisco
San Francisco, California

W. B. Saunders Company, Philadelphia, London, Toronto, 1978

W. B. Saunders Company: West Washington Square
Philadelphia, PA 19105

1 St. Anne's Road
Eastbourne, East Sussex BN21 3UN, England

1 Goldthorne Avenue
Toronto, Ontario M8Z 5T9, Canada

Use and Interpretation of Renal Biopsy ISBN 0-7216-8620-6

© 1978 by W. B. Saunders Company. Copyright under the International Copyright Union. All rights reserved. This book is protected by copyright. No part of it may be reproduced, stored in a retrieval system, or transmitted in any form or by any means, electronic, mechanical, photocopying, recording or otherwise, without written permission from the publisher. Made in the United States of America. Press of W. B. Saunders Company. Library of Congress catalog card number 76-45967.

Last digit is the print number: 9 8 7 6 5 4 3 2 1

To our wives
Carlene Striker, Patricia Quadracci, and
Carol Cutler

FOREWORD

In the relatively few years since the introduction of the renal biopsy, improvements in technique, advances in morphologic diagnostic procedures, and widespread use of this modality have resulted in rapid accumulation of considerable information on the pathologic changes seen in the kidney in a wide spectrum of renal disease. This book represents a major advance in correlating the basic patterns of stress and injury to the kidney with the structural alterations they produce at various stages in the natural history of different renal diseases and in turn with their implications for renal function, therapy, and prognosis.

The method described in this text is the outgrowth of a coordinated team approach to the diagnosis and treatment of patients with renal disease at the University of Washington Hospitals, involving more than 4000 patients over an 18 year period. It represents the product of considerable experience in interpreting light and electron micrographs of the kidney and in clinical nephrology.

This monograph is intended for both the pathologist and the clinician. Typical morphologic changes in each disease process are described in detail and are richly illustrated with light and electron micrographs. A series of excellent diagrams will be an extremely valuable aid to the novice by providing a reference for pattern recognition. The chapter on interpretation of biopsy specimens is particularly helpful; it should be read before the section on specific disease entities because it furnishes a sound approach to the clinicopathologic diagnosis of renal disease.

Clinicians will find the system proposed for classification of renal disease especially useful because it discusses the renal biopsy in terms of assessing prognosis and, in most cases, directing therapy. Moreover, this system of classification is sufficiently flexible to adapt to the continued changes in our concepts of the pathogenesis of renal disease that are inevitable in this rapidly developing field.

JAMES L. BENNINGTON, M.D.

PREFACE

The approach presented in this text is a synthesis of clinical and histologic information obtained from over 4000 biopsies collected between 1959 and 1977. The patient population ranged from children to adults. We also have had the good fortune to be the repository for nearly all of the biopsy material obtained from Washington and adjoining states. These facts, coupled with a reasonably stable patient population and a close liaison between the clinical and laboratory services, provided a unique opportunity to study the evolution of renal disease and to attempt a clinically useful disease categorization. We originally struggled with the available clinical and histologic classifications that had been used for nearly 50 years. They proved to be of little use in communicating with our colleagues and patients. Nearly seven years ago we developed a detailed quantitative method of describing renal biopsies. This proved to be too cumbersome for routine use. This text represents our current working approach to renal disease. We do not presume to assert this practical approach represents a new classification. Rather, our intent is to provide a means of communicating clearly and simply to colleagues and patients the nature, extent, and prognosis of the renal disease process.

The experience necessary to prepare this monograph was aided immensely by biopsy material submitted by our clinical colleagues, including Drs. James Burnell, Robert Hickman, Henry Tenckhoff, Joseph Eschbach, Michael Kelly, and a large number of community nephrologists. The stimulating and challenging discussions with these individuals, many clinical fellows, and visiting scientists, as well as the incisive and intuitive questioning of Dr. Belding H. Scribner, helped us to order our thoughts in this rather confusing field.

Our special gratitude goes to Drs. Earl Benditt and Robert G. Petersdorf for providing interest in and support for our endeavor. Augusta Litwer, Hazel Mehrer, and Vicki Jackson contributed excellent technical assistance and patience in the preparation of endless numbers of drafts.

THE AUTHORS

CONTENTS

SECTION I
GENERAL CONSIDERATIONS 1

Chapter One
HISTORY OF RENAL BIOPSY 3

Chapter Two
CLINICAL EVALUATION OF RENAL DISEASES 6

Chapter Three
INDICATIONS, CONTRAINDICATIONS, AND
COMPLICATIONS OF RENAL BIOPSY 13

Chapter Four
TECHNICAL ASPECTS OF RENAL BIOPSY 16

Chapter Five
INTERPRETATION OF BIOPSY SPECIMENS 28

Chapter Six
CORRELATION OF RENAL STRUCTURE AND
FUNCTION 71

Chapter Seven
CLASSIFICATION OF RENAL DISEASES 80

SECTION II
RENAL DISEASES OF ACUTE ONSET 87

Chapter Eight
GLOMERULAR DISEASE OF ACUTE ONSET 89

Chapter Nine
GLOMERULAR DISEASE OF ACUTE ONSET AND
RAPID PROGRESSION 104

Chapter Ten
TUBULO-INTERSTITIAL DISEASES OF ACUTE
ONSET 118

Chapter Eleven
VASCULAR DISEASES OF ACUTE ONSET
(EXCEPT VASCULITIS) 127

SECTION III
SLOWLY PROGRESSIVE RENAL DISEASES 147

Chapter Twelve
SLOWLY PROGRESSIVE GLOMERULAR DISEASE 147

Chapter Thirteen
SLOWLY PROGRESSIVE TUBULO-INTERSTITIAL
DISEASES 165

Chapter Fourteen
SLOWLY PROGRESSIVE RENAL VASCULAR
DISEASE 182

SECTION IV
NEPHROTIC SYNDROME 193

Chapter Fifteen
INFANTILE NEPHROTIC SYNDROME 195

Chapter Sixteen
PRIMARY NEPHROTIC SYNDROME 201

SECTION V
RENAL DISEASES ASSOCIATED WITH SYSTEMIC SYNDROMES 235

Chapter Seventeen
SYSTEMIC LUPUS ERYTHEMATOSUS 237

Chapter Eighteen
WEGENER'S GRANULOMATOSIS AND POLYARTERITIS NODOSA 253

Chapter Nineteen
HENOCH-SCHÖNLEIN PURPURA 265

Chapter Twenty
HEMOLYTIC UREMIC SYNDROME AND THROMBOTIC THROMBOCYTOPENIC PURPURA 271

Chapter Twenty-One
DIABETIC GLOMERULOSCLEROSIS 284

Chapter Twenty-Two
PROGRESSIVE SYSTEMIC SCLEROSIS (SCLERODERMA) 294

Chapter Twenty-Three
AMYLOIDOSIS 301

Chapter Twenty-Four
MULTIPLE MYELOMA 309

Chapter Twenty-Five
RENAL DISEASE OF PREGNANCY 315

SECTION VI
TRANSPLANTATION 321

Chapter Twenty-Six
TRANSPLANT REJECTION AND RECURRENCE OF THE ORIGINAL DISEASE 323

INDEX 341

Section I

GENERAL CONSIDERATIONS

Chapter One

History of Renal Biopsy

Before 1948 there were only occasional reports of histologic studies on living organs for specific diseases; research before that time was based on open surgical biopsies obtained secondarily during an unrelated surgical procedure in the spirit and enthusiasm of Gwyn, who felt that "a kidney can always suffer the loss of a millimeter of substance; the upper surface of an enlarged liver away from the intestine might spare a sliver." Gwyn (1923) reported on kidney biopsies in two patients, one having the nephrotic syndrome and renal amyloidosis. Since that time, many physicians have used direct visualization to obtain renal tissue for diagnostic purposes or clinical investigation. Russell's classic monograph on Bright's disease (1929), for example, presented data on eight patients with kidney biopsies performed during renal decapsulation.

Percutaneous biopsy of the kidney was first performed by Ball in 1934. He advocated aspiration biopsy to aid in the diagnosis of intraabdominal masses, and in his initial report he described a patient with hypernephroma diagnosed by this means. Not until 1943 was the first systematic study using renal biopsy begun. In that year Castleman and Smithwick obtained kidney tissue from 100 patients during the course of splanchnic sympathectomy for hypertension, then assessed the degree of histologic change in the renal vascular tissue.

The next consistent attempt at biopsy of the kidney appears to be that of Alwall in 1944, although his results were not reported until 1952. He attempted percutaneous aspiration biopsy in 13 patients, but he obtained sufficient kidney tissue from only 10. Unfortunately, one patient with oliguria and uremia died following biopsy, and because of this Alwall temporarily abandoned the procedure. The biggest impetus to use of this method came from the reports of Perez Ara (1950) and Iversen and Brun (1951), which showed that percutaneous renal biopsy can be safe and useful.

The clinical interest and methodological investigations of Alwall, Perez Ara, and Iversen and Brun constituted a strong stimulus and led to the present interest in renal biopsy as a clinical and research tool. Following the initial reports of successful and safe percutaneous renal biopsies, a plethora of papers began to appear describing various techniques of obtaining tissue. Iversen and Brun recommended aspiration biopsy in the sitting position, whereas Perez Ara used the prone position. The use of the Vim-Silverman needle was first advocated in 1953 by Fiaschi and his associates, who biopsied 10 patients in the prone position and obtained sufficient tissue for diagnosis in six. Most reports in this period showed a similar degree of success, with adequate tissue being obtained in only two-thirds of the biopsy attempts.

Muehrcke and his colleagues (1955) made significant advances in improving the yield by their demonstration that probing with a small atraumatic needle was useful in localizing the kidney. In addition, they found that a Franklin modified Vim-Silverman needle secured a better core of tissue. They were successful in obtaining adequate renal tissue in 96 of 100 attempted biopsies with these changes in technique, a remarkable improvement. Most latter investigators have agreed that the probing needle improves biopsy yield, and recommend the prone position for biopsy except for women in late pregnancy.

Little attention was directed to the report by Lusted and associates (1956) regarding the use of image-amplified fluoroscopy during an excretory urogram in order to optimally localize the kidney prior to biopsy, and most renal biopsies during the ensuing decade were obtained by the "blind" technique. It is probable that the lag in utilizing fluoroscopy was based to some degree on the lack of facilities in many centers, as well as the cumbersome fluoroscopic equipment needed at that time. The more recent development of television-monitored fluoroscopic equipment with image intensification and the use of large doses of contrast media now assure that most patients' kidneys can be visualized adequately for a safe renal biopsy, except in cases in which markedly impaired renal function lessens the excretion of radiopaque material.

Radionuclide scans have continued to be useful for localizing the kidney prior to biopsy, and the advent of the gamma camera, which allows dynamic observation of renal function, has increased the value of the technique. This method suffers the same limitations as excretory urography, since adequate scans may not be obtained when renal function is severely reduced. However, the problem of hypersensitivity reactions is minimal compared to that associated with conventional excretory urography because of the small dose of radionuclide given.

Certain medical centers greatly interested in improving yield, however, have abandoned the percutaneous route for direct visualization of the kidney through a subcostal surgical incision followed by aspiration or puncture biopsy. The yield is high by this method, but complications have been as great or greater than by the percutaneous route.

Finally, recent application of ultrasound has proved as reliable for localization as image-amplified fluoroscopy. Ultrasound has particular usefulness in three areas: for patients who are pregnant, those with contrast material sensitivities, and those with nonfunctioning kidneys.

References

1. Alwall, N.: Aspiration biopsy of the kidney. Acta Med. Scand. *143*:430, 1952.
2. Ball, R. P.: Needle (aspiration) biopsy. J. Tenn. Med. Assoc. *27*:203, 1934.
3. Castleman, B., and Smithwick, R. H.: The relation of vascular disease to the hypertensive state. J.A.M.A. *121*:1256, 1943.
4. Fiaschi, E., Ercoli, G., and Torsoli, A.: La biopsia renale mediante agopunctura transcutanea; rilievi anatomo-clinici. Minerva Med. *2*:1851, 1953.
5. Gwyn, W. B.: Biopsies and the completion of certain surgical procedures. Can. Med. Assoc. J. *13*:820, 1923.
6. Iverson, P., and Brun, C.: Aspiration biopsy of kidney. Amer. J. Med. *11*:324, 1951.
7. Lusted, L. B., Mortimore, G. E., and Hopper, J. J.: Needle renal biopsy under image amplifier control. Amer. J. Roentgenol. *75*:953, 1956.
8. Muehrcke, R. C., Kark, R. M., and Pirani, C. L.: Biopsy of the kidney in the diagnosis and management of renal disease. New Eng. J. Med. *253*:537, 1955.
9. Perez Ara, A.: La biopsia-punctural del rinon no megalico—considerationes generales y aportacion de un nuevo metodo. Bol. Liga contra cáncer *25*:121, 1950.
10. Russell, D. S.: A classification of Bright's disease. Med. Res. Council Spec. Rep. Ser. No. 142, 1929.

Chapter Two

Clinical Evaluation of Renal Diseases

Introduction

The study of renal disease requires an objective evaluation of clinical, laboratory, and anatomic information. None of these vantage points should operate independently since the same clinical presentation of renal disease may be associated with a variety of histologic lesions. Failure to understand this fact has led to a confusing array of clinical and pathologic categorizations. The renal biopsy, however, provides a systematic evaluation of the available data, which can be reported in quantitative terms, thus avoiding intuitive, nonobjective interpretations, and which can answer the following questions: (1) What is the primary site of the lesion? (2) What is its type and severity? (3) What is its distribution? The subjective data (obtained from the history) and the objective data (obtained from the physical examination and various laboratory tests) can then be interpreted and integrated with the renal biopsy data to formulate a diagnosis and a therapeutic plan. This approach is shown schematically in the following diagrams:

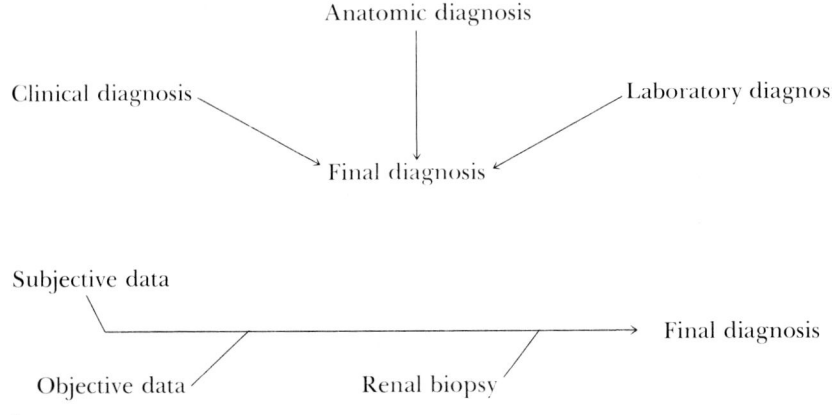

Every component is able to provide data that can be evaluated in light of the other information (lower diagram), rather than each suggesting a diagnosis from a limited vantage point (upper diagram). Such an integrated approach is used in this text; there are no lists of differential diagnoses based solely on histologic criteria.

The following brief outline of various aspects of the subjective and objective data used by the nephrologists in the interpretation of renal disease is intended to acquaint the non-nephrologist with some of the basic aspects of the clinical work-up of renal diseases. For a more thorough discussion of the clinical aspects of kidney disorders, refer to standard textbooks on the subject.

SUBJECTIVE DATA

Constitutional Symptoms

The subjective data, including aspects of the clinical presentation and course, are very useful in understanding the underlying disease process, and especially in estimating the aggressiveness of the renal lesion. The patient who presents with anemia and uremia and only vague constitutional symptoms undoubtedly has a slowly progressive illness which has been in existence for a long period of time, allowing the organ systems to compensate. Patients with the same degree of renal functional impairment who are deathly ill probably have a more rapidly progressive illness, with little opportunity for systemic compensation.

Many signs and symptoms of renal disease are general and nonspecific. When sufficient renal function is lost (glomerular filtration rate less than 10 per cent of normal), producing disturbances of multiple organ systems, the patient is described as having uremic symptoms. These manifestations apparently are related to retention of various metabolic products, and most symptoms can be ameliorated or reversed by adequate dialysis therapy or renal transplantation.

CHANGES IN MICTURITION. Frequent micturition, without concomitant increase in urine volume, suggests a disorder of the lower urinary tract, such as infection or obstruction. Frequent nocturnal voiding is an abnormal symptom, but it is nonspecific. Nocturia may be an early symptom of chronic renal failure, or it may occur with cardiac and hepatic failure in the absence of renal insufficiency.

CHANGE IN URINARY OUTPUT. Mild polyuria is a common symptom of failing renal function in progressive renal insufficiency. It is the result of a concentrating defect and a relative osmotic diuresis in the remaining functional nephrons; it is little influenced by fluid restriction. Oliguria (less than 400 ml daily) occurs in many acute conditions owing to decreased renal perfusion (prerenal), ureteral or bladder outlet obstruction (postrenal), or primary renal disease. It may also be seen in end-stage renal failure. A lesser degree of oliguria may exist (400 to 500 ml) without renal failure, but this is always associated with a severe restriction of solute and water intake and presence of a stimulus for renal absorption of sodium and water.

CHANGE IN URINE COLOR. Depending on the content of pigment and the state of hydration, urine may vary from clear to a deep yellow color. In the absence of drug or food pigment ingestion, an abnormal discoloration of urine is an indication of clinical disease (e.g., hematuria, hemoglobinuria, myoglobinuria, pyuria, porphyria, or melanoma). A cloudy urine frequently indicates pyuria due to a urinary tract infection, but a similar cloudiness is often caused by precipitated ammonium phosphate salts if the urine is alkaline.

The presence of blood in the urine may produce a red to brown discoloration, depending on the amount present and the acidity of the urine. Lesser degrees of hematuria may cause no discoloration and can be detected only microscopically. When hematuria is noted, the presence or absence of pain related to the urinary system is important. Isolated painful hematuria is usually due to bladder or prostatic disease, whereas painless hematuria is most often due to renal or ureteral disease. In addition, the possibility of carcinoma occurring anywhere in the urinary tract should always be considered.

PAIN. The pain related to renal disease is usually situated in the flank or back between the twelfth rib and the iliac crest, with occasional radiation to the epigastrium. The probable cause of the discomfort is stretching of the pain-sensitive renal capsule, and may occur in any condition producing renal swelling, such as acute glomerulonephritis, acute pyelonephritis, nephrolithiasis, polycystic disease, and occasionally renal carcinoma.

Irritation of the renal pelvis or ureter causes pain in the flank and hypochondrium, with radiation into the ipsilateral iliac fossa and often into the upper thigh, testicle, or labium.

EDEMA. Edema is a common manifestation of nephropathy. The complex mechanisms which maintain a constant extracellular volume in health may be upset in similar ways during the course of kidney, liver, or heart diseases. Whatever the cause, edema, which represents retention of sodium and water, is evident initially by an increase in weight, later becoming overt edema. Edema of renal origin often is noticeable first as facial puffiness rather than as ankle swelling, but these characteristics are neither essential nor specific. If fluid retention continues, anasarca with serous effusions may be seen, a condition most often associated with the nephrotic syndrome. Pleural effusions also are fairly common; clinically discernible ascites is less frequent.

PAST MEDICAL HISTORY. A previous history of renal disease is very important; a family history of renal disease, particularly when associated with ear and eye disorders, suggests the diagnosis of hereditary nephropathy. A history of infectious diseases also is helpful in evaluating possible causes of glomerulonephritis.

OBJECTIVE DATA

PATIENT EXAMINATION. Renal disease is the most common cause of hypertension in children and may be a contributing factor in adults as well. The relationship between renal disease and hypertension is complex and poorly understood, despite many clinical and experimental studies. The skin may show pallor, suggesting anemia, or a yellowish-brown pigmentation due to retention of urochromes; excoriatons may be present, suggesting pruritus; and infections, either carbuncles or cellulitis, may occur. Skin lesions, suggesting vasculitis or endocarditis, may provide additional clues to the cause of an observed renal disease. The optic fundi are useful in the evaluation of vascular disease and also should be examined for the presence of hemorrhages, exudates, and papilledema. Examination of the mouth may show a stomatitis or a uriniferous breath. Lessened hearing may suggest the presence of hereditary nephritis. The face, abdomen, or extremities may reveal edema. Palpation of enlarged kidneys would suggest the presence of polycystic renal disease while discovery of bladder or prostatic enlargement should alert one to the possibility of obstruction as the cause of renal disease.

RENAL FUNCTIONAL STUDIES. The kidneys, like most other organs, have a remarkable functional reserve. Considerable structural damage (more than 50 per cent) is necessary before routine chemical functional tests show elevated creatinine or blood urea nitrogen levels. This is true particularly when the disease process is slowly progressive, allowing individual nephron compensation. Tests of tubular and interstitial function (see Chapter 6) are more sensitive, however, and therefore better indicators of early renal damage than the serum creatinine or even creatinine clearance. Maximal urine concentrating ability, for instance, often will be abnormal before the creatinine clearance has begun to fall. This test is performed by injecting pitressin in oil (0.5 ml) subcutaneously and measuring the urine specific gravity, or preferably the urine osmolality, after 8 to 12 hours of water deprivation. A value of 1500 milliOsmoles/liter is normal; levels below 750 mOsm/liter suggest significant structural abnormalities. Evaluation of the concentrating ability provides little additional useful information when other evidence of renal damage is present; it is most helpful if other renal functional tests are normal but renal parenchymal abnormalities are suspected.

STRUCTURAL STUDIES. The most pertinent noninvasive test of intrinsic renal pathology is the urinalysis. Referred to as a "liquid renal biopsy," the usual urine examination involves a qualitative evaluation of certain chemical constituents (pH, glucose, protein), as well as a qualitative microscopic examination of the sediment. If more precise information is desired, measurements should be made using proper test conditions. The customary practice of measuring specific gravity and pH on a randomly voided sample or following a period of overnight dehydration is useful only for indicating good concentrating and acidifying capacity. If results in such samples show lack of concentration or acidification this cannot establish functional impairment.

On the other hand, the finding of significant proteinuria and glycosuria is abnormal, indicative of disease. Glycosuria may signify a primary renal tubular defect, but more often it is caused by hyperglycemia. Serum proteins are retained almost totally by the glomeruli, but those that are filtered are reabsorbed so that the total daily urinary protein is less than 150 mg, undetectable by routine methods. Calculating the total 24 hour protein excretion, or determining the ratio of the protein concentration to creatinine concentration in a single specimen (normal is less than 0.1 mg of protein per milligram of creatinine) is a satisfactory way of quantitating proteinuria. Urinary proteins can be separated and identified by various other chemical and immunologic techniques, and may be of value in the clinical diagnosis or treatment of some renal diseases.

Wide variations in protein excretion may occur with treatment or in association with spontaneous changes in the severity of the renal lesion. Presumably, glomerular permeability, filtration rate, and tubular function are factors influencing the level of proteinuria. Intermittent proteinuria, often moderate in quantity, may indicate renal disease which is mild and nonprogressive. Continuous proteinuria is indicative of renal disease, and when excretion exceeds 2 g per square meter of surface area per day the nephrotic syndrome is diagnosed. It is important to recognize, however, that renal disease can occur in the absence of proteinuria. Nephropathies resulting from hypercalcemia, potassium depletion, and the healing phase of poststreptococcal proliferative glomerulonephritis are examples of this. The character of the protein is often helpful in elucidating the type of renal disease. Bence-Jones proteinuria, or the presence of light chains in the urine, can be found in most gammopathies.

Microscopic examination of the urine sediment is an indispensable part of renal evaluation. For most purposes a qualitative examination is adequate.

Cells are desquamated into urine from any part of the kidney or urinary tract, and uncatheterized samples in women always contain cells from the genital tract as well. Urine usually contains only occasional red and white cells. An increased number of white cells (pyuria) may be seen in diverse renal diseases, but large numbers or clumps of cells indicate inflammation somewhere in the urinary tract or, in women, the genital tract. Recurrent pyuria in women should be evaluated by culture of bladder urine obtained by catheterization or suprapubic aspiration to avoid genital contamination.

The element in urine sediment of greatest importance for diagnosing parenchymal renal disease is the cast. Cellular or granular casts are cylindrical masses of desquamated tubular cells and cellular elements embedded in a protein (mainly mucoprotein) matrix. Casts may be cellular, granular, hyaline, or fatty. Occasional hyaline and granular casts occur in normal states following water deprivation. Although red cell casts may be seen rarely in other renal diseases, they are virtually diagnostic of glomerulonephritis when present in large numbers.

It has been stated that white cell casts are pathognomonic of pyelonephritis. In our experience, however, the finding of white cell casts is indicative only of an inflammatory process and also may be seen in certain stages of proliferative glomerulonephritis and forms of interstitial nephritis unrelated to bacterial infection.

RADIOGRAPHY. A plain film of the abdomen is simple and often one of the most useful procedures in the investigation of renal disease. It can be accomplished irrespective of the degree of renal function, and often the size and shape of the kidneys may be determined. If there is difficulty with routine technique, tomography may be used to facilitate evaluation. Kidney size may be useful, particularly in the investigation of renal failure, because small kidneys suggest the presence of chronic renal disease. Similarly, a unilaterally enlarged kidney may indicate hydronephrosis or compensatory hypertrophy. In addition, excretory urography is helpful in delineating the renal pelvis, ureters, and to some extent, the bladder. The technique depends upon glomerular filtration and concentration of radiopaque contrast media. In the presence of an inadequate glomerular filtration rate, large loading doses or infusions of the contrast chemical may give valuable information even when the rate is 20 per cent of normal. If renal function is too impaired to allow adequate visualization by excretory urography, retrograde pyelography may be used to outline the lower tract.

Role of the Renal Biopsy

The renal biopsy is one parameter of many used in the evaluation of kidney diseases and is of value especially when interpreted in light of other subjective and objective data. The biopsy is done not to establish the diagnosis but to evaluate the injury and help plan therapy; it rarely is helpful in far advanced renal disease. Objective evaluation of the renal biopsy provides information about the type and extent of kidney disease and, therefore, the expected response to treatment. Very few histologic lesions are diagnostic of clinical syndromes. Although a classic "wire loop" lesion may indicate that the patient has systemic lupus erythematosus, this diagnosis is better established by clinical and serologic parameters.

In conclusion, renal biopsy perhaps is analogous to cardiac catheterization, which is performed to provide information on how much the heart is impaired and to what degree the valve is obliterated; it also may confirm clinically suspected aortic stenosis or an unsuspected atrial septal defect. Consequently, a patient who displays symptoms of arthralgia, fever, rash, and positive antinuclear factors, as well as proteinuria and hematuria, may undergo renal biopsy not to establish the diagnosis of lupus erythematosus but to determine the type, distribution, and severity of the renal injury and to plan therapy. Evidence of arteriosclerotic renal disease, which may be suspected clinically, or other, unanticipated lesions, also may be found. Chapter 3 discusses further the usefulness of the renal biopsy in various clinical situations.

References

1. Black, D.: Renal Disease. 3rd Ed. Oxford, England, Blackwell Scientific Publications, 1972.
2. Hamburger, J., and Walsh, A. J.: Nephrology. Philadelphia, W.B. Saunders Co., 1968.
3. Strauss, M. B., and Welt, L. G.: Diseases of the Kidney. 2nd Ed. Boston, Little, Brown & Company, 1971.
4. Brenner, B. M., and Rector, F. C., Jr.: The Kidney. Philadelphia, W. B. Saunders Co., 1976.

Chapter Three

Indications, Contraindications, and Complications of Renal Biopsy

Indications

The indications for performing a renal biopsy vary considerably among clinicians, depending on their past experience with the procedure and their ability to interpret the results. The four most common reasons for performing this technique are (1) it is helpful in establishing the nature of the pathologic process; (2) biopsy frequently is useful in estimating prognosis and the potential for reversibility or progression of the renal lesion; (3) knowledge of the renal histology may suggest whether treatment will be or has been useful; and (4) serial histologic evaluations are necessary to establish the natural history of renal diseases. For the individual patient these indications are interrelated, not independent.

Based on experience, we have categorized various kidney diseases according to the clinical usefulness of renal biopsy (Table 3–1). The procedure is safe and practical, but we would agree with Kark (1968) that the indications for biopsy are "broad and not yet clearly defined." The lack of clinical and pathologic correlation that occurred in the past was related to a paucity of long-term observations and inadequate knowledge of the natural history of renal disease. To a large degree, our previous concepts and biases have impaired, rather than aided, advancement of biopsy interpretation. Ross and Ross (1957), for example, have objected that "some of the claims for renal biopsy in diagnosis are not always well substantiated." This objection should not be used to

TABLE 3-1. Indications for Renal Biopsy

Most Useful
1. Nephrotic syndrome
2. Collagen vascular diseases (systemic lupus erythematosus)
3. Tubulo-interstitial disease of acute onset
4. Proteinuria of unknown etiology
5. Hematuria of unknown etiology
6. Transplantation
7. Research

Probably Useful
1. Glomerular disease of acute onset, with or without rapid progression
2. Slowly progressive tubulo-interstitial disease

Possibly Useful
1. Vascular disease of acute onset
2. Kidney disease of pregnancy
3. Gouty nephropathy
4. Diabetic nephropathy

Not Useful
1. End-stage renal disease
2. Established polycystic lesion
3. Infectious nephropathy
4. Hepatorenal syndrome

fault the technique, but rather to encourage its use in a consistent and scientific fashion.

Contraindications

We accept an uncorrectable bleeding disorder as the only absolute contraindication to renal biopsy. Others also have listed a solitary kidney and an uncooperative patient as absolute contraindications. In our opinion, however, if the information that might be gained is valuable enough, the biopsy of a solitary kidney is only a relative contraindication because the incidence of complications is so low. Biopsies of a single functioning transplanted kidney, for instance, have been done frequently to diagnose and study possible graft rejections. Uncooperative patients also are rare, since an adequate explanation of the procedure combined with prebiopsy sedation usually permits safe biopsy.

Other relative contraindications include conditions that are associated with an increased morbidity following biopsy, such as renal tumors, large renal cysts, hydronephrosis, perinephric abscesses, severe reduction in blood or plasma volume, severe hypertension, and advanced renal failure with symptoms of uremia. Some of these conditions are correctable, at least temporarily. Before biopsy, however, we would suggest correction of a severe anemia or reduced plasma volume, reduction of hypertension with drugs, and several dialyses to alleviate uremia.

Complications and Their Management

Mortality from percutaneous renal biopsy is very low. White (1963), for example, was able to find only 17 deaths in over 10,000 biopsies in his review of the literature. We have had one biopsy-associated death in over 3000 biopsies.

Hematuria is the most common complication of renal biopsy; microscopic hematuria is in evidence following virtually all successful biopsies. Gross hematuria occurs in about 5 per cent of cases. In our experience, however, the hematuria clears with rest, and surgical intervention is required only in rare instances, including nephrectomy. In persistent cases, the use of ϵ-aminocaproic acid has been useful.

Perinephric hematoma is another complication that usually is associated with changes in vital signs, as well as falling hematocrit levels and flank pain, with typical radiation into the groin. Surgical intervention is indicated only for persistent bleeding with an inability to maintain blood volume with transfusion.

Finally, rare complications include laceration of some other viscus, infection, arteriovenous fistulas, and pneumothorax. Surgery may be necessary in these cases.

References

1. Kark, R. M.: Renal biopsy. J.A.M.A. 205:220, 1968.
2. Kark, R. M., Muehrcke, R. C., Pollak, V. E., et al.: An analysis of five hundred percutaneous renal biopsies. Arch. Int. Med. 101:439, 1958.
3. Kincaid-Smith, P.: The clinical value of renal biopsy. Proceedings of the Third International Congress of Nephrology, Washington, D.C., Vol. 2. Morphology, Immunology, Urology. New York, S. Karger, 1967.
4. River, G. L., Dovenbarger, W. V., Nikolái, T. F., and Moffat, N. A.: Unusual complications of kidney biopsy. J. Urol. 103:15, 1970.
5. Ross, J. H., and Ross, I. P.: The value of renal biopsy. Lancet 2:559, 1957.
6. Takacs, F. J., Dodd, J. B., and Zinman, L.: The liberal approach to renal biopsy. Lahey Clin. Foundation Bull. 18:1, 1969.
7. White, R. H. R.: Observations on percutaneous renal biopsy in children. Arch. Dis. Child. 38:260, 1963.
8. Haygood, T. A., Atkins, R., Kennedy, J. A., and Cutler, R. E.: Aminocaproic acid treatment of prolonged hematuria following renal biopsy. Arch. Intern. Med. 127:478, 1971.

Chapter Four

Technical Aspects of Renal Biopsy

THE TECHNIQUE OF PERCUTANEOUS RENAL BIOPSY

The success and safety of percutaneous renal biopsy is related directly to the experience of the operator and careful attention to patient preparation and technique.

PREBIOPSY PROCEDURE. The patient's permission is obtained after explanation of the procedure. At this time, it is important to check the clinical history for possible hemorrhagic tendencies, to measure the prothrombin time, platelet count, hematocrit, and serum creatinine level, and to examine the urine carefully. Although this is seldom necessary, if there is any question of a bleeding disorder, a more elaborate clotting screen should be done (i.e., bleeding time, clotting time, partial thromboplastin time), and any abnormalities should be corrected prior to biopsy. Routinely, except for small children, we do not type and cross-match blood prior to biopsy.

Technique of "Blind Biopsy"

The kidneys can be localized satisfactorily by a flat film of the abdomen or from an excretory urogram. When difficulty in adequate visualization is encountered, tomography or a double-dose excretory urogram, or a combination of both, frequently is helpful in obtaining a satisfactory roentgenographic examination.

A relaxed and cooperative patient is mandatory in order to obtain an adequate biopsy specimen safely. Mild sedation and analgesia are obtained with an intramuscular injection of meperidine hydrochloride

(1 mg/kg) and promethazine hydrochloride (1 mg/kg) 30 to 60 minutes prior to the biopsy. One relative contraindication to biopsy is an uncooperative patient. Infants and most small children, for example, are not candidates for biopsy unless they can be sedated adequately. General anesthesia is seldom required (exception: occasionally in a small child). Although each operator develops his or her own modifications, the initial report by Kark and Muehrcke (1954) is still an adequate description of the general biopsy technique:

> The patient empties his bladder and then lies on his abdomen on a firm-surfaced table or cart. A long sausage-shaped sandbag 4 inches thick is placed under him and across the lower abdomen. The lateral border of the right kidney at either the twelfth or the eleventh rib is marked on the radiographs, and the distance from the vertebral spinous process to the lateral border of the right kidney is measured (x centimeters). The surface markings of the vertebral spinous processes of the lower back, the right twelfth rib, and the right superior spinous process of the ilium are marked on the skin of the back parallel to the line of the vertebral spinous processes and x centimeters from it. These lines with the lower border of the twelfth rib form a triangle in which the puncture is made, usually 1 inch medial to the lateral line and ½ inch below the twelfth rib, or 1 inch below the eleventh rib if the twelfth rib is missing.
> The patient is asked to take a deep breath. The kidney is then palpated from the back as it moves with respiration. Palpation confirms the position, mobility, and size of the kidney and indicates roughly its depth from the surface. Naturally the kidney cannot be felt in very obese patients.
> One per cent procaine is injected into the skin at the puncture site, and a 7 inch long, 20 gauge exploring needle is passed downwards and obliquely towards the kidney. The needle can be felt going through the back muscles, the deep lumbar fascia, the perinephric fat, and the kidney capsule. The patient is next asked to take several deep breaths. If the exploring needle is in the kidney, a characteristic movement is seen: the hub of the needle swings through a wide arc, moving towards the head during inspiration and towards the buttocks during expiration. If the needle is not in the kidney tissue, it is advanced slightly until it penetrates the capsule and moves smoothly on deep breathing. The depth of kidney below the skin is measured on the stem of the needle, and procaine is injected into the tissues of the back as the needle is withdrawn.
> A small nick is made in the procainized skin weal with a bistoury scalpel. The modified Vim-Silverman needle and stylet are pushed through the nick in the skin and down the track of the infiltrating needle to the measured depth. Again one can feel the structures of the back being penetrated, and the kidney capsule is located exactly. The patient is again asked to take a deep breath. When the characteristic swing of the needle is seen, the cutting prongs are inserted to their full depth in the kidney tissue. The needle sheath is then advanced over the cutting prongs to make it bite tissue. While this is being done, the prongs must not be moved lest they be pushed through the kidney. These maneuvers secure a fragment of kidney 1 to 2 cm long without twisting the needle. The prongs and needle sheath are now withdrawn, and the tissue is examined under a hand lens to make sure that both cortex and medulla have been taken. The tissue is immediately fixed, and the needle is swirled in a liquid medium for culture. Should extra tissue be required for the inoculation of laboratory animals, for additional histological examinations (special tissue stains, radioautographs or enzyme studies), or for biochemical analysis, a fresh biopsy needle is reintroduced through the puncture site and down through the

infiltrated tract, but the point of the needle is moved somewhat laterally before the second piece of tissue is taken.

The patient is asked to hold his breath, and should be quite still whenever the needles or prongs are advanced into or withdrawn from the kidney. Moreover, the operator must not handle the needles while they are swinging during the deep-breathing maneuvers. If these precautions are neglected, the needles might tear the kidney.

Technique of Biopsy With Television-Monitored Fluoroscopy

Although the blind percutaneous renal biopsy technique previously described has served nephrologists well for many years, a significant contribution to the biopsy technique was made by Lusted and his colleagues (1956) with the introduction of visual identification of the kidney and biopsy needle by image-amplified fluoroscopy. With the current availability of television-monitored fluoroscopy, biopsy can be done by visual control in an illuminated room, offering the distinct advantage of greater patient safety, close to 100 per cent yield of renal tissues, and an ideal setting for the training of other operators interested in the basic technique. The patient lies prone on the fluoroscopy table on a foam rubber pillow for abdominal compression. An intravenous solution (containing 1.5 to 2.0 ml/kg of 50 per cent diatrizoate sodium or 60 per cent meglumine iothalamate in an equal volume of 5 per cent dextrose) is infused rapidly (10 to 15 minutes) through a large-bore needle. About 10 to 15 minutes later, perhaps somewhat longer if renal function is significantly impaired, the opacified kidney and the renal pyelocalyceal system can be identified readily on the television screen.

Depending on the position of the kidney, respiration is stopped at the end of inspiration or expiration, and the operator places the tip of a pointer on the skin overlying the desired area of renal biopsy, usually the lower pole. This may be repeated through several respiratory cycles until the desired degree of accuracy and consistency is obtained. The skin site is then marked with an indelible pen, and after surgical cleansing and draping, the area is infiltrated with a local anesthetic. A 6 inch, 20 gauge needle is inserted as an exploratory needle and for further anesthesia of the deeper tissues. As the needle is advanced to a point within range of the kidney, fluoroscopy is used to examine the relationship of the needle tip to the kidney. If, on respiration, the lower pole of the kidney moves independently under the tip of the needle, the needle is still superficial to the renal parenchyma. When the tip of the needle moves in unison with the desired section of kidney to be biopsied, satisfactory placement has been accomplished. The exploring needle is then removed, the kidney depth noted and a small skin incision made to allow for the larger biopsy needle. The procedure is repeated in the positioning of the biopsy needle, and after satisfactory placement, the biopsy is obtained in the standard manner. A new disposable renal biopsy needle* has been developed whose design and sharpness facilitate the obtaining of nonfragmented cores of kidney tissue.

We concur with Haddad and Mani (1967), however, in several important technical points regarding this method: (1) the contrast dose must assure adequate visualization, (2) perpendicular needle positioning should be used whenever possible, (3) careful judgment of needle depth is necessary, and (4) the oscillation of the needle with respiration cannot be depended on to insure accurate placement. Seemingly appropriate respiratory swings can occur with the tip in either lumbar or perinephric tissue and also be present if the needle has passed through the kidney. Conversely, a poor swing may be meaningless because of a short needle or excessive kidney depth in obese or very muscular patients. With the ready availability of television-monitored fluoroscopic equipment in most hospitals, we recommend this technique for obtaining percutaneous renal biopsies. Although it is not used frequently, other groups have found retrograde pyelography, radionuclide renal scanning, or ultrasonic studies to be of benefit in localizing the kidneys prior to biopsy. These three techniques usually give adequate localization even in the presence of severely impaired renal function. In addition, ultrasound has the advantage of allowing accurate measurement of renal depth below the skin surface.

Biopsy in Children

Percutaneous renal biopsies can be performed in small children with minor modifications of the procedure performed in adults, by changing only the degree of sedation required in order to maintain patient immobility during the procedure. (A combination of promethazine [1 mg/kg], chlorpromazine [1 mg/kg], and meperidine hydrochloride [0.5 mg/kg] given approximately 30 to 40 minutes prior to the procedure produces adequate sedation and analgesia for most children. If the patient still is not sedated adequately, diazepam [10 mg/m^2] may be given intravenously just prior to the procedure.)

Biopsy of Transplanted Kidneys

Since the transplanted kidney lies in the pelvis in a superficial and easily palpable location, biopsy is relatively simple. Sedation is not

---

*Travenol Tru Cut Disposable Biopsy Needle, Travenol Laboratories, Inc., Morton Grove, Illinois 60053.

required in most instances. The upper pole is palpated, and the skin is infiltrated over the pole with local anesthetic. Because the kidney lies approximately 1 cm below the surface of the skin, the needle tract and perinephric tissue can be anesthetized at the same time. A nick is made in the skin with a sharp scalpel, and a 2½ inch, 20 gauge needle is used to ascertain kidney depth. The biopsy needle is introduced to the depth of the kidney and the biopsy obtained as previously described.

Postbiopsy Measures

Immediately after the biopsy, pressure is exerted at the biopsy site for 3 to 5 minutes until superficial bleeding has ceased. A small bandage is applied to the site of biopsy and the patient is changed to the supine position and should remain quietly in bed for approximately 12 hours. Pulse and blood pressure are monitored during this same period, and each voided urine sample is observed for blood.

If gross hematuria is found, bed rest is continued as long as it persists. The patient should be carefully examined in the perirenal area for a hematoma or unusual pain. In addition, abundant fluid should be taken orally or infused to initiate a mild diuresis, minimizing the colic and obstruction from blood clotting within the renal pelvis. The hematocrit should be monitored, as significant perinephric blood loss may not be apparent.

PROCESSING BIOPSY SPECIMENS FOR LIGHT AND ELECTRON MICROSCOPY

The hospital surgical pathology laboratory can be expected to encounter renal biopsy specimens on a semi-routine basis. In contrast to some other biopsy tissues, in which patterns and overall organization are sufficient, kidney specimens require clear definition of individual cells and subcellular structure and extracellular materials such as basal lamina and deposits. Proper interpretation of renal biopsy tissue therefore requires that the specimen be rapidly and completely fixed, that the sections be thin enough to allow high resolution of structural detail, and that a variety of special stains be applied. There are a limited number of embedding media that satisfy the latter two criteria, and which are applicable in the routine hospital pathology laboratory.

Since 1881, paraffin has been very useful as an embedding medium. The requirements for ultrathin sections and preservation of cell structure stemming from the development of electron microscopy have led to exploration of various plastics as embedding media. The following paragraphs outline the methods using methacrylate embedding for renal biopsies and compare this method with the standard paraffin technique.

Fixation for Light and Electron Microscopy

Immediately after biopsy, specimens for light microscopy are placed in cold 6.25 per cent glutaraldehyde solution for at least 2 to 3 hours. Other fixatives, such as 10 per cent freshly prepared paraformaldehyde or formaldehyde, also are satisfactory. The latter is the poorest choice for preservation of cellular detail.

For paraffin embedding, the tissues are dehydrated in a graded series of alcohols, immersed in xylene, placed in melted paraffin for 30 minutes under vacuum, and then embedded in paraffin. For methacrylate embedding, the tissues are dehydrated in a graded series of alcohols, then infiltrated and embedded in glycol methacrylate, as described by Agodoa and associates (1975).

The embedded tissues can be sectioned with any microtome which will accept a glass knife. A microtome setting of 2 micrometers (μm) is used for paraffin- and 1 μm for methacrylate-embedded tissue. Sections are stained with hematoxylin and eosin (H&E), periodic acid–Schiff (PAS), Gomori's trichrome, and a modified methenamine silver nitrate technique (AgBS). The new glycol methacrylate preparation has necessitated staining methacrylate sections in a water bath at 65° Celsius.

Appearance of Structures with Methacrylate or Paraffin Embedding

GLOMERULI

METHACRYLATE EMBEDDING. The overall glomerular architecture is well defined in the methacrylate-embedded tissues (Fig. 4–1). The capillary basal lamina is poorly stained by the H&E technique and thus appears as a refractile, hyaline substance. Deposits in or on the basal lamina appear as dark-staining material on the negatively stained background. PAS and AgBS stain the basal lamina. Deposits are not apparent with the PAS stain. Subepithelial intramembranous deposits are identified in the AgBS stain as lucent areas between spikes of glomerular capillary basal lamina projecting toward the epithelial surface. Mesangial sclerosis in methacrylate-embedded tissues stained with H&E appears as an increased amount of basal lamina-like material in the mesangial area. This correlates well with findings by electron microscopy. The mesangial cell cytoplasm stains pink with H&E. There is thus a very clear differentiation between true mesangial sclerosis and increased mesangial cell cytoplasm. Increased mesangial matrix (sclerosis) appears as grayish to black material with the AgBS stain, whereas the mesangial cell cytoplasm appears as a lighter color.

Epithelial cell processes are clearly seen at higher magnifications

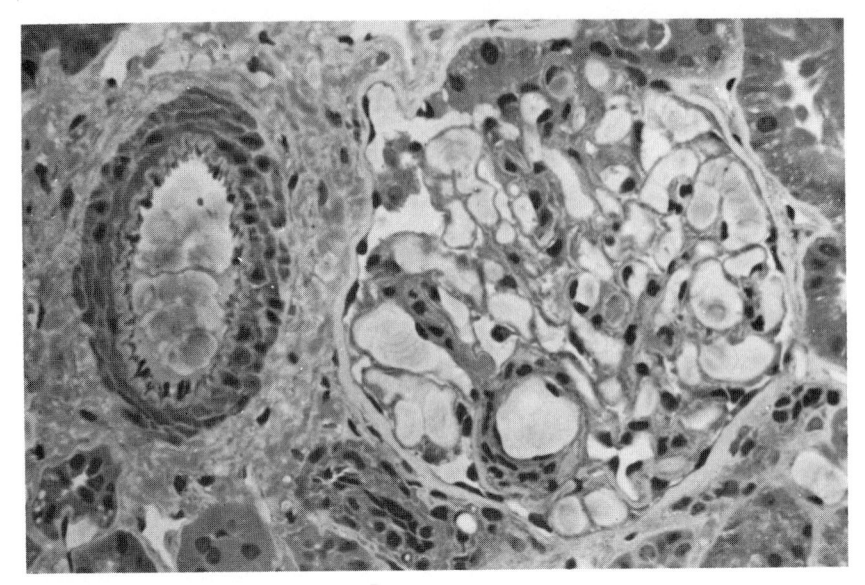

Figure 4-1 Methacrylate-embedded tissue, sectioned at 2 μm thickness. The basal lamina of Bowman's capsule and of the glomerulus is unstained. Note that this is also true of the internal elastic lamella and the basal lamina of the smooth muscle cells of the blood vessel on the left. The cell cytoplasm stains darkly with this stain. Nuclei are clearly visible. (H&E, × 300.)

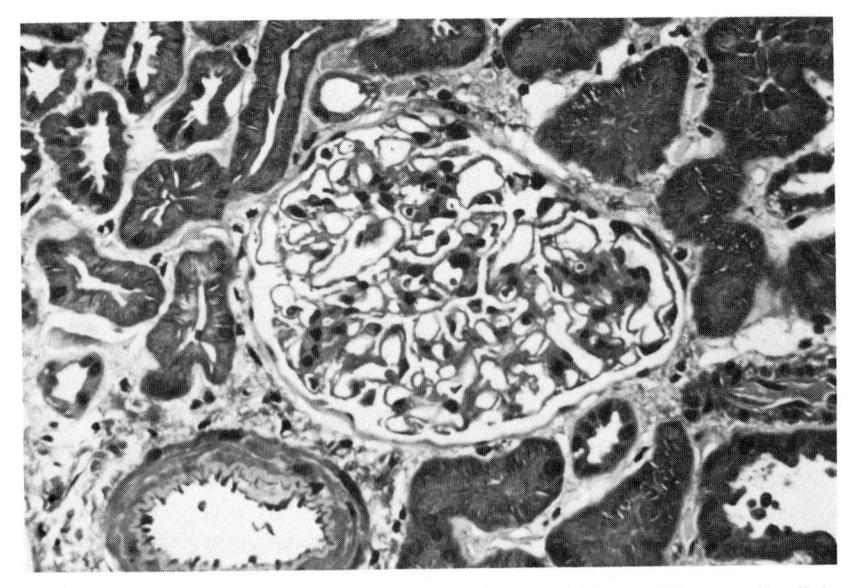

Figure 4-2 A paraffin-embedded section of 2 μm thickness. The overall cellular detail is not as clear as in the previous photomicrograph. Note also that the cells in capillary spaces appear to be somewhat "shrunken." (H&E, × 300.)

(× 1000 to 1250), and loss of the normal architecture can be identified with all three stains.

PARAFFIN EMBEDDING. At a microtome setting of 2 μm, thicker sections are obtained with paraffin-embedded tissues than with methacrylate. The basal lamina, cell cytoplasm, and deposits all stain a similar pink color with the H&E technique, and thus mesangial sclerosis, deposits, and cell cytoplasm cannot be clearly differentiated (Fig. 4-2). Epithelial cell processes likewise cannot readily be identified. Basal lamina and mesangial sclerosis stain deep purple with the PAS technique; deposits are not identified by this stain. With the AgBS stain the basal lamina appears black, mesangial sclerosis is grayish to black, and the cell cytoplasm is pink. Subepithelial and intramembranous deposits appear as clear zones between darkly stained segments of basal lamina. With the trichrome technique, deposits are chromatrope 2R positive and therefore appear as red substances on or in the green-staining basal lamina; mesangial matrix appears as green material in the mesangial area.

TUBULES

METHACRYLATE EMBEDDING. The epithelial cell brush border of the proximal tubules is very clearly defined with all three stains (Fig. 4-3), as are the cell nuclei, lysosomes, and intercellular channels. The basal lamina is unstained with H&E, appears light purple on PAS, and stains black with AgBS.

PARAFFIN EMBEDDING. The main point of difference lies mainly in the greater thickness of the section, resulting in a poorly defined epithelial cell brush border and cellular details that are less clear than in the methacrylate-embedded material (Fig. 4-4).

INTERSTITIUM

METHACRYLATE EMBEDDING. Collagen appears pink with H&E, light purple with PAS, and gray to black with AgBS. Inflammatory, mononuclear, and polymorphonuclear cells are easily identifiable with all three stains. The interstitial capillary space is well maintained.

PARAFFIN EMBEDDING. The only significant difference seems to be in the smaller size of the capillary lumen in the interstitium of the paraffin-embedded as compared with methacrylate-embedded tissues.

VESSELS

METHACRYLATE EMBEDDING. The internal elastic lamella appears unstained with H&E and light purple with PAS (Fig. 4-5). AgBS stains

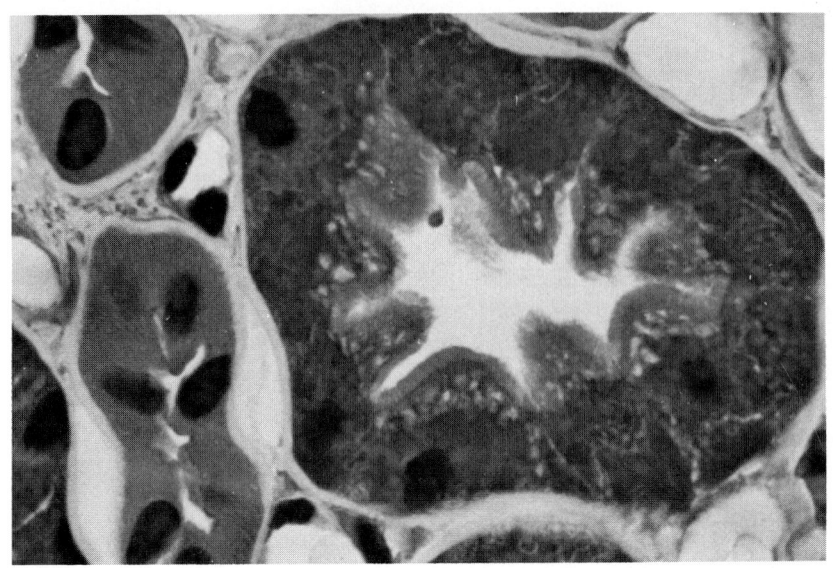

Figure 4–3 Methacrylate-embedded specimen of proximal and distal tubules. The brush border of the proximal tubule is clearly identified, as are the apical vacuoles and the intercellular spaces. To the left of the photomicrograph are sections of two distal tubules. The smooth epithelial surface is apparent. Note that here also the basal lamina of the tubules is unstained. (H&E, × 1200.)

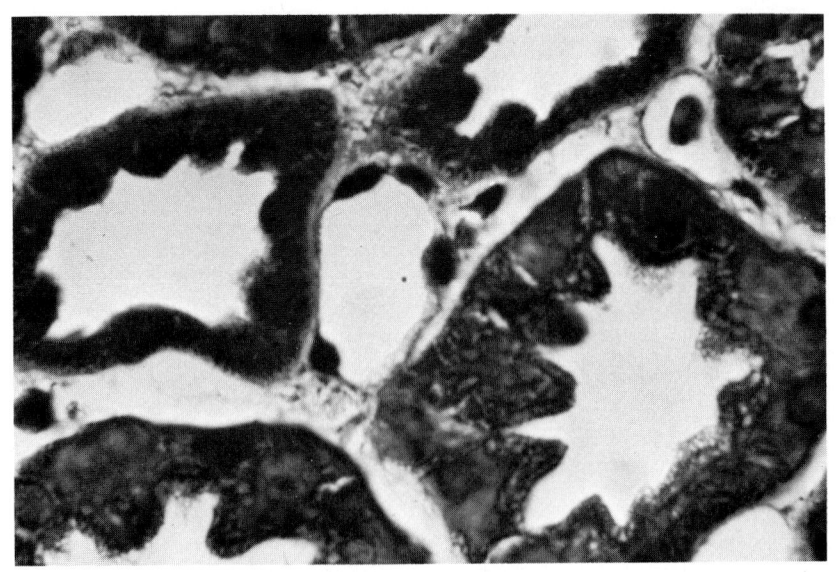

Figure 4–4 Paraffin-embedded specimen showing proximal and distal tubules. The brush border can be outlined in the proximal tubules. Note that the lumina of both proximal and distal tubules are considerably larger than in the methacrylate-embedded tissues. The cell details are somewhat obscured, owing to the thickness of the section. Note also that the cytoplasm of the distal tubules appears to be somewhat shrunken around the nuclei, in contrast to the methacrylate-embedded material. (H&E, × 1200.)

the basal lamina of the endothelial and smooth muscle cells black. The smooth muscle cells are clearly outlined. Hyaline deposits and sclerosis in the vessel wall appear as unstained areas.

PARAFFIN EMBEDDING. The main difference evident with the H&E technique is that there is poor differentiation between the cellular and extracellular components of the vessel (Fig. 4–6). With the AgBS stain, the elastic lamella stains black, and the cytoplasm of the endothelial and muscle cells appears pink.

Comparison of Methacrylate and Paraffin Techniques

Methacrylate embedding of renal tissues obtained at biopsy appears to offer several advantages over paraffin embedding. The process is more rapid (the time required for embedding of tissue and staining with H&E is approximately 2 hours for methacrylate and 4½ hours for paraffin), tissue architecture is less distorted, and thinner sections can be obtained (1 μm compared with 2 to 4 μm). Methacrylate also offers several cost benefits since it is a relatively inexpensive plastic, is readily available, is easy enough to use in most routine histology laboratories, and greatly reduces technician time. H&E and AgBS stains alone most often are sufficient for elucidation of structural alterations, in comparison to paraffin-embedded tissues, which require H&E, PAS, and trichrome stains. The main disadvantage of methacrylate-embedded tissues is their poor staining with Gomori's trichrome.

The final and most important advantage of methacrylate embedding is that the resolution is at such a level that only in unusual instances is it necessary to resort to electron microscopy to thoroughly evaluate the tissue. Thus, for the routine biopsy, a methacrylate-embedded specimen examined at high power, coupled with careful immunofluorescence microscopy, provides a rapid and inexpensive analytical approach to the interpretation of renal disease.

Processing Biopsy Specimens for Fluorescence Microscopy

The specimen should be kept moist, but not immersed in saline. The tissue should be frozen rapidly and sectioned shortly thereafter.

Approximately 20 fresh frozen sections, no thicker than 5 to 6 μm, are required for immunofluorescence staining for IgG, IgA, IgM, and C3. Two slides should be stained with each specific fluoresceinated antibody, and an additional slide should serve as a blocking control. The

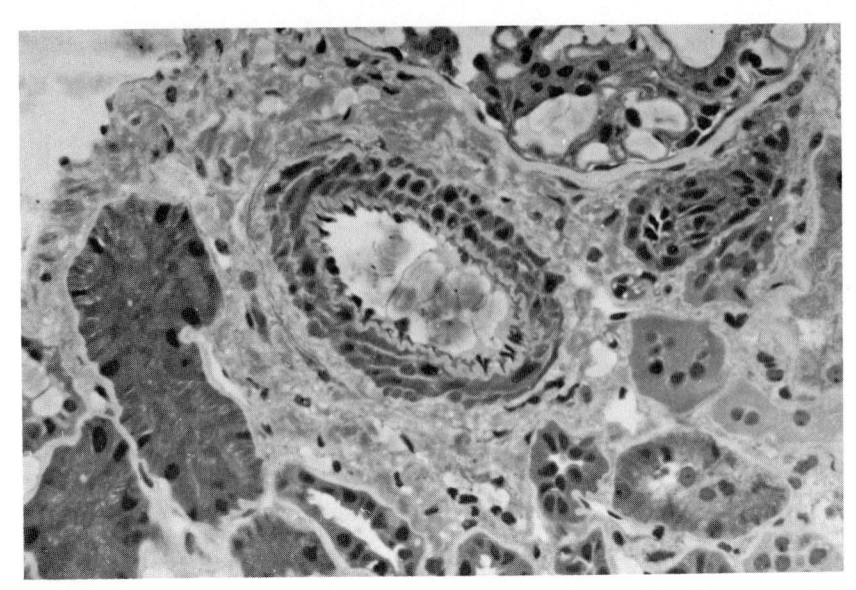

Figure 4-5 A methacrylate-embedded specimen. The vessel in the center of the photomicrograph is a small artery. In this stain the medial cells are clearly identifiable as separate entities outlined by a lucent basal lamina. The endothelium is represented by a thin layer of continuous cytoplasm. Note the increased amount of connective tissue around the vessel, which represents a normal feature of the "skeleton" of the kidney. (H&E, × 300.)

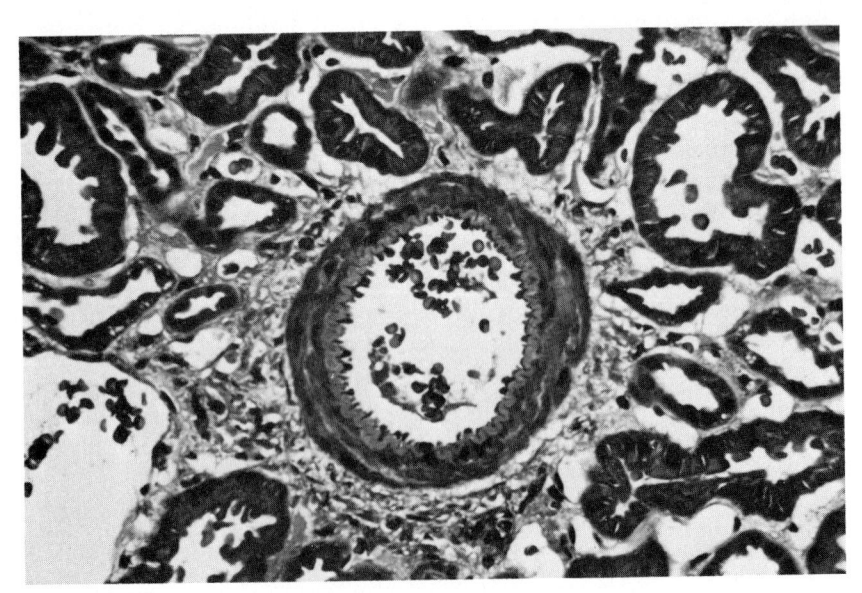

Figure 4-6 Paraffin-embedded specimen containing a vessel in the center of the photomicrograph. As was previously noted, the thickness of the section makes cellular details more difficult to discern in paraffin-embedded tissues. There is shrinkage of the tissue as well. (H&E, × 300.)

slides are immersed in normal saline for 15 minutes to remove extraneous serum proteins. All slides except the blocking control are placed in Coplin jars containing fluoresceinated antisera. A small drop of unfluoresceinated antibody with the same specificity as the fluoresceinated antiserum is added to the blocking control slide. Care is taken to assure that the antibody completely covers the frozen sections. All slides are incubated for 30 minutes at room temperature in the Coplin jars for the fluorescent staining or in a humidified petri dish for the blocking control. Following this incubation period, the antibody is removed by immersing the slides successively in three changes of saline. A further 30 minute incubation with specific fluoresceinated antiserum is necessary for the blocking controls. The slides are then dehydrated by immersing them successively in 35 per cent, 75 per cent, 95 per cent, and 100 per cent ethanol, followed by immersion in xylene. Coverslips are then affixed with low fluorescence mounting media. The stained slides should be stored under refrigeration in the dark. Under these conditions, fluorescence will be maintained for up to 6 months.

The specimen may be viewed with either transmitted or epi-illumination. The latter provides greater definition and lower background fluorescence. It does, however, require a relatively expensive attachment to the regular fluorescence microscope.

References

1. Agodoa, L. Y., Striker, G. E., Chi, E.: Glycolmethacrylate embedding of renal biopsy specimens for light microscopy. Am. J. Clin. Pathol. 64:655, 1975.
2. Bolton, W. K., Tully, R. J., Lewis, E. J., and Ranninger, K.: Localization of the kidney for percutaneous biopsy. Ann. Int. Med. 81:159, 1974.
3. Colgan, J. R., Bischel, M., and Morrow, J. W.: Retrograde catheter localization for percutaneous renal biopsy. J.A.M.A. 217:824, 1971.
4. Haddad, J. K., and Mani, R. L.: Percutaneous renal biopsy. An improved method using television monitoring and high-dose infusion pyelography. Arch. Int. Med. 19:157, 1967.
5. Kark, R. M.: Renal biopsy. J.A.M.A. 217:824, 1971.
6. Kark, R. M., and Muehrcke, R. C.: Biopsy of kidney in prone position. Lancet 1:1047, 1954.
7. Keller, H. I., Malloy, J. P., and Sauer, G. F.: The renal scan. An aid to renal biopsy. J.A.M.A. 188:1085, 1964.
8. Koehler, J. K.: Advanced Techniques in Biological Electron Microscopy. Berlin, Springer-Verlag, 1973.
9. Lee, B.: Microtomist's Vade-Mecum. 9th Ed. Edited by J. B. Gatenby and E. V. Cowdry. Philadelphia, Blakiston, 1928.
10. Lillie, R. D.: Biebrich scarlet–Picro aniline blue: A new differential connective tissue and muscle stain. Arch. Pathol. 29:705, 1940.
11. Lusted, L. B., Mortimer, G. E., and Hopper, J. J.: Needle renal biopsy under image amplifier control. Amer. J. Roentgenol. 75:953, 1956.
12. Newman, S. B., Borysho, E., and Swerdlow, M.: Ultramicrotomy by a new method. J. Res. National Bureau of Standards 43:183, 1946.
13. Telfer, N., Ackroy, D. A. E., and Stock, S. L.: Radio-isotopic localisation for renal biopsy. Lancet 1:132, 1964.

Chapter Five

Interpretation of Biopsy Specimens

Introduction

This chapter is designed to aid in understanding the kidney's responses to diverse stimuli in terms of the basic pathologic processes. Rather than catalogue a list of exotic diseases which have unknown causes and uncertain prognoses, however, we are providing a framework on which to place current and future observations and data in a useful perspective.

Clinical recognition of renal disease depends on interpretation of changes in the urine and plasma. The type and magnitude of variations reflect the site and severity of the lesion. This concept can be applied to each anatomic and functional component of the kidney. Excluding the production and modification of specific hormones, the major tasks performed by the kidney are ultrafiltration of the plasma, selective reabsorption of parts of the filtrate, and secretion of various substances into the tubular lumina. All these processes are regulated within rather narrow limits, and aberrations are reflected by a change in the quality or quantity of the end product—urine.

For instance, when protein is present in excessive quantities in the urine, which is an abnormality in the segment of the nephron that normally excludes protein from the filtrate, the glomerulus should be suspected. The presence of proteinuria is, in fact, a reliable laboratory indicator of glomerular disease. Although this approach can be criticized as being too simplistic, it allows some sense to be made from the multiple histopathologic, functional, and clinical presentations of renal disease.

Interpretation

GLOMERULAR DISEASE

GENERAL CONSIDERATIONS. A clear understanding of glomerular disease rests on a consideration of the normal glomerular structure and the basic pathologic changes which may happen. The glomerulus consists of cells and extracellular material (Figs. 5–1 and 5–2). The possible cellular changes are (1) an increase in number (hyperplasia), (2) a change in cell function, and (3) exudation (infiltration by neutrophils) (Table 5–1). The extracellular changes which are likely to occur include (1) an increase in amount of extracellular material (sclerosis or scarring) (Table 5–2), and (2) accumulation of foreign proteins in the form of deposits (Table 5–3).

Various cellular and extracellular changes may coexist in one patient; the extent and severity correlate with immediate renal function and long-term prognosis. Tables 5–1 to 5–4 summarize these changes and their characteristics. The following discussion will consider the determination and description of each compartment.

The normal structure and function of each of the glomerular elements is basic to the interpretation of changes as a result of disease processes. The function of the glomerulus is to form an ultrafiltrate of plasma and to deliver it to the attached tubular segment. The structure is suited ideally for this function, consisting of a network of capillaries with an extensive filtration surface area. The skeleton (glomerular basal lamina and mesangial matrix) is an important element of the glomerulus, and it is sturdy enough to withstand higher pressures than are present in other capillary beds. Recent studies also suggest that the internal aspect of the glomerular basal lamina is a prominent component of the filtration barrier.

The cells likewise are well suited to their location. The mesangial cells, for example, are thought to be contractile. This capability suggests that they might monitor and adjust the flow to individual capillary loops. These cells also appear to gather circulating materials such as immune complexes and other particulate matter. The endothelial cells, on the other hand, have a thin, attenuated cytoplasm, and their membranes are highly fenestrated over the peripheral portions of the capillary. The epithelial cells, however, have a large number of cell processes (pedicels) which rest on the glomerular basal lamina and interdigitate extensively with adjacent cells. The junction between these cells is a modified desmosome which effectively excludes proteins of greater size than 50,000 molecular weight from the filtrate, while allowing relatively free passage of low-molecular-weight solutes and water. The extensive interdigitation of the epithelial cell processes greatly increases the surface area occupied by these cell junctions and thus the area for filtration.

Text continued on page 63

30 Interpretation of Biopsy Specimens

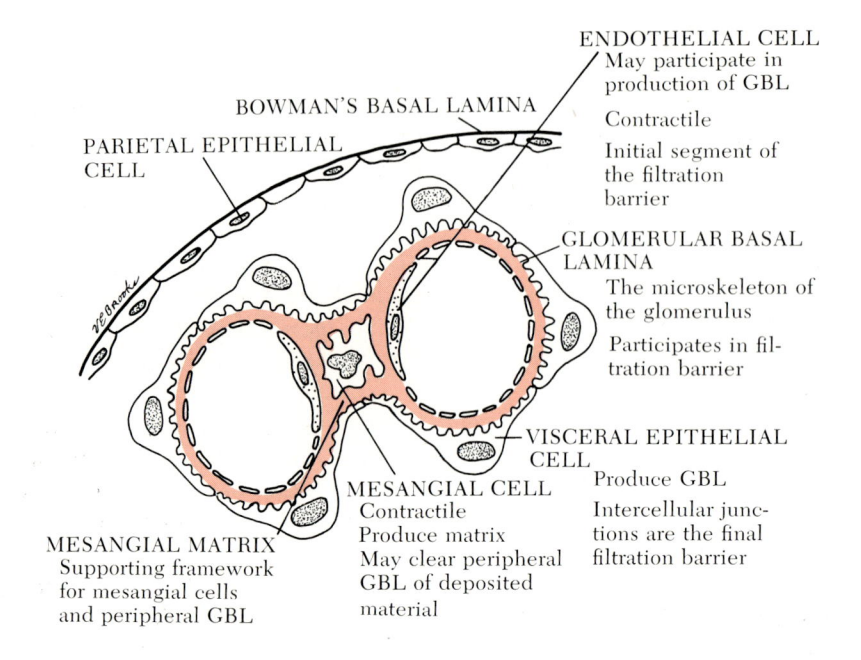

Figure 5-1 Diagrammatic representation of a normal glomerulus.

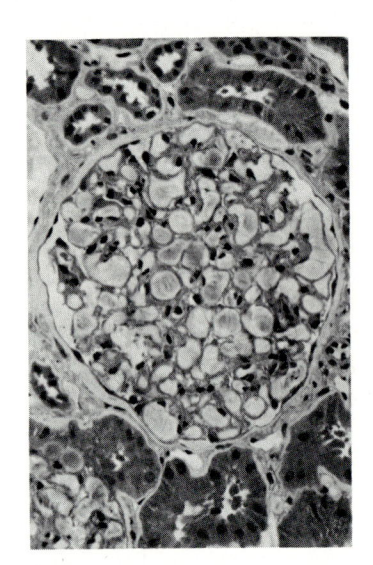

Figure 5-2 Normal glomerulus (H&E, ×300).

TABLE 5–1 Glomeruli: Cellular Change

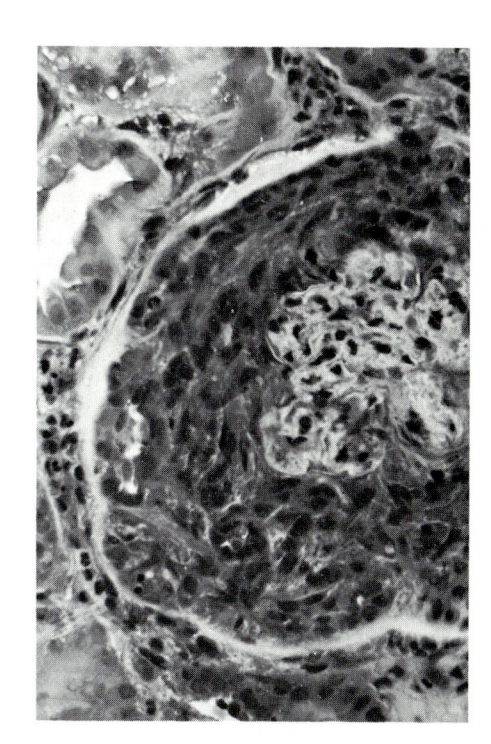

Structural Abnormality

Epithelial Cells
  Diffuse hypercellularity

Functional Abnormality

Occlusion of urinary space; damage to capillary wall, leading to leakage of cells and protein into filtrate

Renal Syndrome

Glomerular disease of acute onset and rapid progression (Chapter 9)
Arteritis (Chapter 18)

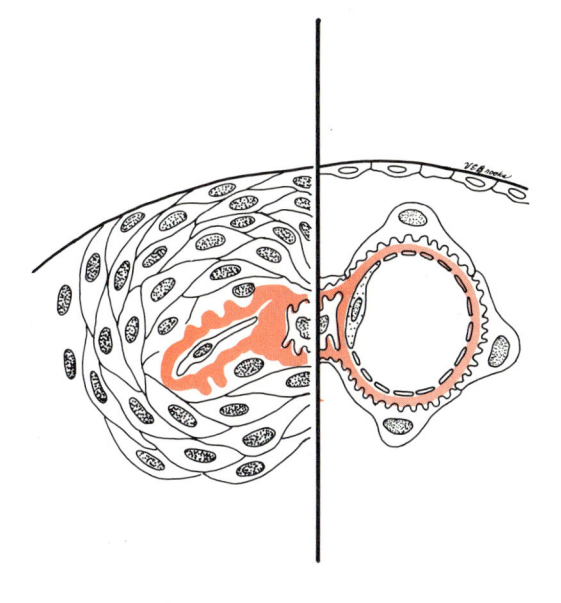

Table 5–1 continued on following page

32 INTERPRETATION OF BIOPSY SPECIMENS

TABLE 5-1 Glomeruli: Cellular Change (*Continued*)

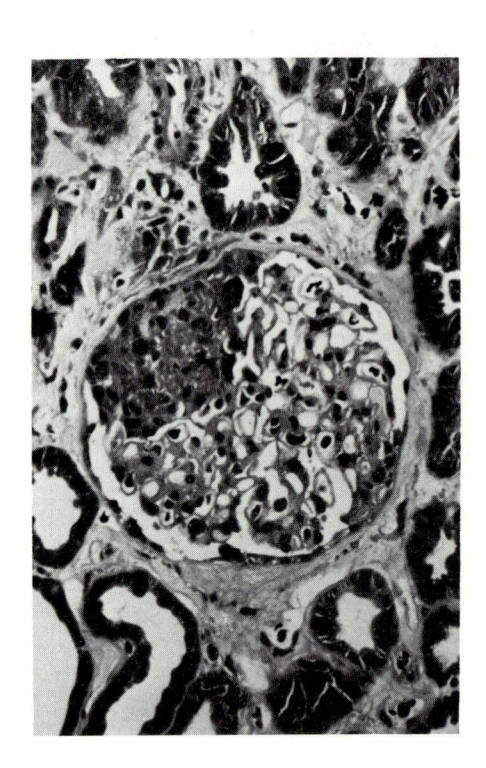

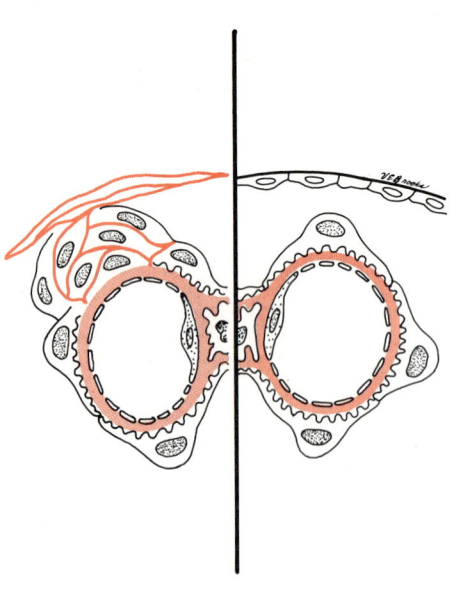

Structural Abnormality

Segmental hypercellularity

Functional Abnormality

Damage to the GBL, with leakage of cells and protein into filtrate

Renal Syndrome

Glomerular disease of acute onset (Chapter 8)
Benign recurrent hematuria (Chapter 12)
Various systemic syndromes (Section V, Chapters 16 to 20)

TABLE 5-1 Glomeruli: Cellular Change (*Continued*)

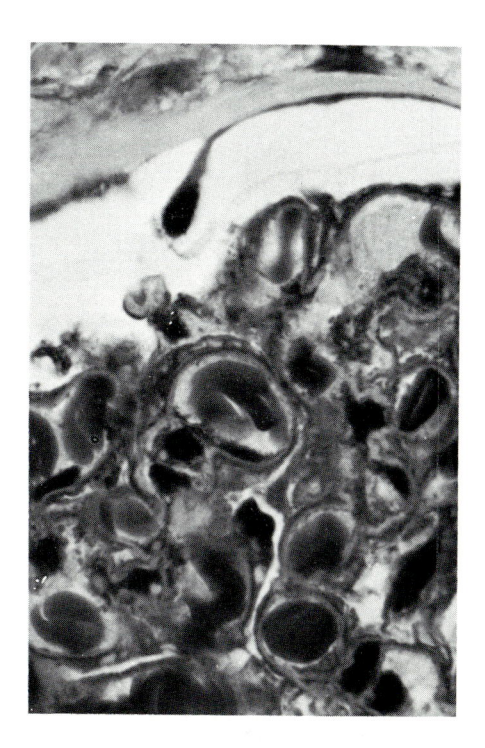

Structural Abnormality
Fusion of foot processes

Functional Abnormality
Leakage of protein into filtrate

Renal Syndrome
Nephrotic syndrome (Section IV)

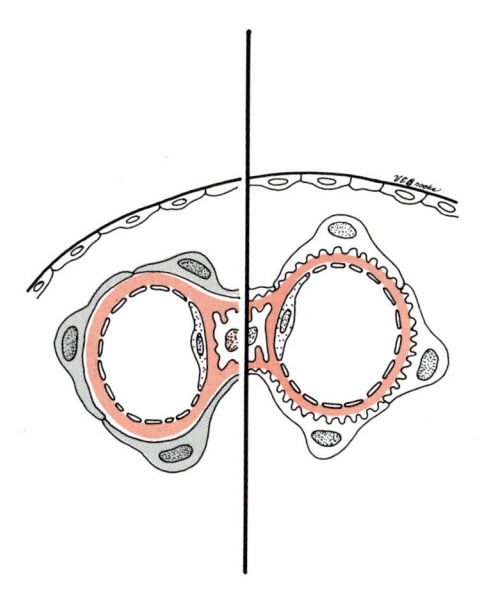

Table 5-1 continued on following page

34 Interpretation of Biopsy Specimens

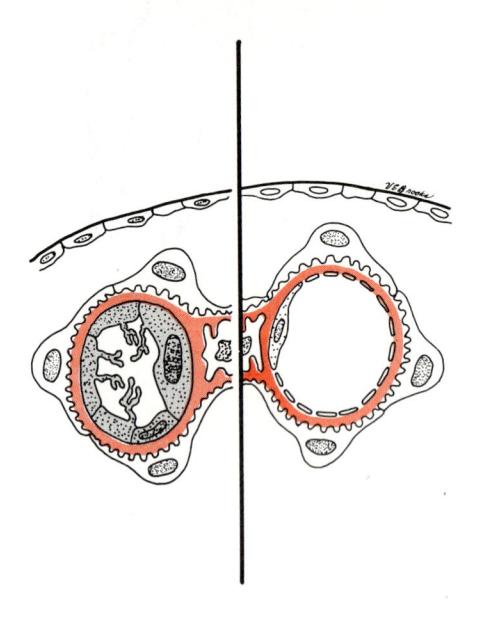

TABLE 5-1 Glomeruli: Cellular Change (*Continued*)

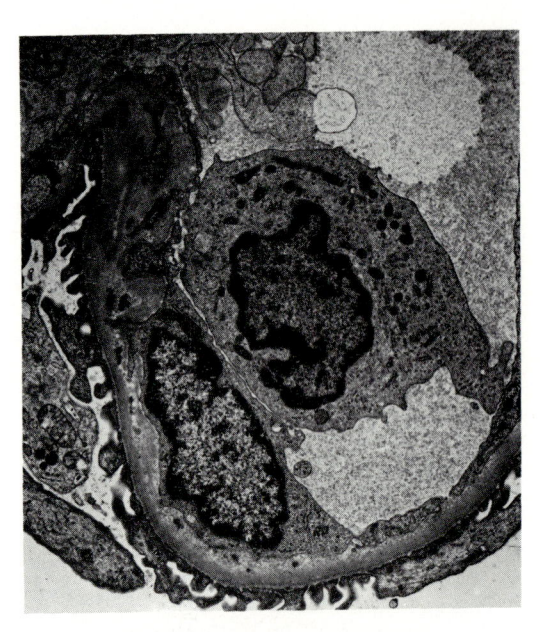

Structural Abnormality

Endothelial Cells
  Hypercellularity and swelling

Functional Abnormality

May precipitate platelet and RBC destruction, proteinuria, hematuria

Renal Syndrome

Toxemia of pregnancy (Chapter 25)

Vascular disease of acute onset (Chapter 11)

TABLE 5-1 Glomeruli: Cellular Change (*Continued*)

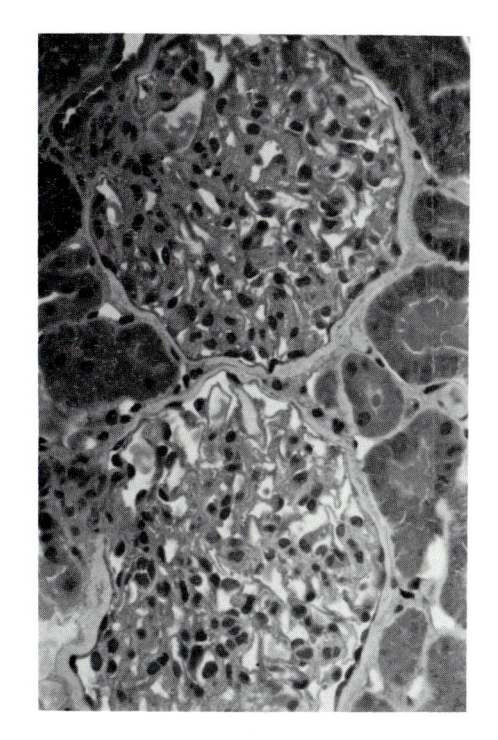

Structural Abnormality

Mesangial Cells
  Hypercellularity

Functional Abnormality

Abnormalities in turnover or composition of mesangial matrix and possibly GBL, leading to decreased filtration surface and proteinuria

Leakage of protein into the filtrate

Renal Syndrome

Slowly progressive glomerular disease (Chapter 12)

Nephrotic syndrome (Section IV)

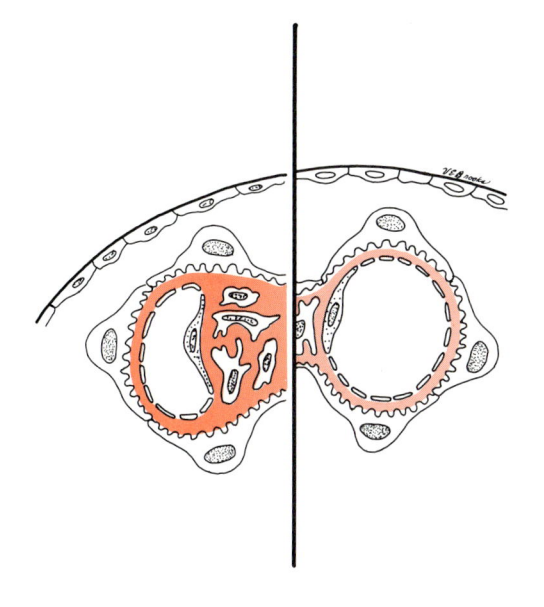

Table 5-1 continued on following page

TABLE 5-1 Glomeruli: Cellular Change (*Continued*)

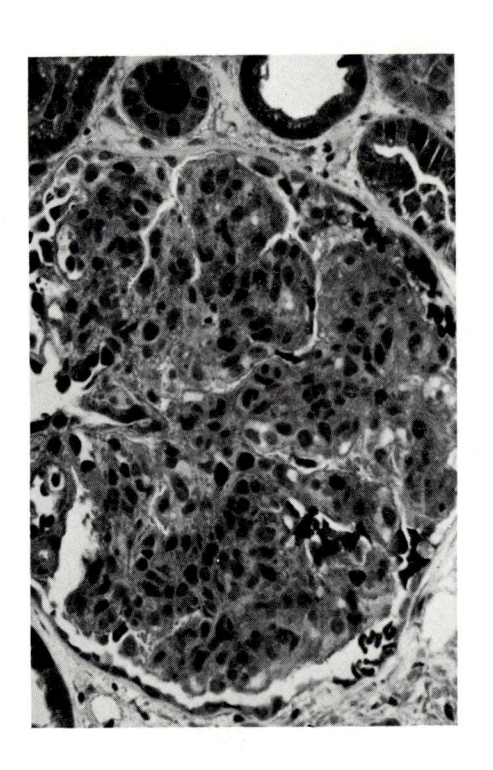

Structural Abnormality

Inflammatory Cells

Functional Abnormality

Inflammation and release of proteolytic enzymes may damage cells and GBL, cause local thrombosis, hematuria, proteinuria, decreased filtration surface

Renal Syndrome

Glomerular disease of acute onset (Chapter 8)
Systemic lupus erythematosus (Chapter 17)

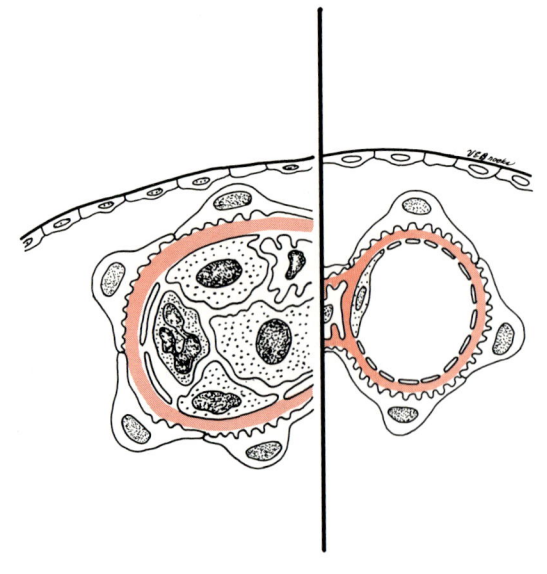

TABLE 5-2 Glomeruli: Extracellular Material

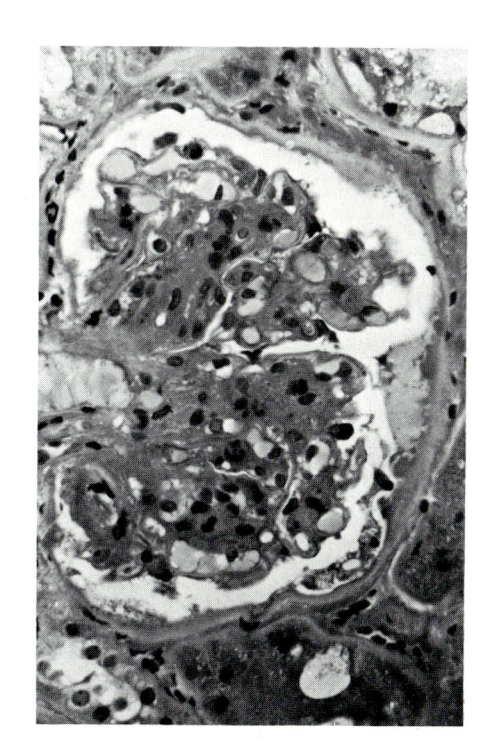

Structural Abnormality

Glomerular Basal Lamina
  Diffuse thickening

Functional Abnormality

Decreased filtration surface, proteinuria

Renal Syndrome

Diabetic glomerulosclerosis (Chapter 21)

Nephrotic syndrome (Chapter 16)

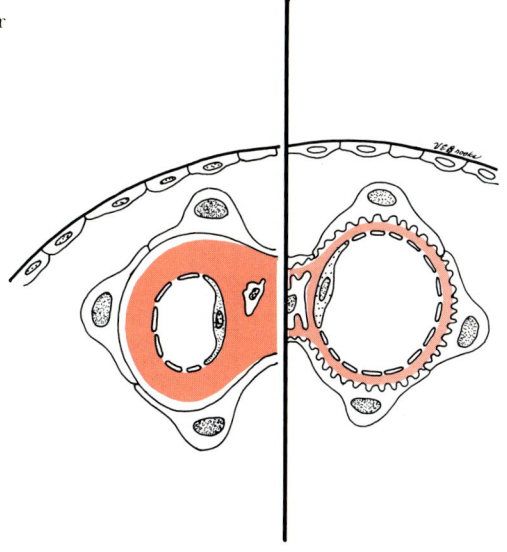

Table 5-2 continued on following page

38   Interpretation of Biopsy Specimens

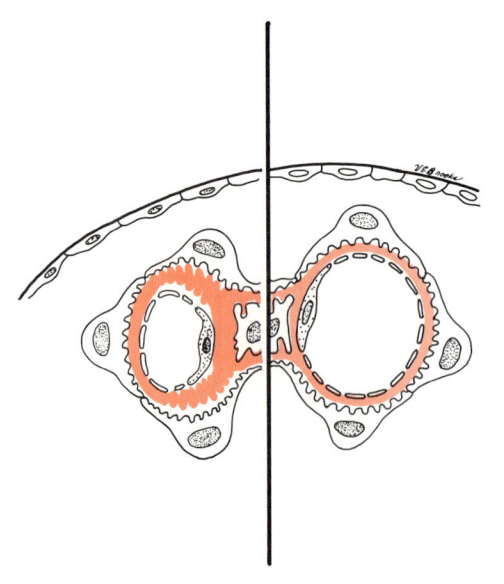

TABLE 5–2   Glomeruli: Extracellular Material (*Continued*)

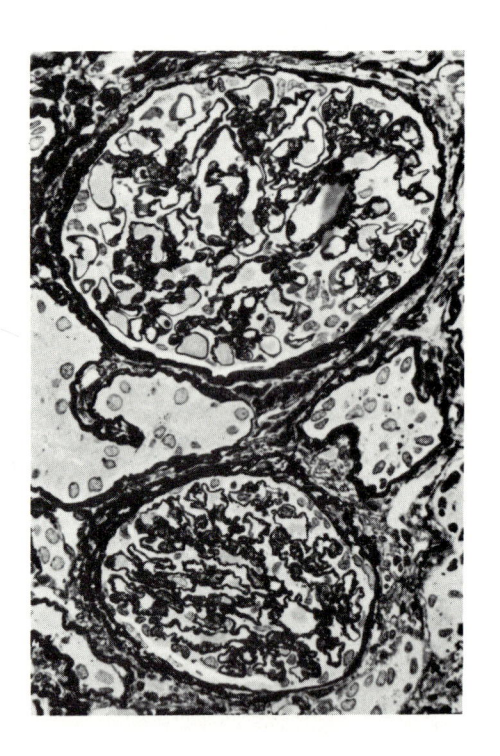

Structural Abnormality
GBL Collapse

Functional Abnormality
Decreased filtration surface

Renal Syndrome
Slowly progressive renal vascular disease (Chapter 14)

TABLE 5-2 Glomeruli: Extracellular Material (*Continued*)

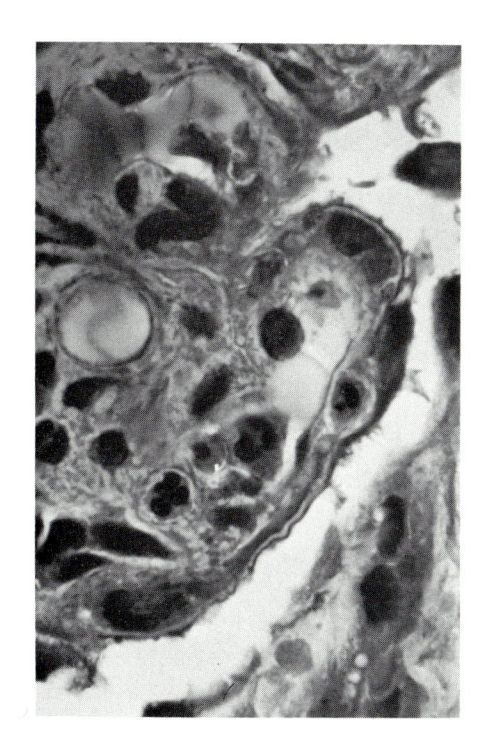

Structural Abnormality
Reduplication or splitting

Functional Abnormality
Proteinuria and decreased filtration surface

Renal Syndrome
Slowly progressive glomerular disease (Chapter 16)

Infantile nephrotic syndrome (Chapter 15)

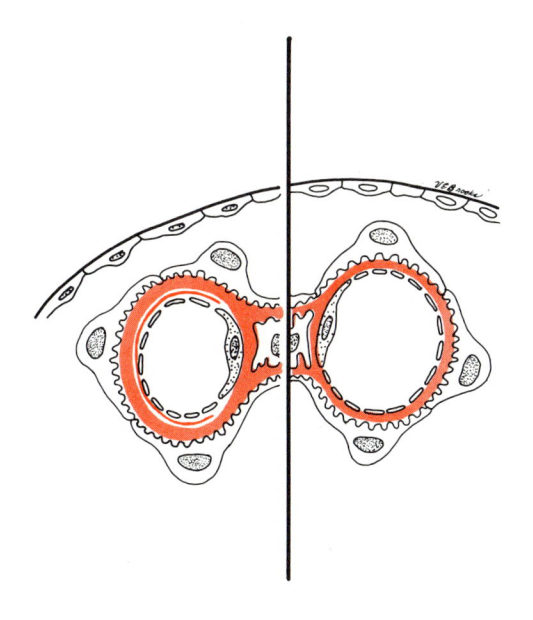

Table 5-2 continued on following page

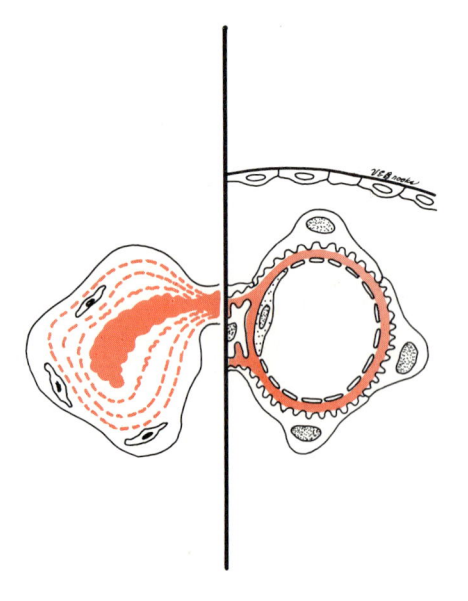

TABLE 5-2   Glomeruli: Extracellular Material (*Continued*)

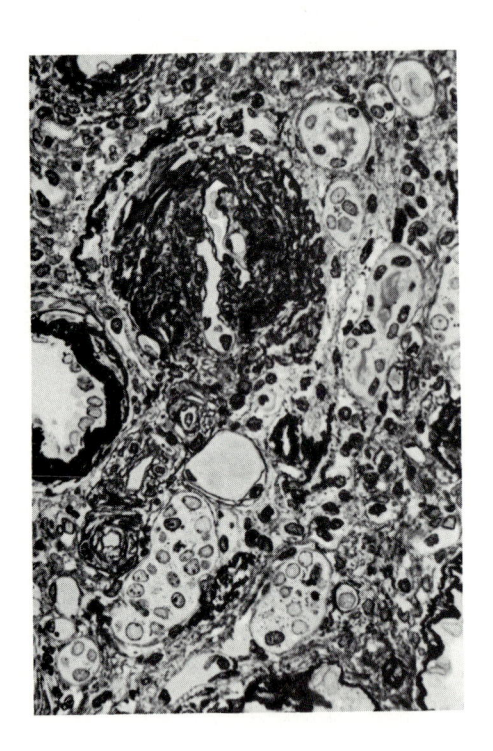

Structural Abnormality

Obsolescence

Functional Abnormality

Decreased number of functioning nephrons

Renal Syndrome

Slowly progressive glomerular disease (Chapter 12)

End-stage renal disease of any cause

TABLE 5-2   Glomeruli: Extracellular Material (*Continued*)

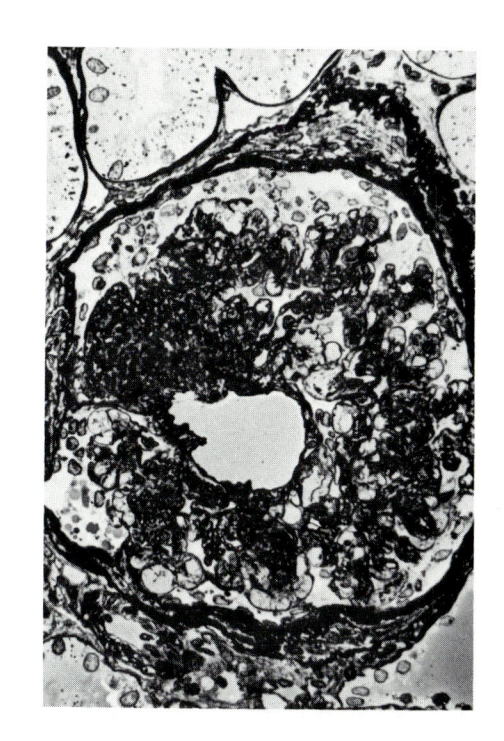

Structural Abnormality

Mesangial Matrix
  Increase

Functional Abnormality

Decreased mesangial function

Decreased filtration surface

Renal Syndrome

Slowly progressive glomerular disease (Chapter 12)

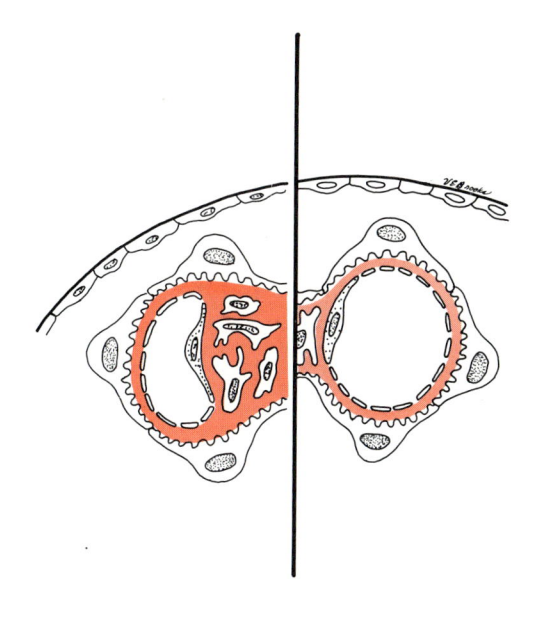

TABLE 5-3 Glomeruli: Deposits

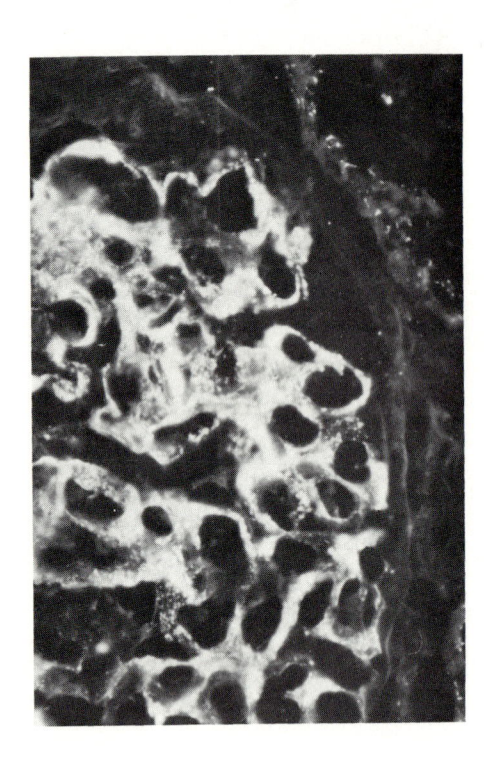

Structural Abnormality

Subendothelial Deposits
  Predominantly immunoglobulin
  Diffuse and irregular

Functional Abnormality

Glomerular inflammation, proteinuria, hematuria

Decreased filtration surface

Renal Syndrome

Systemic lupus erythematosus (Chapter 17)

Glomerular disease of acute onset associated with endocarditis (Chapter 8)

TABLE 5-3 Glomeruli: Deposits (*Continued*)

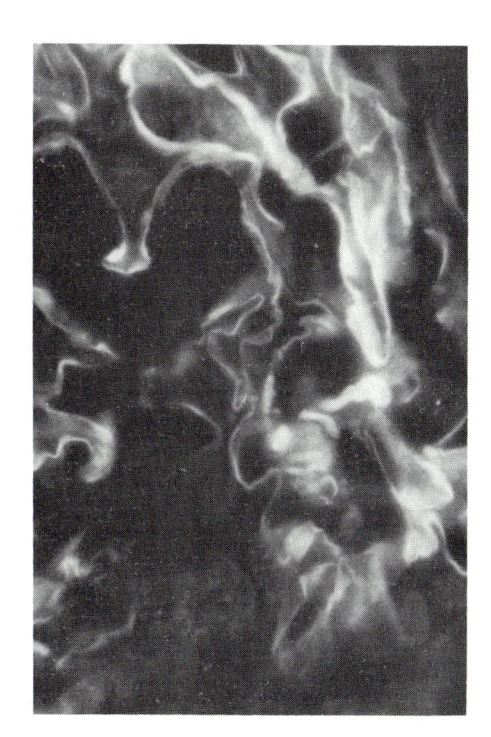

Structural Abnormality

Subendothelial Deposits
  Diffuse and linear

Functional Abnormality

Epithelial cell proliferation and obstruction of urinary space

Renal Syndrome

Glomerular disease of onset and rapid progression (Chapter 9)

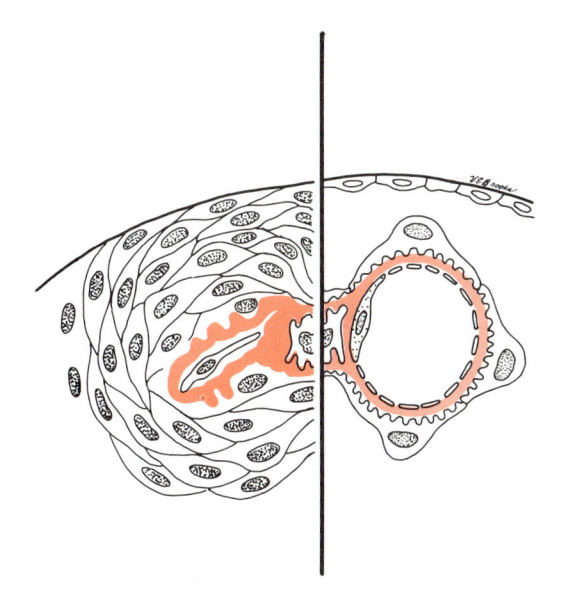

Table 5-3 continued on following page

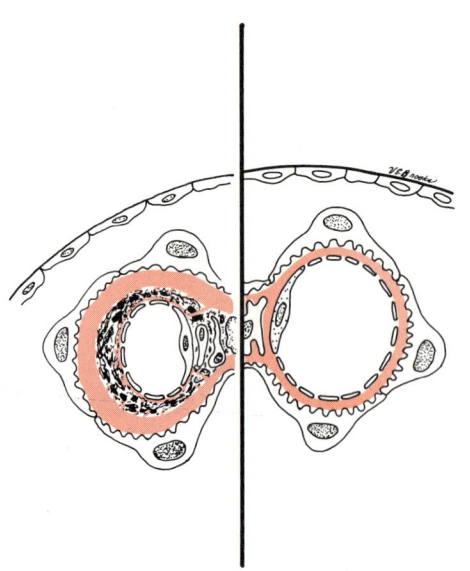

TABLE 5-3   Glomeruli: Deposits (*Continued*)

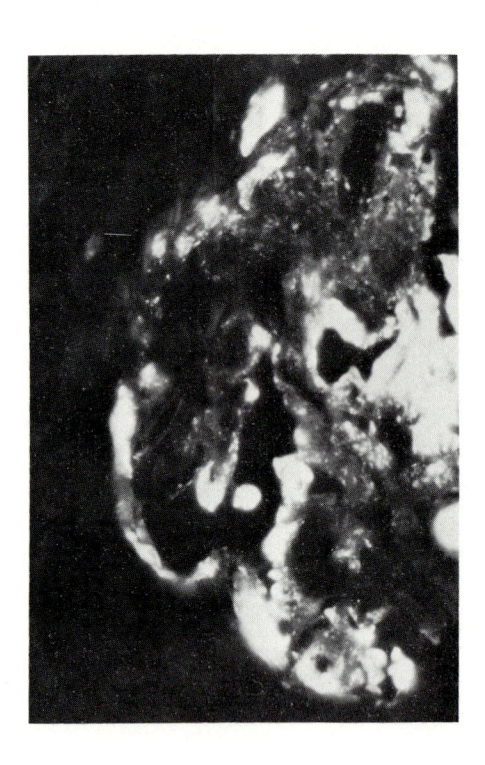

Structural Abnormality

Predominantly complement in thickened GBL

Functional Abnormality

Decreased filtration surface, proteinuria, hematuria

Renal Syndrome

Subset of membranoproliferative glomerulonephritis with subendothelial deposits (Chapter 16)

TABLE 5-3 Glomeruli: Deposits (*Continued*)

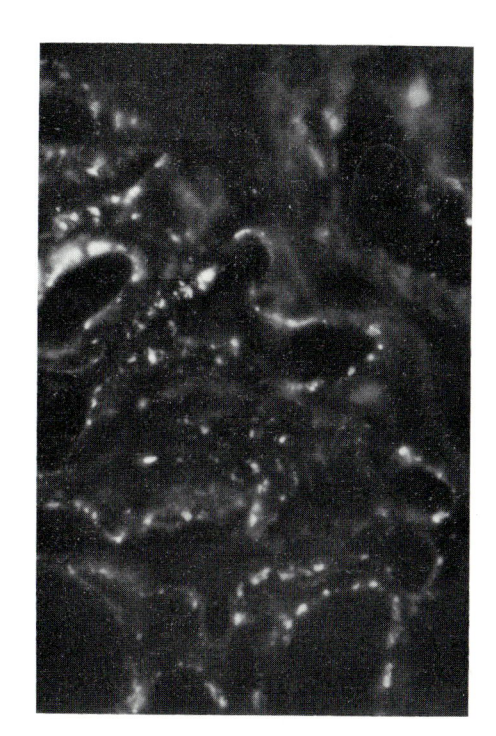

Structural Abnormality

Intramembranous Deposits
  Predominantly immunoglobulin in thickened GBL

Functional Abnormality

Basal laminar thickening leading to proteinuria and decreased filtration surface

Renal Syndrome

Nephrotic syndrome — membranous lesion, Stages III and IV (Chapter 16)

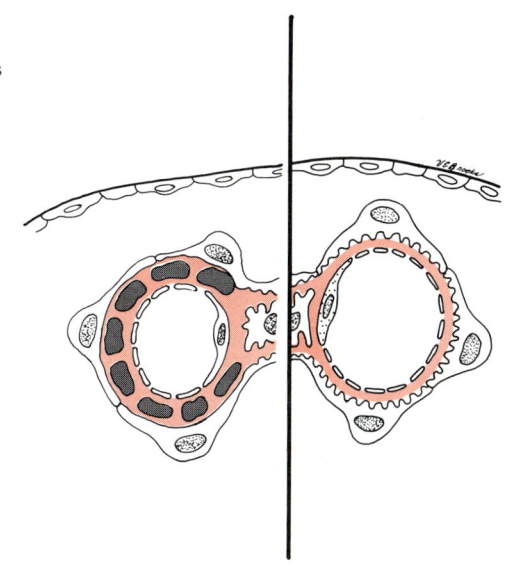

Table 5-3 continued on following page

46 Interpretation of Biopsy Specimens

TABLE 5–3 Glomeruli: Deposits (*Continued*)

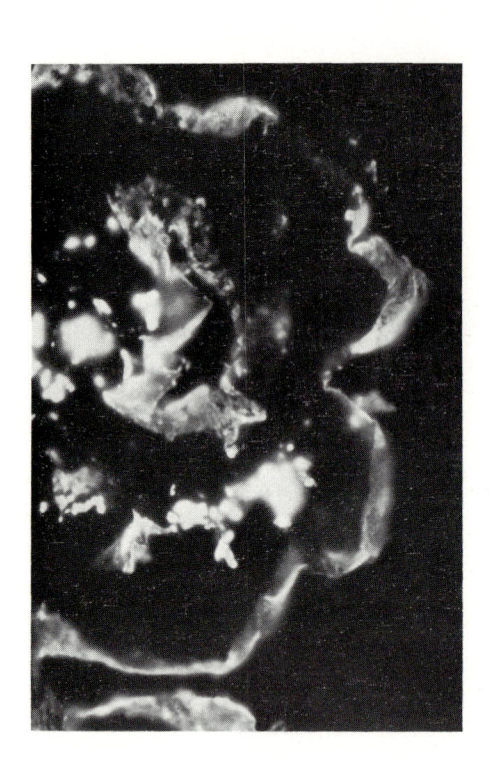

Structural Abnormality

Intramembranous Deposits
Predominantly complement in thickened GBL

Functional Abnormality

Glomerular inflammation, proteinuria, hematuria, decreased filtration

Renal Syndrome

Subset of membranoproliferative glomerulonephritis with dense intramembranous deposits (Chapter 12)

TABLE 5-3 Glomeruli: Deposits (*Continued*)

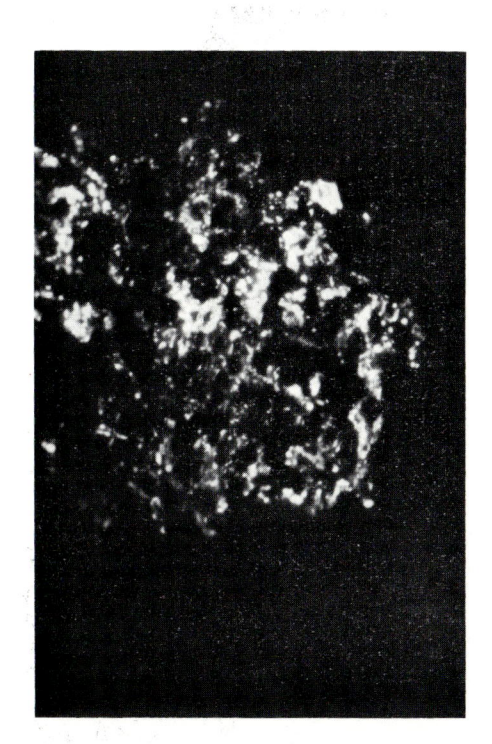

Structural Abnormality

Subepithelial Deposits
  Diffuse and irregular

Functional Abnormality

Glomerular inflammation, proteinuria, hematuria, decreased filtration surface

Renal Syndrome

Glomerular disease of acute onset (Chapter 8)

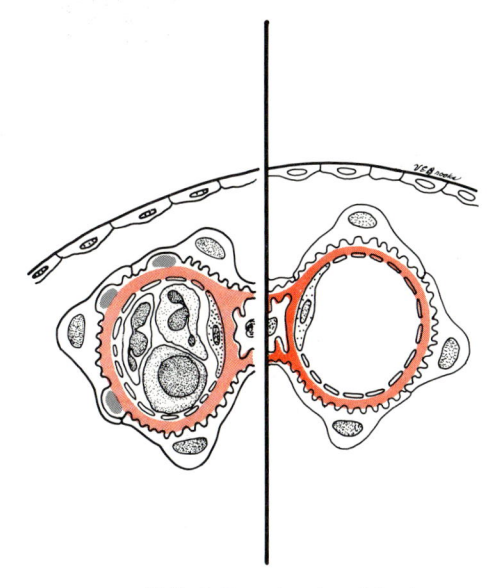

Table 5-3 continued on following page

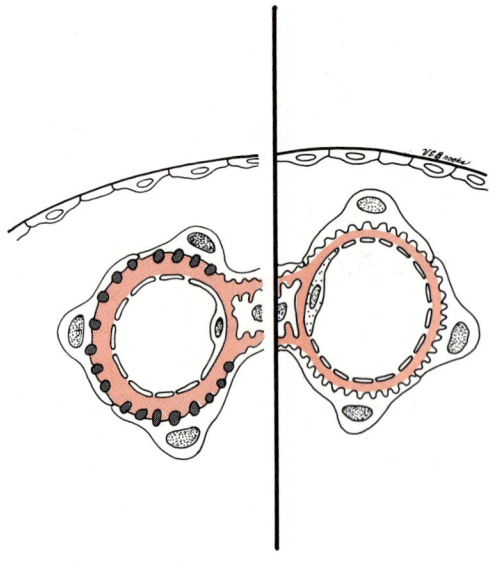

TABLE 5-3 Glomeruli: Deposits (*Continued*)

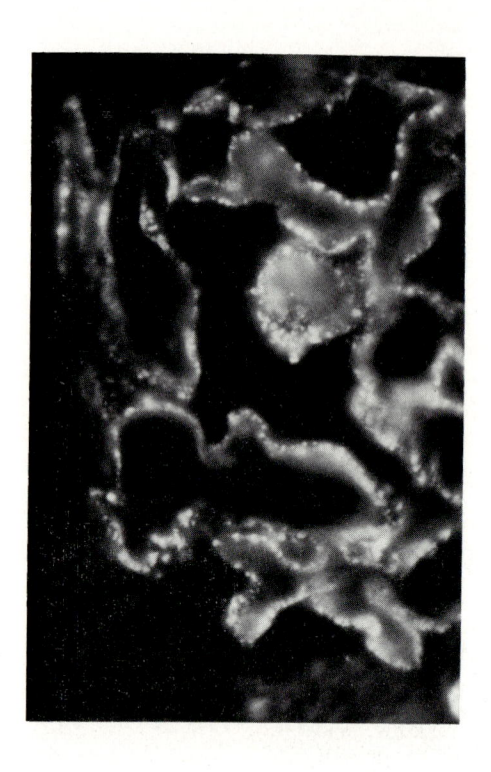

Structural Abnormality

Subepithelial Deposits
  Diffuse and regular

Functional Abnormality

Basal laminar thickening proteinuria and decreased filtration

Renal Syndrome

Nephrotic syndrome — membranous lesions, Stages I and II (Chapter 16)

TABLE 5-3 Glomeruli: Deposits (*Continued*)

Structural Abnormality

Mesangial Deposits
 Predominantly immunoglobulin and diffuse in nature

Functional Abnormality

Mesangial sclerosis, decrease in filtration surface, hematuria and proteinuria

Renal Syndrome

Seen in association with heavy immunoglobulin deposits elsewhere in the glomeruli

IgA deposits — benign recurrent hematuria (Chapter 12)

IgM deposits — focal sclerosing lesion of nephrotic syndrome (Chapter 17)

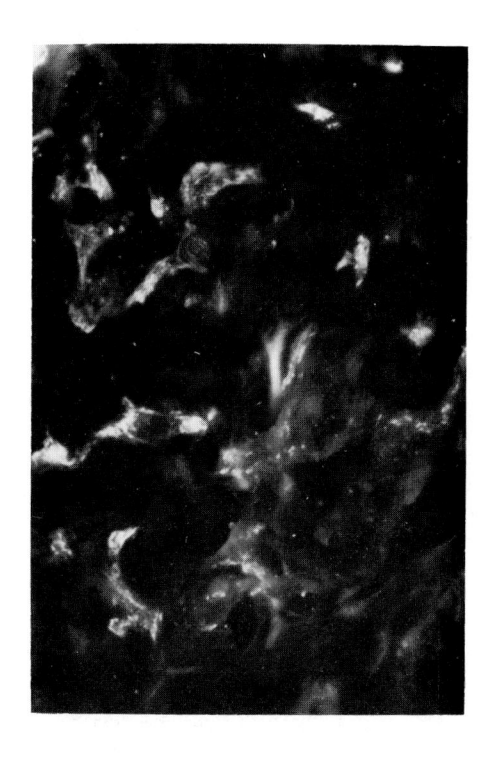

50 INTERPRETATION OF BIOPSY SPECIMENS

TABLE 5-4 Tubulo-Interstitial Compartment: Cellular Change

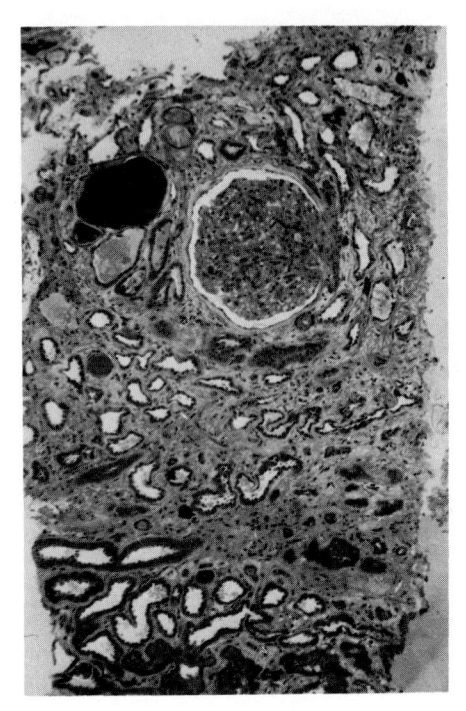

Structural Abnormality

Tubular Epithelium
  Atrophy

Functional Abnormality

Inability to concentrate and acidify the urine maximally, decreased GFR, and abnormal sodium handling

Renal Syndrome

Slowly progressive renal disease (Section III)

TABLE 5-4 Tubulo-Interstitial Compartment: Cellular Change (*Continued*)

Structural Abnormality

Tubular Epithelium
From cytoplasmic swelling to frank necrosis

Functional Abnormality

Variable degrees of acute renal insufficiency

Renal Syndrome

Tubulo-interstitial disease of acute onset (Chapter 10)

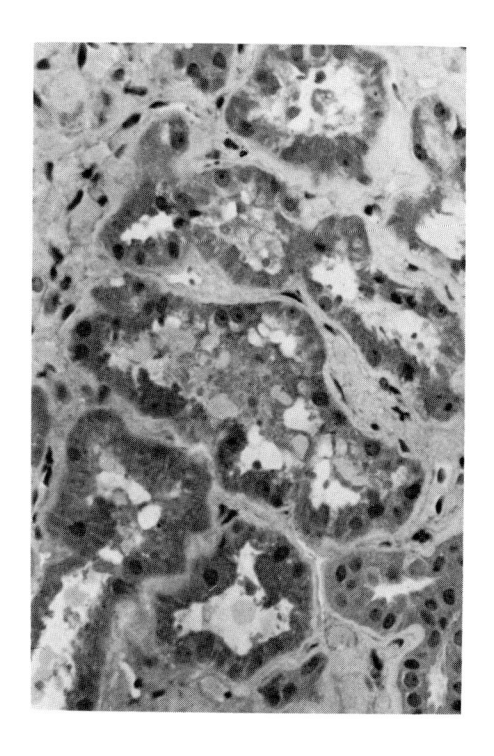

Table 5-4 continued on following page

TABLE 5-4 Tubulo-Interstitial Compartment: Cellular Change (*Continued*)

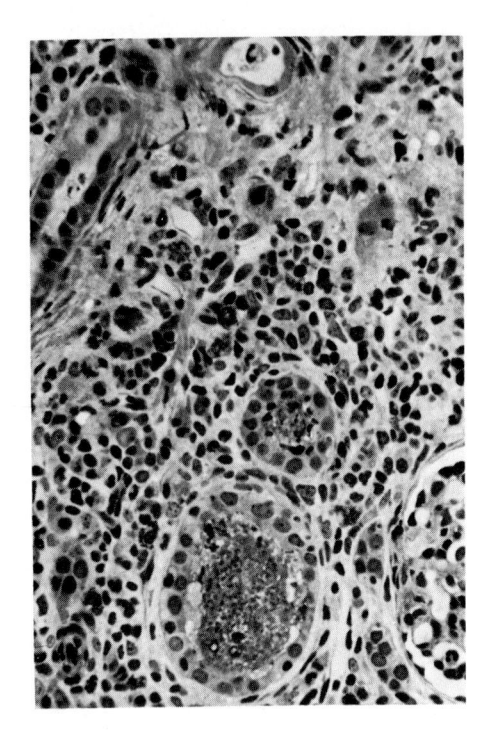

Structural Abnormality

Interstitium
  Inflammatory cells

Functional Abnormality

Tubular dysfunction and, with protracted injury, nephron loss

Renal Syndrome

Tubulo-interstitial disease of acute onset (Chapter 10); transplantation rejection (Chapter 26); any renal disease of acute onset (Section II)

TABLE 5-5 Tubulo-Interstitial Compartment: Extracellular Material

Structural Abnormality
Edema

Functional Abnormality
Interference with blood flow and transport leading to variable degrees of dysfunction

Renal Syndrome
Tubulo-interstitial diseases of acute onset (Chapter 10)

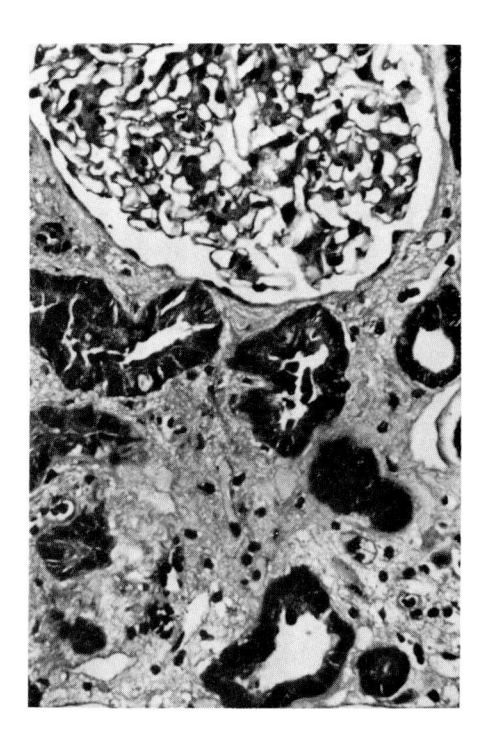

Table 5-5 continued on following page

TABLE 5-5 Tubulo-Interstitial Compartment: Extracellular Material
(*Continued*)

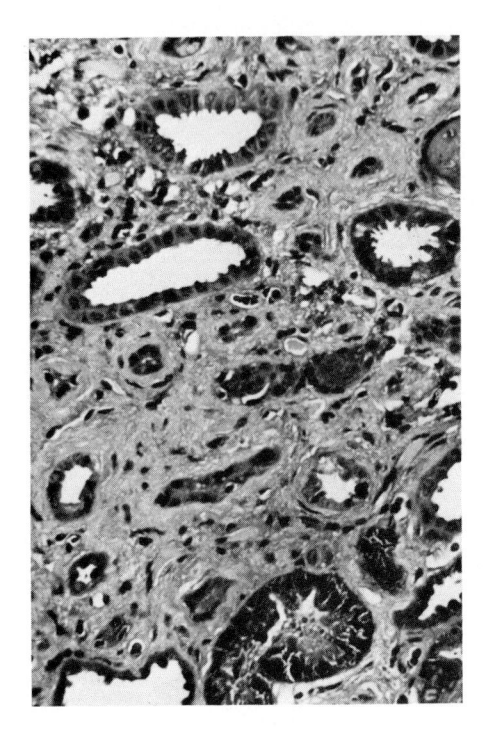

Structural Abnormality

Interstitial Fibrosis

Functional Abnormality

Progressive nephron loss and renal failure; always accompanies tubular atrophy

Renal Syndrome

Slowly progressive renal disease (Section III)

INTERPRETATION OF BIOPSY SPECIMENS   55

TABLE 5-5   Tubulo-Interstitial Compartment: Extracellular Material
(Continued)

Structural Abnormality
Basal Laminar Thickening

Functional Abnormality
Unknown; may interfere with transport

Renal Syndrome
Slowly progressive tubulo-interstitial disease (Chapter 13)

Diabetes mellitus (Chapter 21)

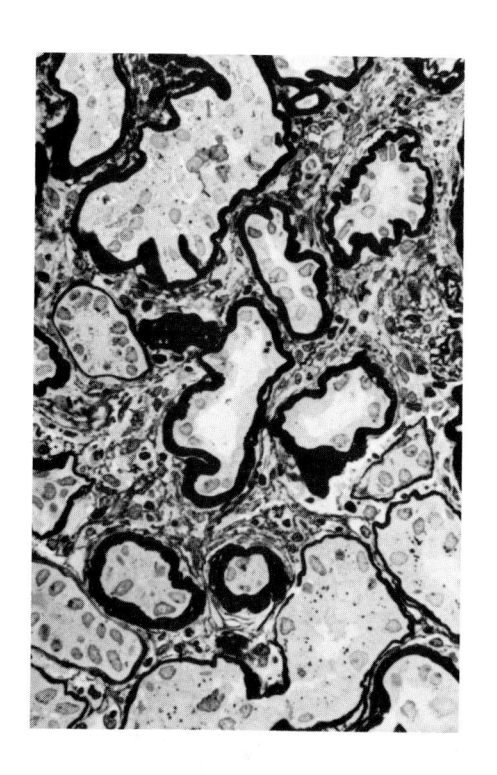

Structural Abnormality
Deposits

Functional Abnormality
Unknown; may initiate inflammatory process and injury

Renal Syndrome
Acute interstitisl nephritis (Chapter 10)

Membranoproliferative glomerulonephritis (Chapter 12)

Systemic lupus erythematosus (Chapter 17)

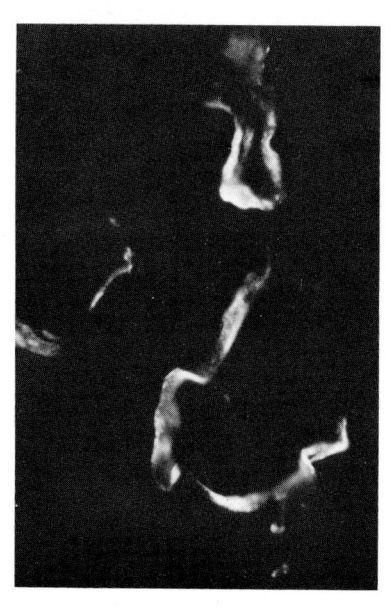

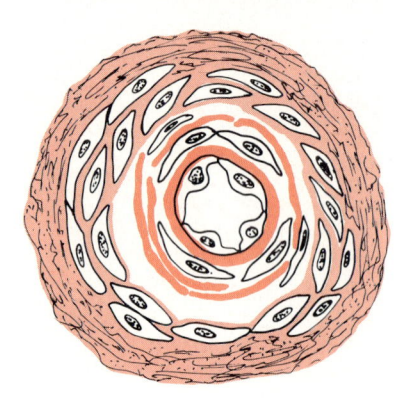

TABLE 5-6   Vascular Compartment: Cellular Change

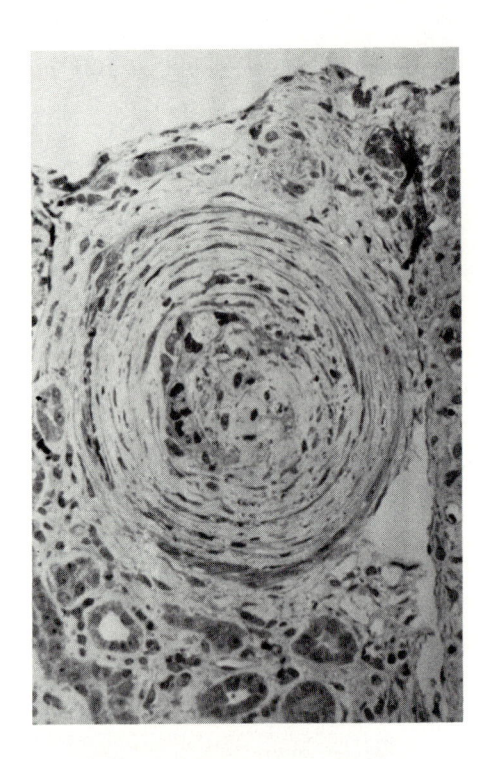

Structural Abnormality
Intimal Hypercellularity

Functional Abnormality
Acute decrease in blood flow

Renal Syndrome
Malignant nephrosclerosis (Chapter 11)

Scleroderma (Chapter 22)

Transplant rejection (Chapter 26)

INTERPRETATION OF BIOPSY SPECIMENS 57

TABLE 5–6 Vascular Compartment: Cellular Change (*Continued*)

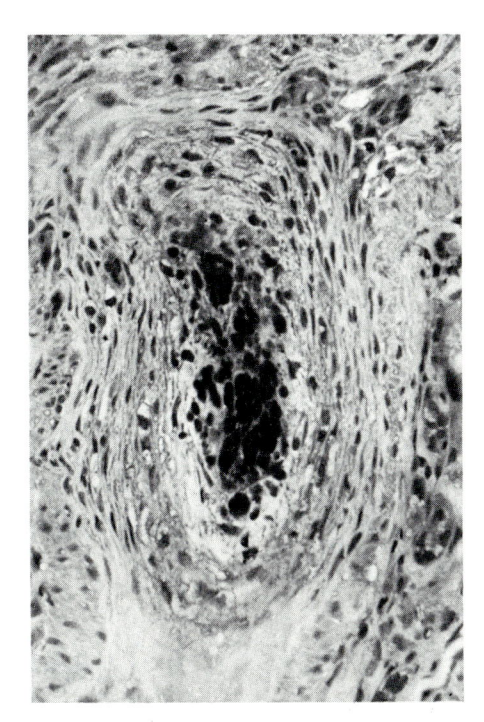

Structural Abnormality
Medial Hypercellularity

Functional Abnormality
Decrease in blood flow

Renal Syndrome
Slowly progressive renal vascular disease (Chapter 14)

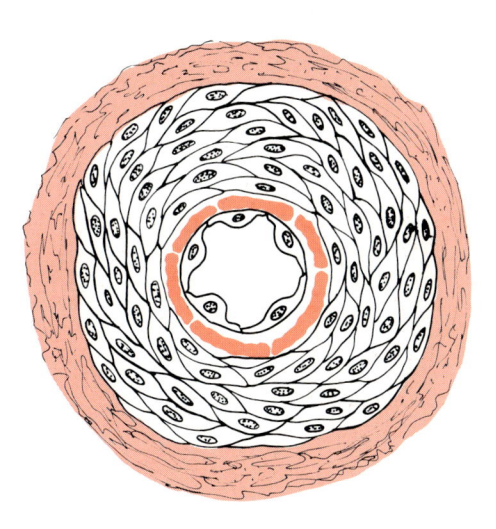

Table 5–6 continued on following page

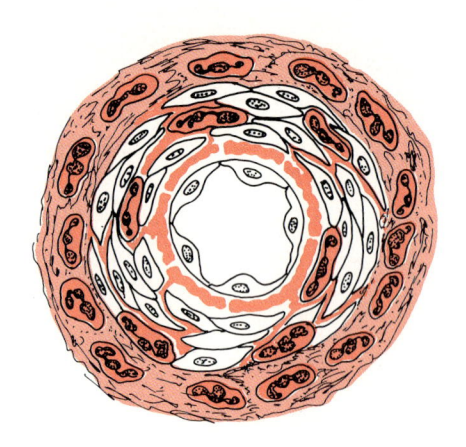

TABLE 5-6 Vascular Compartment: Cellular Change (*Continued*)

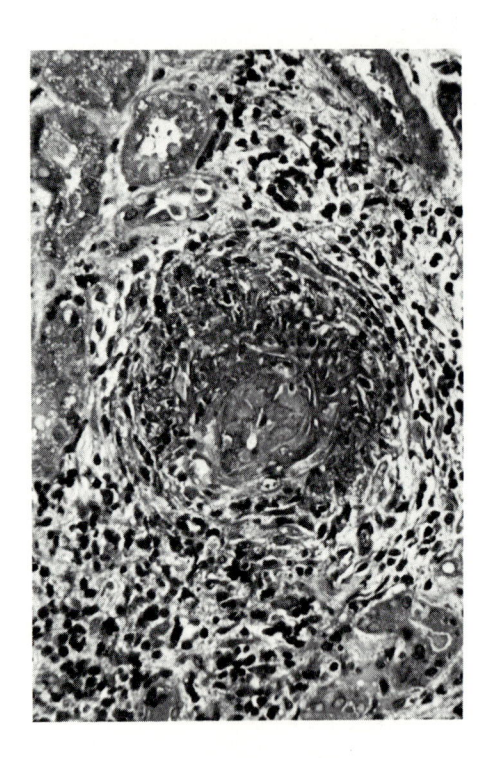

Structural Abnormality

Inflammatory Infiltrate

Functional Abnormality

Damage to the vascular wall and obstruction of blood flow

Renal Syndrome

Arteritis (Chapter 18)

Transplant rejection (Chapter 26)

TABLE 5–7   Vascular Compartment: Extracellular Material

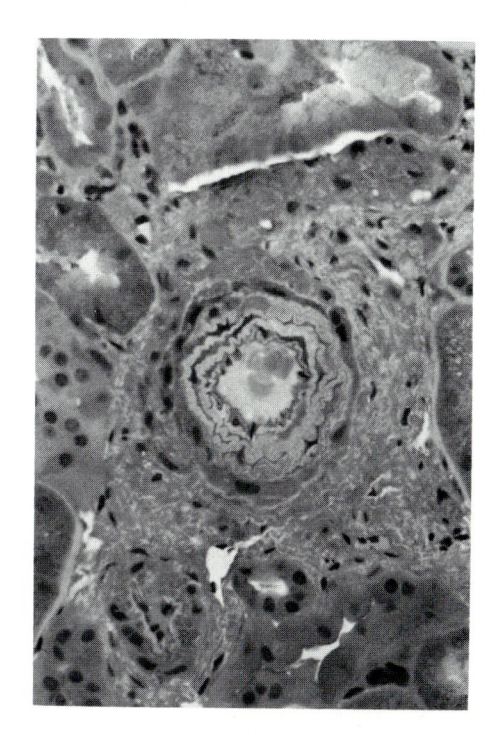

Structural Abnormality

Elastic Laminar Thickening and Reduplication

Functional Abnormality

Loss of normal vessel resilience

Renal Syndrome

Slowly progressive vascular disease (Chapter 14)

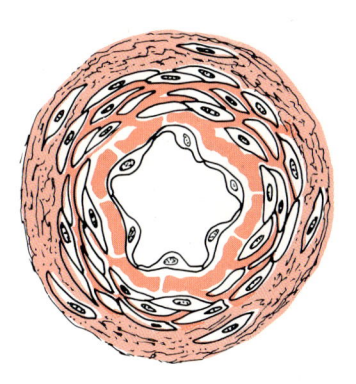

Table 5–7 continued on following page

60 Interpretation of Biopsy Specimens

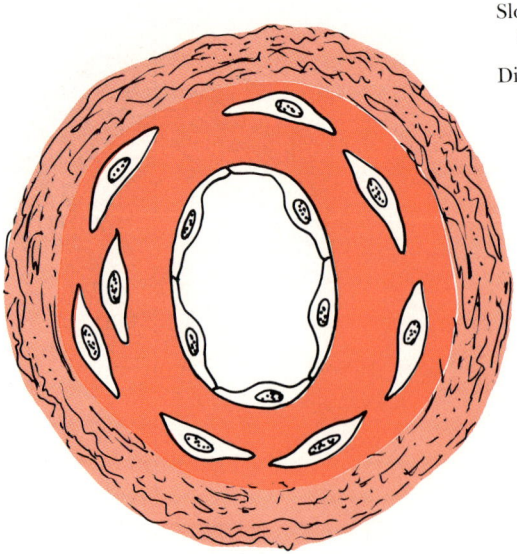

TABLE 5–7 Vascular Compartment: Extracellular Material (*Continued*)

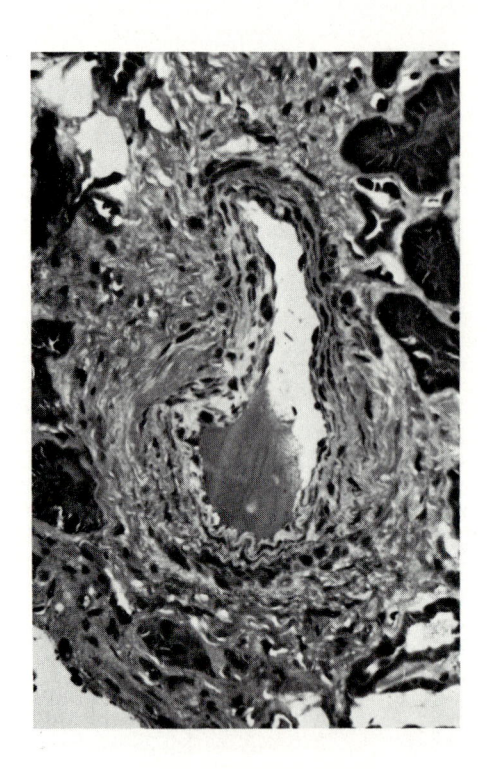

Structural Abnormality

Basal Lamina Increase of Intimal and Medial Cells

Functional Abnormality

Loss of resilience and narrowing of lumen

Renal Syndrome

Slowly progressive vascular disease (Chapter 14)

Diabetes (Chapter 21)

TABLE 5–7   Vascular Compartment: Extracellular Material (*Continued*)

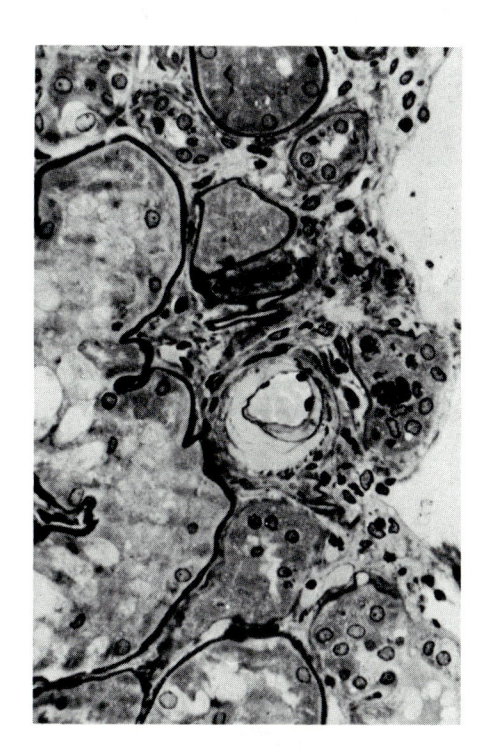

Structural Abnormality

Deposits
  Hyaline

Functional Abnormality

Decrease in flow, or change in flow characteristics

Renal Syndrome

Slowly progressive vascular disease (Chapter 14)

Diabetes mellitus (Chapter 21)

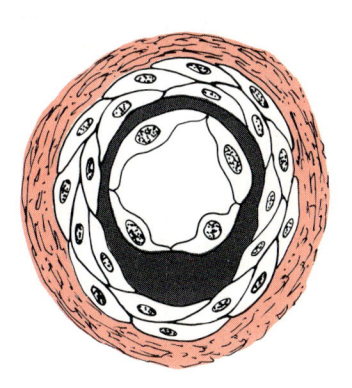

Table 5–7 continued on following page

TABLE 5-7 Vascular Compartment: Extracellular Material (*Continued*)

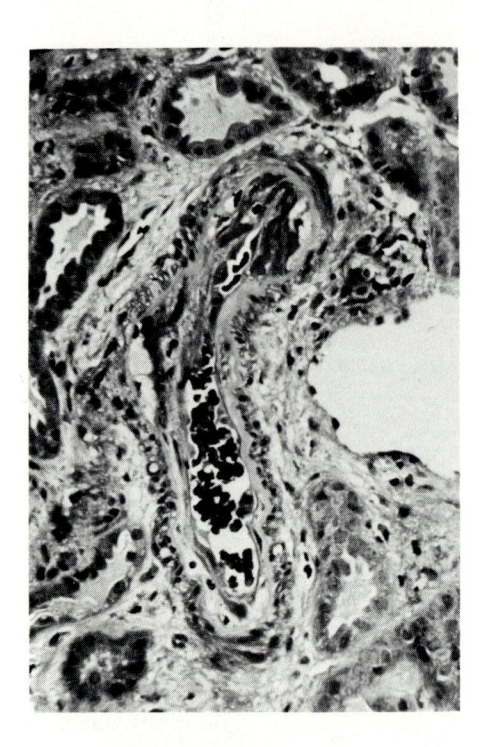

Structural Abnormality

Fibrin

Functional Abnormality

Acute inflammation and obstruction of blood flow

Renal Syndrome

Vascular disease of acute onset (Chapter 11)

Arteritis (Chapter 18)

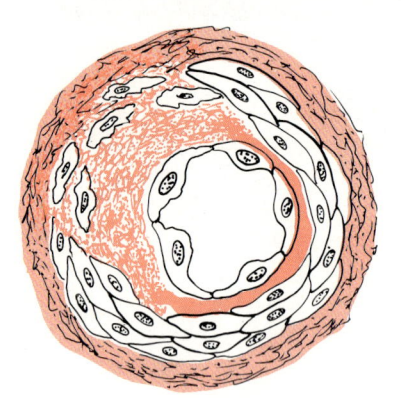

Structural Abnormality

Immunoglobulin

Functional Abnormality

Acute inflammation and obstruction of blood flow

Renal Syndrome

Arteritis (Chapter 18)

CELL CHANGES. Glomerular cells respond to injury in a limited number of ways; these responses may be manifested as a variation in the cell number or function (Table 5–1). The exact function of the individual cell types is not known with certainty, and it is apparent immediately that there are serious gaps in the current data.

Epithelial Cells. The significance of epithelial cell proliferation became clear when it was found that these cells produce the glomerular basal lamina, which contains a collagenous backbone. The accumulation of this material results in formation of a "scar." If Bowman's space becomes obliterated, the glomerulus ceases to function, and the attached tubular segment will atrophy. It is important to note that if this process is limited to the glomeruli, no change in renal function save proteinuria may be apparent until many glomeruli are destroyed and glomerulosclerosis is far advanced. Consequently, measurements of clearance rates do not allow an accurate estimate of the severity of primary glomerular disease.

In certain diseases, cell numbers remain normal, but their function is altered. An illustration of a change in epithelial cell function while the cell number remains stable, for example, is found in patients who have proteinuria and anatomic changes that can only be demonstrated by electron microscopy (Table 5–1, page 33). The alteration in this condition is simply loss of the normal pedicel architecture; the cell junctions (desmosomes) between the pedicels of adjacent podocytes are the sites through which most of the filtrate passes. Alterations in this structure often result in a change in the composition of the filtrate, variations which are roughly proportional to the degree of injury. For instance, if only the pedicellar anatomy is altered, protein appears in the filtrate in large amounts, but relatively low-molecular-weight species predominate—so-called selective proteinuria. More severe glomerular injury is reflected in the appearance of larger-molecular-weight species of proteins in the urine—so-called nonselective proteinuria.

Little is known about the regulation of glomerular basal lamina synthesis; it is thought, however, that the epithelial cell contributes substantially to this process. Prolonged or irreversible injury to the epithelial cells might result in abnormalities in the amount (thickening or duplication) or composition of the glomerular basal lamina. These changes could be reflected in the structural integrity, elasticity, antigenicity, or filtration properties of the structure. Thickening of the glomerular basal lamina, for example, would seem to impede the appearance of high-molecular-weight solutes in the filtrate, whereas, in fact, the opposite appears to be the case. Proteinuria and the increased thickness of the glomerular basal lamina often occur together, suggesting that both are results of injury-induced epithelial cell changes. The former is caused by abnormalities in the synthesis or degradation of the glomerular basal lamina, and the latter is due to altered cell function or intercellular junctions.

Endothelial Cells. Endothelial cells are the first component of the filtration barrier. Their membranes are extensively fenestrated and they ordinarily have a smooth luminal surface. They have been noted to be phagocytic and contractile in vitro. In other capillary beds these cells synthesize a basal lamina, but it is not known what contribution they make to the glomerular basal lamina.

Little attention has been paid to changes of glomerular endothelial cells except in pregnancy. It is known that the cells' response to injury consists of swelling, formation of multiple surface projections, proliferation, and production of a new layer of glomerular basal lamina. The swelling and surface projections are associated with (or cause) red cell and platelet destruction (Table 5-1, page 34).

Ordinarily, when an injury is sufficiently severe to be associated with endothelial cell proliferation, the architecture of the glomerulus is so distorted that it is difficult to identify endothelial cells. Renal diseases with chronic injury to the cells, however, are associated with a widened subendothelial space and production of a new basal lamina immediately adjacent to the endothelial cell. An example is the nephrotic syndrome associated with hypocomplementemia (page 000).

Mesangial Cells. The existence of mesangial cells was established in the late 1950's. Soon after their discovery the mesangial region was noted to be one of the sites of accumulation for circulating macromolecules, and it was hypothesized that mesangial cells are phagocytic and may be a functional component of the reticuloendothelial system. More recently, their contractile capabilities have been demonstrated. A modest increase in cell number is associated with what is thought to be a relatively mild glomerular injury which often accompanies accumulations of immunoglobulins in the surrounding matrix (Table 5-1, page 35). As in the case of the endothelial cell, pronounced proliferation may render it difficult to detect the exact cell type involved. Mesangial cells also produce extracellular material; thus, persistent proliferation may be associated with an increased quantity of mesangial matrix.

EXTRACELLULAR MATERIAL CHANGES

Increase in Amount (Table 5-2). The extracellular material consists of both glomerular basal lamina and mesangial matrix. The composition of the intact structure suggests that nearly half is composed of collagen. In addition, a collagenous protein has been isolated by partial digestion of the intact structure, as well as from cultures of glomerular cells.

Although the exact role of the basal lamina in the filtration barrier is not clear, one of its prime functions is to serve as the microskeleton of the glomerulus. The peripheral basal lamina may show changes in contour, thickness, or lamination, and, in common with collagenous proteins elsewhere in the body, turnover is very slow and the lamina is quite resistant to enzymatic degradation. Consequently, when laid down in excess quantities or in abnormal locations, it is removed slowly or not at all, resulting in sclerosis or scarring. Little is known of the composition of the glomerular basal lamina in disease, but it is probably altered under these conditions. The result could be changes in permeability, elasticity, or antigenicity. An increase in mesangial matrix also is associated with prolonged mesangial hypercellularity and slowly progressive glomerular diseases.

Deposits. Deposits of proteins commonly are noted in the region of the extracellular material. Proteins, such as antigen-antibody complexes which localize in capillary walls, may form quite conspicuous "deposits." The location, distribution, and composition of deposits is of considerable importance (Table 5-3). Immunoglobulin G (IgG) in combination with antigen and complement components, for instance, can localize in any position; but when the lattice size (number of molecules) is small, most frequently they are demonstrated in a subepithelial location. On the other hand, immunoglobulins M (IgM) and A (IgA), as isolated proteins or in combination with IgG and complement components, frequently are found in a mesangial or subendothelial position. The description used to identify the location of deposits varies among institutions; for example, deposits which are found scattered over glomerular loops in a random or irregular distribution and size have been called "granular," "lumpy-bumpy," and so forth. The deposits found on the epithelial aspect of the glomerular basal lamina, which have a regular distribution and size, sometimes are referred to as epimembranous, while those on the endothelial side of the glomerular basal lamina have been called endomembranous or subendothelial. Such confusion in terminology could be avoided if a description is used which states the location, size, and distribution in strict anatomic terms. Abbreviated descriptions could become useful when uniform definitions are agreed upon.

Distribution of Changes. Cellular and extracellular processes noted previously may involve all of every glomerulus (diffuse changes), all of a few glomeruli (focal changes), or different parts of the glomeruli (segmental changes). "Local and "focal" have been used interchangeably in the past. It is more precise, however, if the actual number involved in each process can be used. The description that 14 of 28 glomeruli are involved, for instance, leaves no room for doubt about extent of the disease.

TUBULO-INTERSTITIAL DISEASE

GENERAL CONSIDERATIONS. The tubular compartment is complex in terms of both its structure and its function (Table 5-4). Four segments of the compartment are distinguishable: proximal convoluted tubule, loop of Henle, distal convoluted tubule, and collecting duct. The coordination and intactness of the cells' functional capabilities in each of these regions determines the final composition and volume of the bladder urine. Since the total number of nephrons greatly exceeds that required to maintain adequate renal function, a lesion must involve a large number of nephrons or a specific metabolic sequence in all structures before it becomes clinically apparent.

The structural integrity of the renal cortex depends on the interstitial connective tissue surrounding the blood vessels (Figs. 5-3 and 5-4). This structural component is continuous with the thin, filamentous collagen bundles which connect to the basal lamina and give spatial organization to the glomeruli, tubules, and peritubular capillaries. With the exception of the areas immediately adjacent to blood vessels, the interstitium of the renal cortex contains only capillaries, a scattering of so-called interstitial cells, and a sparse number of collagen fibers.

The interstitium of the medulla, on the other hand, contains a large quantity of mucopolysaccharides and connective tissue, as well as a sizeable number of cells with an ordered and easily identifiable relationship to the adjacent tubules and vessels. In addition, it is the probable site for production of prostaglandins and erythropoietin, and the metabolism of vitamin D.

CELL CHANGES (TABLE 5-4)

Tubular Atrophy. Renal biopsy is not yet a clinically useful method of assessing tubular injury unless the lesion is severe. For this reason, little is known about tubular response to injury except in cases in which the lesion is such that renal function ceases almost entirely, or the tubules atrophy or contain unusual luminal contents, such as casts. Certain uncommon metabolic disorders such as cystinosis, homocystinuria, and oxalosis lead to specific changes, but these are the exceptions. More sensitive measurements probably would allow increased recognition of segmental dysfunction.

Cytoplasmic Swelling and Necrosis. Acute injury, most commonly from derangement of renal blood flow, leads to varying degrees of tubular ischemia and injury. Rarely, tubular cell poisons, such as heavy metals or ethylene glycol, produce similar results. The histologic lesions vary from mild swelling of the tubular cell cytoplasm, which may be difficult to distinguish from fixation artifact in paraffin-embedded sections, to frank cellular necrosis.

Proliferation (Interstitial Cells). As an isolated event, proliferation of interstitial cells is probably rare. An increased number of interstitial cells admixed with other cells in an inflammatory infiltrate, however, occurs frequently. These are recognizable by their stellate shape and rich cytoplasmic content of dilated rough endoplasmic reticulum.

INFLAMMATORY CELL INFILTRATE

Diffuse. The composition, distribution, and sites of an inflammatory infiltrate may be useful indicators of the type of injury.

Interpretation of Biopsy Specimens

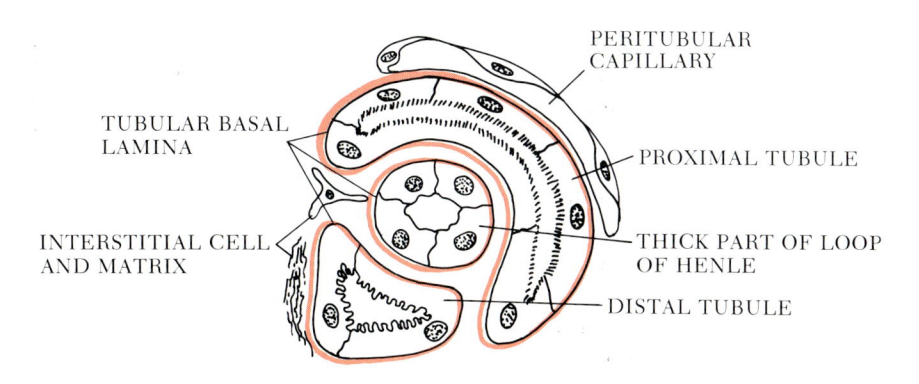

Figure 5-3 Diagrammatic representation of the tubulo-interstitial compartment.

In systemic lupus erythematosus, for example, the presence of a diffuse inflammatory cell infiltrate (plasma cells and lymphocytes) is considered to be a more accurate indicator of renal disease activity than many other histologic parameters. The presence of eosinophils and neutrophils connotes an acute inflammatory reaction which is often a response to cell death, as in tubular injury, bacterial invasion, or hypersensitivity reaction. Lymphocytes and plasma cells are commonly seen in the case of acute homograft rejection episodes, the invading cells often infiltrating the tubules as well.

Figure 5-4 Normal tubules and interstitium (H&E, ×1200).

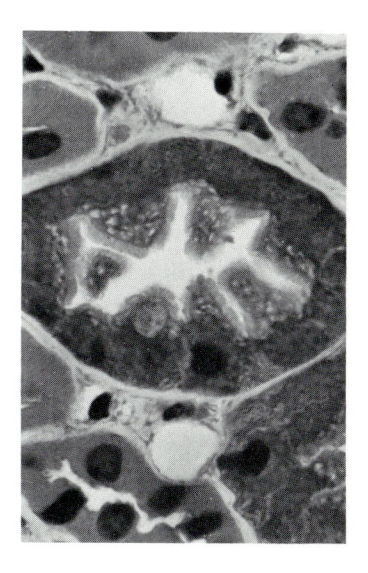

Focal. Localized collections of inflammatory cells are often seen in areas of cell injury. Examples include the infiltrate present around glomeruli with epithelial cell proliferation or in the region of veins and lymphatics in chronic homograft rejection. In addition, small collections of lymphocytes often are found in areas of fibrosis containing atrophied tubules and obsolescent glomeruli, typified in the fibrotic foci of nephrosclerosis.

EXTRACELLULAR MATERIAL CHANGES (TABLE 5–5)

Edema. Indicators of edema include increased distance between tubules and absence of recognizable capillaries and cells, or extracellular material in the intervening space. Fixation in formalin, Zenker's solution, and other fixatives of this type tends to obscure edema, however, since they cause considerable tissue shrinkage.

Fibrosis. "Fibrosis" refers to widened interstitial spaces with an increased number of collagen bundles. This matrix also contains an increased quantity of mucopolysaccharides, remnants of tubular and vascular basal lamina, as well as other, unspecified components. Chapter 6 will detail normal tubular function, which depends on the close opposition of tubules to adjacent capillaries and other structures.

BASAL LAMINA THICKENING

This change accompanies interstitial fibrosis and tubular atrophy. Since the tubular basal lamina is easy to visualize and ordinarily is abundant, minor changes may be quite apparent. Thus chronic mild injury, leading ultimately to atrophy of the nephron, may first be manifest as mild thickening of the tubular basal lamina.

The basal lamina is often multilaminate as well as thickened. Since this disease process most commonly is seen as an accompaniment of tubular atrophy, the profiles are wrinkled and shrunken as well as thickened and duplicated.

VASCULAR DISEASE (TABLE 5–6)

GENERAL CONSIDERATIONS. The arterial supply to the kidney is an endarterial system, and the arteries present in a renal biopsy specimen generally are the size of arcuate vessels or smaller (Figs. 5–5 and 5–6). Since the blood flow to the cortex passes through glomerular capillaries before reaching the peritubular capillaries, it is technically a portal system. The tubules supplied by a postglomerular capillary vary with the capillary's position in the cortex. For the most part, however, the blood flow through a glomerulus supplies segments from multiple other nephrons, but, depending on its location in the cortex, a glomerulus may not contribute to the blood supply of any part of its attached nephron. The most distal part of the cortical capillary network is the blood supply to the cortical segments of the medullary ray.

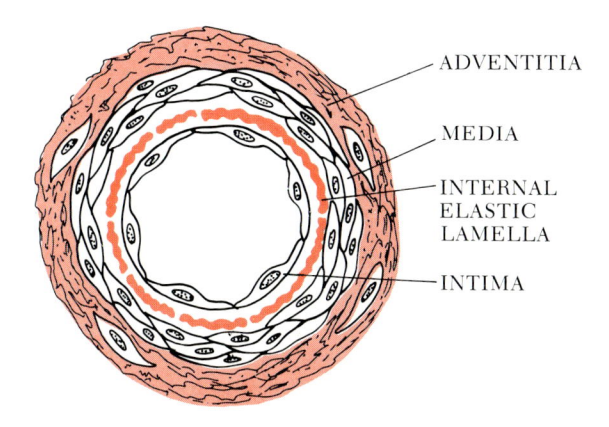

Figure 5-5 Diagrammatic representation of a normal artery.

The difficulty of obtaining larger blood vessels for histologic examination by invasive techniques is related to their relative inaccessibility from the cortical surface. Noninvasive external techniques, for example, such as xenon washout or injected microspheres, are not sufficiently refined or complete to be helpful. The widespread clinical use of renal homografts and the high incidence of hypertension, both of which are associated with vascular lesions, makes this area of great importance. (See Table 5-6.)

Figure 5-6 Normal artery (H&E, ×300).

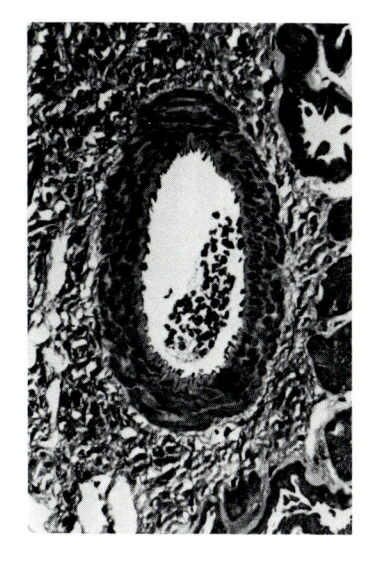

CELL CHANGES

Intimal Cells. Endothelial cellular changes include swelling (or thickening) and hypercellularity. The endothelium of the arteries and arterioles is nonfenestrated, forming a thin layer over the basal lamina. Severe injury induced by intravascular coagulation, for example, or deposition of antigen-antibody complexes, leads to separation of the cells from their basal lamina. The result is aggregation of platelets at the site, with leakage of serum proteins out of the lumen into the wall. The extent of this change is related directly to the severity of the insult.

Less severe injury leads to endothelial cell proliferation. The change may involve the entire circumference or only one portion of the wall. It is often quite localized and tends to occur near bifurcations. Inflammatory cells are often present in the zone of intimal cell necrosis or proliferation. Since this alteration represents a severe, acute injury, neutrophils are commonly found.

The peripheral capillary loops of the glomerulus, on the other hand, are lined by a fenestrated endothelium. There has been controversy over whether these fenestrations are closed by membranes. Injury to the cells results in swelling and loss of fenestrae. Villous transformation of the surface also occurs, and the result of this change appears to be local destruction of platelets and possibly red blood cells. Although the peritubular capillary endothelium is nonfenestrated, the cells respond similarly.

Medial Cells. These are smooth muscle cells that maintain the vessel caliber at a prescribed diameter. They are surrounded by a basal lamina which interconnects with that of adjacent medial cells, the intima, and the adventitial connective tissue. The alterations include a change in number of cells and development of vacuoles, as well as necrosis and infiltration with inflammatory cells.

Since their number normally varies with the vessel size, it is difficult to determine whether the vessel in question is hypercellular or a normal but larger vessel. Atrophy or decrease in cell number is somewhat easier to detect, since there is usually an associated increase in connective tissue. Likewise, necrosis is associated either with transudation of plasma proteins or infiltration with inflammatory cells.

EXTRACELLULAR MATERIAL CHANGE. The extracellular material consists of the basal lamina, which is adjacent to all cells, and an elastic lamina found between intimal and medial cells. The basal lamina is thickened as a result of chronic, slowly advancing injury, an easily recognized reaction combining an increase in the amount of both basal lamina and elastic lamella occurring in a lamellar pattern internal to the media. These "myointimal" cells share many ultrastructural characteristics of smooth muscle cells, but are located in the region of the intima.

Deposits of protein also are present in this region. Large masses may exist either circumferentially or as a nodule in one area. On electron microscopy, cell debris and amorphous material are observed. Fluorescence microscopy also reveals many serum proteins.

Chapter Six

Correlation of Renal Structure and Function

A basic element of the study of an organ is appreciation of the relationship between its structural and functional characteristics. Although these relationships have been found in the normal kidney, analyses in renal disease have been fraught with difficulties because, as Oliver (1961) has noted, the damaged kidney is a collection of "thousands of fantastically altered organs of strange design and anomalous behavior." The development of percutaneous biopsy, however, has not only improved our understanding of the anatomic features of renal disease, but also has allowed a simultaneous comparison of its clinical and histologic aspects.

GLOMERULAR FILTRATION RATE (GFR)

The clearance of both inulin and creatinine shows a high correlation to both interstitial and tubular damage regardless of diagnosis (Fig. 6-1). The total interstitial compartment damage correlates better with GFR than any of the individual interstitial components. Interstitial fibrosis and infiltration with inflammatory cells also correlate highly with the glomerular filtration rate. Edema, on the other hand, shows no significant correlation, which may be related to the difficulty in quantitating edema on a biopsy specimen. All patients whose inulin clearance is below 60 ml/min have moderate to severe interstitial or tubular abnormalities, but we have been unable to demonstrate this lesion in patients with a clearance above 100 ml/min (Figs. 6-1 and 6-2).

In contrast to the previous findings, there is only a rough correlation between inulin or creatinine clearance and histologic abnormalities

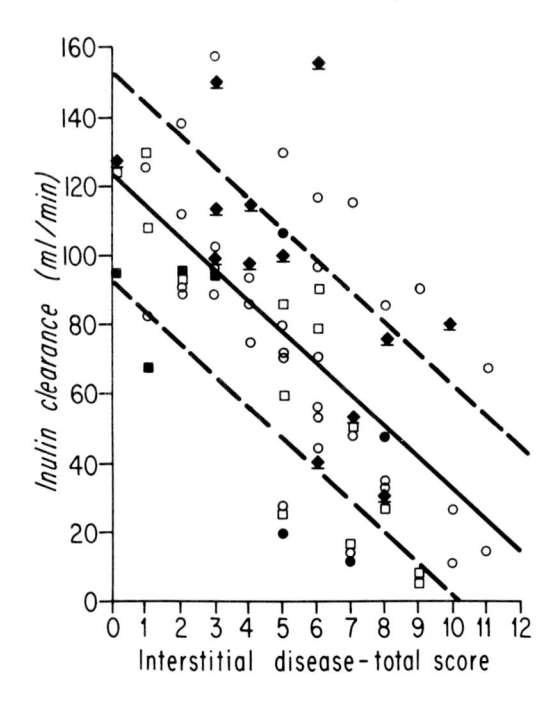

Figure 6-1. Relationship between inulin clearance and interstitial disease. The regression line (solid line) is y = 122 − 8.8x and S.E.E. (dashed line) is 31. Symbols refer to cases belonging to conventional diagnostic groups: ♦, acute glomerulonephritis; ○, chronic glomerulonephritis; ●, interstitial nephritis; ■, nephrosclerosis; □, miscellaneous. In this and the following figures (Figs. 6-2 to 6-5) note that the distribution of patients is without regard to the conventional categorization of diseases. (From Schainuck et al., 1970.)

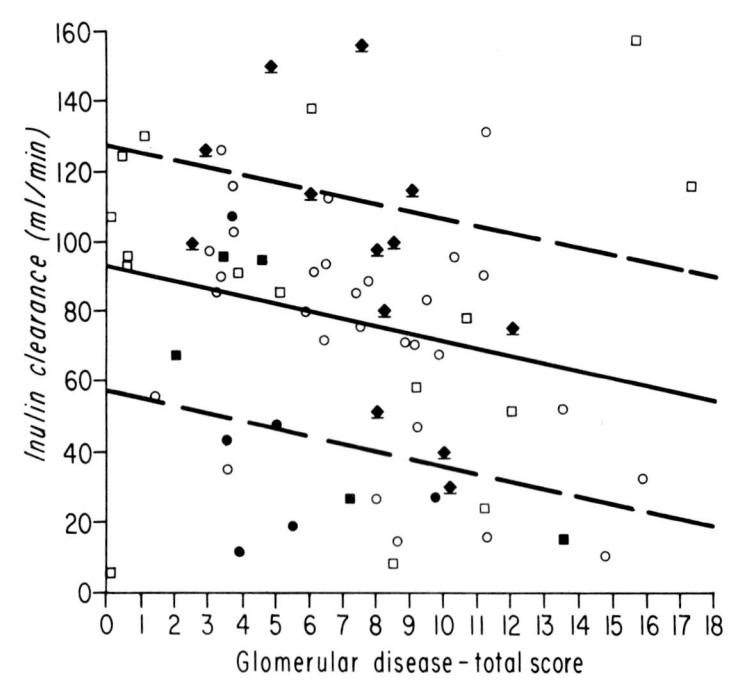

Figure 6-2. Relationship between inulin clearance and glomerular disease. Regression line (solid line) is y = 92 − 0.02x and S.E.E. (dashed line) is 39. The poor correlation is apparent. The symbols are the same as in Figure 6-1. (From Schainuck et al., 1970.)

of the glomeruli (Fig. 6–2). A clearance rate within the normal range, for instance, is compatible with severe glomerular changes, whereas markedly impaired clearance often occurs when minimal glomerular alterations are present. Even when the primary lesion is a form of glomerulonephritis, however, diminished inulin clearance does not always signify severe glomerular disease; rather, it indicates abnormal tubules and interstitium.

Although we have emphasized the relationship between the glomerular filtration rate and tubulo-interstitial disease, it should be noted that the glomerular filtration rate also correlates well with the degree of vascular disease. Creatinine clearance correlates with tubulo-interstitial disease as well, but not with glomerular disease, and patients whose creatinine clearance rate is less than 80 ml/min will generally have mod-

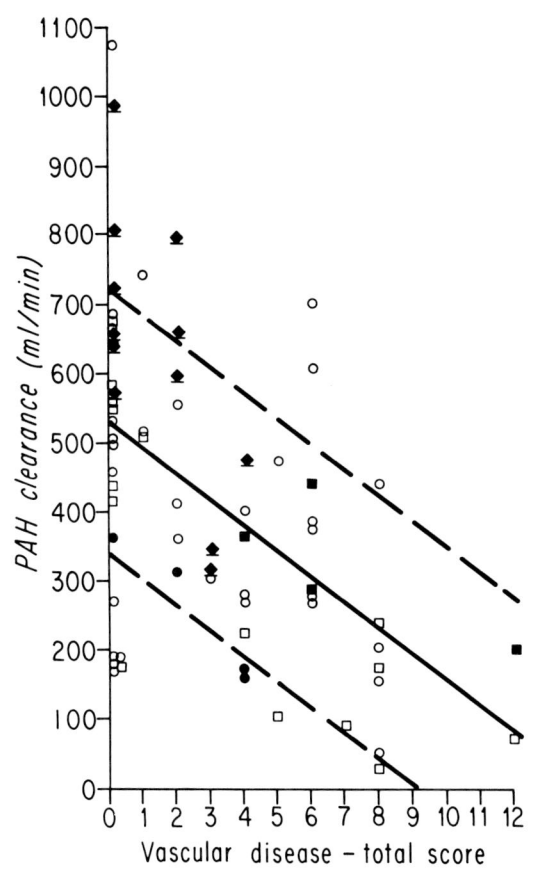

Figure 6–3. Relationship between PAH clearance and vascular disease. Regression line (solid line) is y = 533 − 38x and S.E.E. (dashed line) is 193. Although wide variation is seen in patients with no vascular abnormalities, all but two patients with more than minimal disease have decreased PAH clearance. The symbols are the same as in Figure 6–1. (From Schainuck et al., 1970.)

erate to severe tubulo-interstitial disease. Thus, because of its simplicity, creatinine clearance rate remains the clinical test of choice in evaluating the glomerular filtration rate.

RENAL BLOOD FLOW

The renal blood flow rate shows a high correlation with tubular and interstitial disease in addition to the degree of vascular disease (Fig. 6-3). For example, patients whose para-amino-hippuric acid (PAH) clearance is above 500 ml/min rarely have histologic vascular disease. On the other hand, PAH clearance of under 200 ml/min may

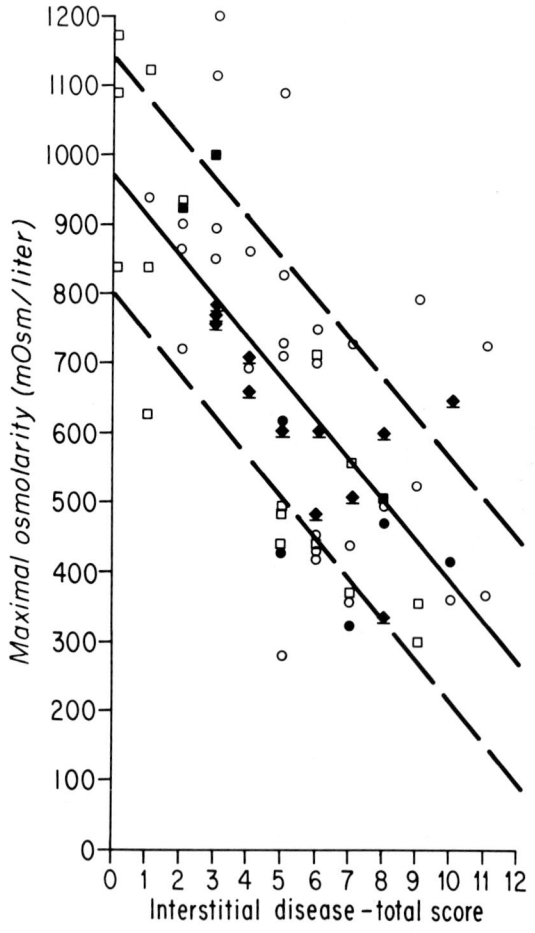

Figure 6-4. Relationship between maximal urinary osmolarity and interstitial disease. Regression line (solid line) is $y = 975 - 59x$ and S.E.E. (dashed line) is 179. The symbols are the same as in Figure 6-1. (From Schainuck et al., 1970.)

be seen in the absence of vascular disease, indicating that plasma flow can be decreased without significant morphologic abnormalities in renal arteries.

CONCENTRATING ABILITY

The concentrating ability is a very sensitive indicator of the presence or absence of tubular and interstitial abnormalities (Fig. 6-4). It is the degree of tubulo-interstitial damage, and not the basic disease process, that appears to determine the degree of impairment in concentrating ability. Maximal urinary osmolarity of less than 600 mOsm/liter indicates moderate to severe tubulo-interstitial disease, whereas the ability to concentrate over 800 mOsm/liter is associated with minimal abnormalities (Fig. 6-4). In addition, there is a significant relationship between concentrating ability and glomerular disease.

ACIDIFYING ABILITY

A high degree of correlation is found between ammonium excretion following an acute acid load and the amount of interstitial, tubular, and glomerular damage (Fig. 6-5). Patients whose ammonium excretion is less than 40 μEq/min, for instance, have moderate to severe tubulo-interstitial disease, whereas patients whose excretory rate is above 60 μEq/min seldom demonstrate severe tubulo-interstitial abnormalities. Ability to excrete titratable acid also correlates well with interstitial and tubular disease, and to a lesser degree with glomerular changes. On the other hand, the minimal urinary pH obtainable bears no relationship to any aspect of renal pathology, nor does it appear to be related to any other area of renal function.

INTERPRETATION

There are several possible explanations for the poor correlations found between functional impairment and the glomerular abnormalities. First, a variety of glomerular lesions may have little or no functional consequences. Although there is general agreement that an atrophic or sclerotic glomerulus is probably incapable of contributing to urine formation, the functional significance of marked basal lamina thickening or proliferation of cellular elements is uncertain. Second, studies of experimental renal disease, as well as observations on patients who have undergone nephrectomy, have shown that residual nephrons are capable of increasing function rapidly without observable change in structure. These data suggest that the relatively normal glomeruli seen on biopsy may undergo compensatory functional hyper-

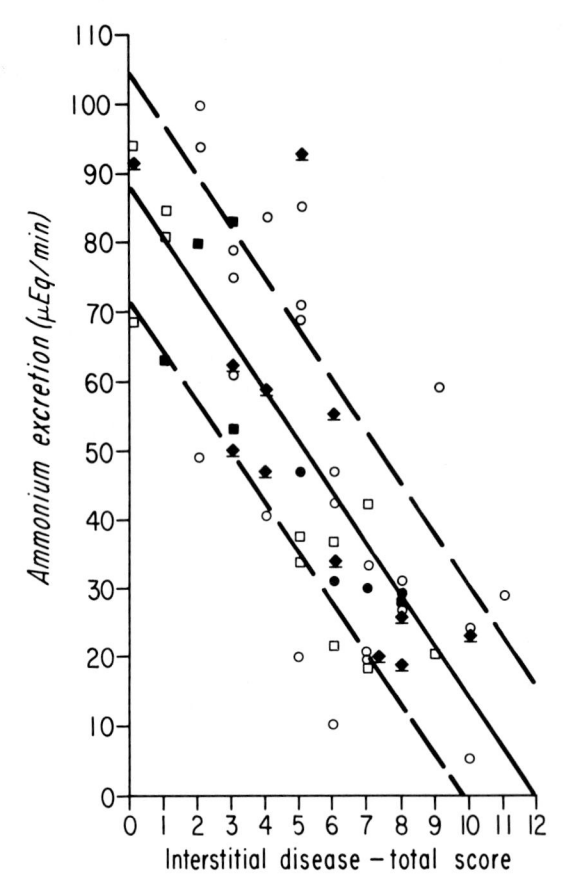

Figure 6–5. Relationship between ammonium excretion following an acute acid load and interstitial disease. The regression line (solid line) is $y = 90 - 7.6x$ and S.E.E. (dashed line) is 20. The symbols are the same as in Figure 6–1. (From Schainuck et al., 1970.)

trophy. Third, microdissection studies have documented the presence of atubular glomeruli in renal disease that may appear normal on section, but which do not contribute to urine formation. Fourth, the most severely atrophied glomeruli may merge with the surrounding interstitium and become unrecognizable or might be removed by inflammatory cells.

It may appear paradoxical that abnormalities of the interstitial tissue show a close correlation with abnormalities of renal physiology. Far from being merely a supporting structure, however, the normal interstitium consists of a network of capillaries constituting about 25 per cent of the total renal mass. This capillary network arises from the postglomerular (efferent) arterioles and provides the blood supply to the tubules. Exchange of water and solute between tubules and blood occurs via this network as well. Interruption of blood flow through these capillaries immediately would abolish glomerular filtration pressure and eventuate in ischemic tubular (and, therefore, nephron) atrophy. In a precise microangiographic study of renal arterial patterns, Ljungquist (1963) has shown that these peritubular capillaries are markedly decreased in areas of interstitial inflammation, edema, or fibrosis.

Disease in various anatomic compartments could lead to decreased blood flow through the peritubular capillaries and consequently to a decreased glomerular filtration rate. Glomerular disease may interfere with blood flow through the glomerular capillaries, whereas arteriolonephrosclerosis would diminish flow in the arterioles. When widespread interstitial inflammation occurs, on the other hand, compression or obliteration of this capillary network could be expected, with a profound effect on renal blood flow. Interference with the peritubular blood flow by any of these processes would lead to tubular degeneration and atrophy, and thus the entire nephron would cease to exist as a functioning entity.

The final stage of many types of renal disease may be the dissolution of all or part of the nephron, with replacement by interstitial fibrosis. Studies have shown that during the development of renal failure, the glomeruli atrophy and are submerged in interstitial tissue. Thus, interstitial inflammation and fibrosis associated with renal dysfunction appear to be a reflection of nephron atrophy. Furthermore, as parenchymal elements are destroyed, they are replaced by inflammatory cells, edema, and ultimately fibrosis. The interstitial abnormalities recognizable on renal biopsy appear to be sensitive indicators of this process, and therefore correlate with functional impairment.

The correlation between concentrating ability and tubulo-interstitial disease is striking, despite the fact that the specimens analyzed represent renal cortical tissue. Of the three parameters used to test the kidney's ability to excrete acid, the maximal rate of ammonium excretion appears to correlate most closely with tubulo-interstitial disease. The majority of patients who are unable to excrete 40 μEq/min or more of ammonium after an acute acid load show moderate to severe interstitial and tubular disease. Decreased ammonium and titratable acid excretion is probably related to decreased nephron mass.

The correlation between glomerular disease and both ammonium excretion and concentrating ability might appear fortuitous; however, both of these functions depend upon maintenance of a complex interaction between glomerular filtration rate, tubular transport mechanisms, and peritubular blood flow. Maximal concentrating ability may be modified by abnormal spatial configuration of medullary loops of Henle, decrease in medullary hypertonicity, preferential destruction of juxtamedullary glomeruli, tubular unresponsiveness to antidiuretic hormone, or increased osmotic load per functioning nephron. Ammonium excretion, on the other hand, may be altered by decreased delivery of substrate to tubular cells, deficiency of enzymes crucial to acid production, as well as diminished tubular mass. Thus, minimal renal damage in any of the anatomic segments of the tubulo-interstitial compartments might be expected to interfere with these functions before defects in inulin or PAH clearance become apparent.

Ammonium excretion and maximal urinary osmolarity appeared to be the most sensitive indicators of renal disease.

SUMMARY

In conclusion, the available renal function tests are considered to be imprecise indicators of renal damage. The main contributors to this dilemma are the tremendous functional reserve of the kidney and the lack of a means of stressing the system.

Proteinuria remains the best indicator of glomerular change, but it provides little precise information concerning the distribution or severity of the lesion. Generally, minor abnormalities result in loss of proteins of low molecular weight (albumin), whereas more severe lesions result in the appearance of high-molecular-weight proteins in the urine. This information is of use in establishing the presence or absence of glomerular lesions in patients with the nephrotic syndrome, but does not allow further definition of glomerular pathology.

Finally, the most useful index of tubulo-interstitial disease is concentrating ability. Fortunately, this is an easy test to perform, but as with proteinuria, provides information on the presence or absence of renal disease rather than its extent. Thus, if a more exact prognosis is desired, or if a treatment program is contemplated, renal biopsy becomes of significant value.

References

1. Bricker, N. S., Klahr, S., and Rieselbach, R. E.: The functional adaptation of the diseased kidney. J. Clin. Invest. 43:1915, 1964.
2. Brod, J., and Benesova, D.: A comparative study of functional and morphologic renal changes in glomerulonephritis. Acta Med. Scand. 157:23, 1957.
3. Jorgensen, K.: Titrimetric determination of the net excretion of acid-base in urine. Scand. J. Clin. Lab. Invest. 9:287, 1957.
4. Ljungquist, A.: The intrarenal arterial pattern in the normal and diseased human kidney. Acta Med. Scand. Suppl. 174:5, 1963.
5. Kellow, W. F., Cotsonas, N. J., Jr., Chomet, B., and Zimmerman, J. J.: Evaluation of the adequacy of needle-biopsy specimens of the kidney on autopsy study. Arch. Int. Med. 104:353, 1959.
6. Maxwell, M. H., and Kleeman, C. R.: Clinical Disorders of Fluid and Electrolyte Metabolism. New York, McGraw-Hill Book Company, 1962.
7. Oliver, J.: The antithesis of structure and function in renal activity. Bull. N. Y. Acad. Med. 37:81, 1961.
8. Parrish, A. E., Kramer, N. C., Hatch, F. E., Watt, M. F., and Howe, J. S.: Relation between glomerular function and histology in acute glomerulonephritis. J. Lab. Clin. Med. 58:197, 1961.

9. Risdon, R. A., Slopper, J. C., and de Wardener, H. E.: Relationship between renal function and histological changes found in renal-biopsy specimens from patients with persistent glomerular nephritis. Lancet 2:363, 1968.
10. Rosenbaum, J. L., Mikail, M., and Wiedmann, F.: Further correlation of renal function with kidney biopsy in chronic renal disease. Am. J. Med. Sci. 254:156, 1967.
11. Striker, G. E., Schainuck, L. I., Cutler, R. E., and Benditt, E. P.: Structural-functional correlations in renal disease. I. A method for assaying and classifying histopathologic changes in renal biopsies. Hum. Pathol. 1:615, 1970.
12. Schainuck, L. I., Striker, G. E., Cutler, R. E., and Benditt, E. P.: Structural-functional correlations. Hum. Pathol. 1:632, Dec., 1970.
13. Wrong, O. M., and Davis, H. E. F.: The excretion of acid in renal disease. Quart. J. Med. 110:259, 1959.

Chapter Seven

Classification of Renal Diseases

The term "glomerulonephritis" literally means inflammation of the glomeruli and tubules (the nephron), and usually refers to a nonspecific inflammatory response of the kidney thought to affect primarily the glomeruli, although the tubules and interstitium are also affected. Through common usage, however, any change presumed to affect primarily the glomeruli, even sclerosis (scarring), has been called glomerulonephritis. Thus, the glomerular lesion characterized by uniform, glomerular basal lamina thickening and glomerular hypocellularity, is called "membranous glomerulonephritis." Although they are incorrect, such usages of the term are too deeply ingrained in medical literature to be discarded easily. The term glomerulopathy has been suggested for conditions which are not clearly inflammatory in origin.

Characteristically, the major urinary findings associated with the glomerular change reflect its inability to handle the normal function of excluding cells and large molecular weight proteins from the filtrate. Thus, red cells (hematuria) and protein (proteinuria) are found in the urine. Red blood cells mixed with protein (red blood cell casts) are thought to be pathognomonic of glomerular disease. Their presence, in fact, is referred to as "glomerular bleeding."

The current nomenclature of renal disease was developed gradually over the past two centuries. Morgagni, in the 18th century, was the first physician to systematically study and record the relationships between structure and function. The father of the modern investigation of renal disease, however, was Richard Bright. He convincingly demonstrated that those with constant "albuminous urine" had diseased kidneys. The eponym "Bright's disease" was then given to any kidney malady associated with proteinuria. In 1914, Volhard and Fahr, taking advantage of the advances in medicine since Bright's time, carefully followed patients with renal diseases, and noted that they could be

TABLE 7-1 Classification of Renal Diseases According to Volhard and Fahr

	Clinical Findings		Prognosis	Laboratory Findings	Anatomic Findings	
	Onset	*Physical Findings*			*Gross*	*Histologic*
Acute	Rapid	Edema, mild hypertension	Excellent	Proteinuria, RBC, RBC casts	Enlarged kidneys	Diffusely hypercellular, enlarged, bloodless glomeruli containing many neutrophils (proliferation and exudation)
Subacute	Insidious	Edema, mild hypertension	Rapid progression to renal failure	Proteinuria, RBC, RBC casts (patient may have renal failure when first seen)	Enlarged kidneys	Glomerular hypercellularity (primarily epithelial cells—crescents)
Chronic	Insidious	Hypertension, edema, polyuria	Slow progression to renal failure	Proteinuria, RBC, casts (granular and occasional RBC)	Small and scarred	End-stage; that is, scarring has so affected the architecture that the original process is not discernible

divided into a limited number of categories, depending on clinical presentation and evolution of renal function. They also found that the gross and histologic anatomic findings at autopsy could be classified according to a scheme based on the primary pathologic processes (see Table 7–1).

These observations formed the foundations for their classification of renal disease, under which we labor today. The first category, characterized by rapid onset with good prognosis, was called acute glomerulonephritis. Patients who appeared with glomerulonephritis of rapid onset but who had a rapid and progressive decrease in renal function were placed in the category of subacute (nonhealing or rapidly progressive) glomerulonephritis. When the initial diagnosis depended on a chance finding of proteinuria, and the clinical course to renal failure was measured in decades, the process was called chronic glomerulonephritis. The designations acute, rapidly progressive, and chronic, therefore, suggest a temporal sequence of disease.

This classification, although representing a major advance in the understanding of renal disease at the turn of the century, has not sufficed for modern medicine. At present, the classification of renal disease is very complex. None of the categories stands alone, and there is considerable confusion within and among institutions as to the exact meaning of terms. In developing this text, however, we have chosen a descriptive approach which includes the appropriate information from any of the affected categories. Although this method is wordy and somewhat redundant, with considerable overlap between groups, it is the least restrictive approach, allowing for the expression of quantitative results best fitting the status of our current information on renal disease.

For a patient with kidney disease, for example, who has systemic lupus erythematosus, the description might be as follows: systemic lupus erythematosus with chronic glomerulonephritis and stable but reduced renal function, which is characterized histologically by diffuse mesangial sclerosis and uniform subepithelial deposits of IgG.

The topics covered by the chapters of this book are divided into those conditions in which the kidney is the site of the primary disease (Table 7–2), and those in which the kidney is only one of several significantly affected organs. The former are subgrouped on the basis of their clinical course (i.e., resolution, rapid progression, slow progression) and major site of intrarenal disease (i.e., glomeruli, tubules, and so forth).

GLOMERULONEPHRITIS: EVOLUTION AND ASSOCIATED LESIONS

Most of the histologic reactions considered characteristic of glomerulonephritis commonly are thought to involve only the glomeruli.

TABLE 7-2 Classification of Primary Glomerular Diseases

Proposed Classification of Glomerular Disease	Other Clinical Classifications	Associated Pathologic Classification	Examples of Etiologies
Glomerular disease of acute onset	Acute nephritic syndrome Ellis Type 1 — acute GN Acute poststreptococcal GN	Diffuse *proliferative* and *exudative* GN	Immune complex disease Postinfectious GN
Glomerular disease of acute onset and rapid progression	Rapidly progressive GN Subacute GN Ellis Type 1 — rapidly progressive Goodpasture's syndrome	Extracapillary GN (80% Crescents) Focal necrotizing GN	Antiglomerular basement membrane antibody
Slowly progressive glomerular disease	Chronic glomerulonephritis Ellis Type 2 Subchronic GN	Proliferative GN Sclerosing GN	Unknown ? Immunologic ? Inherited abnormalities in extracellular material turnover
Primary nephrotic syndrome	Nephrosis	Minimal lesion Proliferative lesion Membranoproliferative lesion Sclerosing lesion	Unknown Unknown Abnormal complement activation through the alternate pathway Chronic immune complex disease

In fact, the glomeruli are but one part of a large renal capillary system. Recently it has been discovered that many capillary beds exhibit response to injuries similar to those seen in the glomeruli. Consequently, if a diffuse reaction of great severity occurs in the glomerular capillary bed, interstitial capillaries also may be affected, and interstitial inflammation might be expected as well. Similarly, "capillaritis" may be manifest in other capillary beds (muscles, resulting in myalgia; central nervous system, resulting in seizures; and so forth).

The course of renal disease, as outlined in Figure 7-1, is overly

84   CLASSIFICATION OF RENAL DISEASES

```
                        GLOMERULONEPHRITIS
                              Injury
                             /      \
                        Acute        Chronic
                       /     \              \
   Proliferation, focal ---- Proliferation, diffuse    Sclerosis
                    |         /        \              (scarring or
                    |        /          \             "hyaline" change,
                    |   Intracapillary   Extracapillary   which may be focal
                    |   (endothelial     (epithelial)     or diffuse)
                    |   and/or
                    |   mesangial and/or
                    |   exudative)
                    |       |                  |
                  remove              continued
                  injury                 injury
                    |                       \
                 Recovery              Renal failure
```

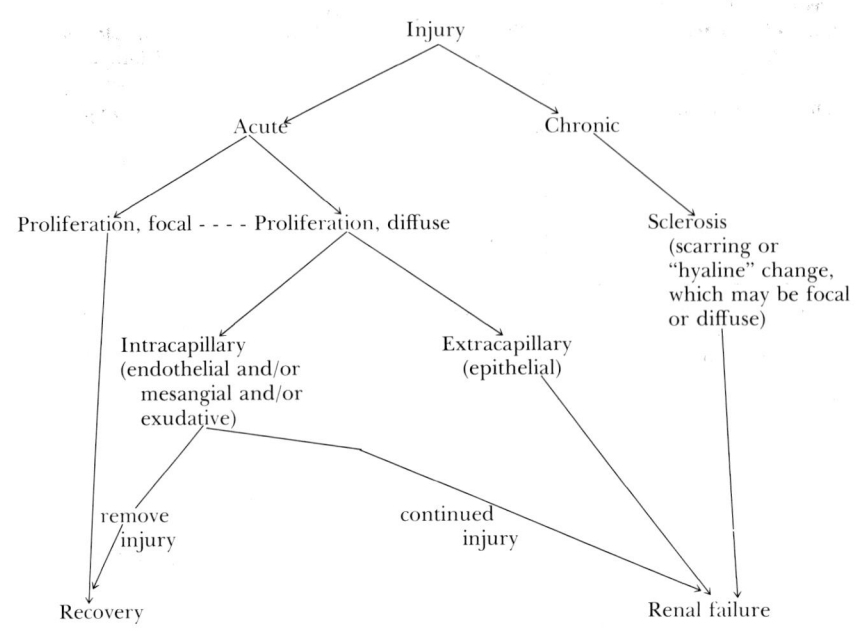

Figure 7–1   Evolution of glomerular injury.

simplified, but serves to illustrate the important issues. If the stimulus is acute and transitory or acute and focal, the process tends to resolve. If the stimulus to the acute change persists, the process may result in sclerosis and loss of renal function. In addition, if diffuse proliferation involves the epithelial cells, the end result is sclerosis or obsolescence of glomeruli, with subsequent atrophy of the tubular segments. Finally, if the stimulus is low-grade and unresolved, slowly accumulating sclerosis and gradual loss of nephrons and renal functions will occur.

These syndromes can be caused by various factors, and although the kidney has but a few ways of responding to an injury, the response in the individual patient is not stereotyped. For example, an agent may cause mild, reversible nephritis in one patient but produce either rapid progression or slow progression to renal failure in another. Therefore, although poststreptococcal nephritis is discussed in Chapter 8 as a glomerular diease of acute onset, one must be aware that in rare cases it may also progress rapidly to renal failure, as discussed in Chapter 9, or enter a slowly progressive course, as outlined in Chapter 12.

The syndromes discussed in Sections II, III, and IV are those in which the kidney is primarily affected. Section V deals with diseases in which the kidney is significantly involved as part of a systemic illness, while Section VI deals with the unique situation of renal transplantation.

References

1. Black, D. A. K.: Diagnosis in renal disease. Brit. Med. J. 2:315, 1970.
2. Cameron, J. S.: A clinician's view of the classification of glomerulonephritis. *In* Glomerulonephritis, Part II, P. Kincaid-Smith, T. H. Mathew, and E. L. Becker (eds.). New York, John Wiley & Sons, 1972.
3. Churg, J., and Duffy, J. L.: Classification of glomerulonephritis based on morphology. *In* Glomerulonephritis, Part II, P. Kincaid-Smith, T. H. Mathew, and E. L. Becker (eds.). New York, John Wiley & Sons, 1972.
4. Habib, R.: Classification of glomerulonephritis based on morphology. *In* Glomeruloneprhitis, Part II, P. Kincaid-Smith, T. H. Mathew, and E. L. Becker (eds.). New York, John Wiley & Sons, 1972.
5. Volhard, F., and Fahr, T.: Die Brightsche Nierenkrankheit. Berlin, Springer, 1914.

Section II

RENAL DISEASES OF ACUTE ONSET

Chapter Eight

Glomerular Disease of Acute Onset

Introduction

Although the causes of glomerular disease of acute onset are varied, they often produce similar clinical manifestations and histologic changes (Table 8-1). Only those in which the kidney is the primary site of injury, however, will be covered in this chapter. The remainder have prominent primary systemic manifestations and will be discussed later in the book.

The classic example of glomerular disease of acute onset is poststreptococcal glomerulonephritis. Strong evidence exists that this is an immune complex disease in which streptococcal antigens provoke an antibody response; the subsequent antigen-antibody complexes in the circulation are deposited in the glomerular capillary walls. These complexes activate the complement pathway with liberation of chemotactic factors, causing polymorphonuclear leukocytic infiltration. The release of lysosomal enzymes, in addition to further activation of the complement system, leads to damage of the capillary wall, including the glomerular basal lamina.

There is considerable controversy regarding the exact nature of the complexes. For example, certain streptococcal antigens have been shown to cross react with the glomerular basal lamina, while other investigators have demonstrated the presence of streptococcal antigen in the deposits. All would agree, however, on the presence of a host antibody and complement in irregular subepithelial deposits. Furthermore, the histologic pattern of immune complex deposition in poststreptococcal glomerulonephritis is similar to that seen in a variety of human and animal immune complex diseases. The activation of the complement system, with significant lowering of C_3 and C_4 which

TABLE 8-1 Glomerular Diseases of Acute Onset

I. Immune complex disease
  A. Exogenous antigen
    1. Postinfectious
    2. Serum sickness
  B. Endogenous antigen
    1. Systemic lupus erythematosus (Chapter 17)
    2. Tumors
    3. Thyroiditis
    4. ?Polyarteritis nodosa, ?Wegener's granulomatosis (Chapter 18)
II. Vasculitis
  A. Henoch-Schönlein purpura (Chapter 19)
  B. Hemolytic uremic syndrome, thrombotic thrombocytopenic purpura (Chapter 20)
III. Idiopathic

---

occurs in immune complex disease, can also be demonstrated in poststreptococcal glomerulonephritis and in most other examples of postinfectious glomerulonephritis.

Glomerulonephritis has also been found to be of "immune complex" origin in other infectious diseases, including bacterial endocarditis, "shunt nephritis" (infected ventriculo-atrial shunts), varicella, Australian antigen positive hepatitis, syphilis, and malaria. The latter three may cause a sclerosing lesion and excessive proteinuria (the nephrotic syndrome) rather than acute glomerular disease. This may be due to the persistence of antigens in the circulation.

Clinical Data

PRESENTATION. Patients with acute glomerulonephritis usually complain of edema, oliguria, and dark urine. If fluid retention is marked, circulatory congestion and hypertension with headaches as well as visual disturbances occur. In addition, a history of sore throat, impetigo, or culture-proved β hemolytic streptococcus infection one to two weeks prior to onset of these symptoms, and/or elevated serum antibody titers to streptococcal antigen (antistreptolysin O and antistreptolysin-hyaluronidase) are helpful in documenting the etiology. The course is by no means stereotyped, and in many patients the first clue to poststreptococcal glomerulonephritis is the incidental discovery of gross hematuria. The disease may also present with anuria, severe circulatory congestion, and hyperkalemia, and it may lead to death in the initial phases, although in the majority of instances the signs and symptoms gradually abate over a matter of days.

Other forms of postinfectious glomerulonephritis do not cause as great a diagnostic problem as poststreptococcal glomerulonephritis because the organism often can be cultured from the site of infection or from the blood when nephritis becomes apparent. The nephritis of subacute bacterial endocarditis, however, may present a diagnostic enigma, since it often is difficult to detect, and the systemic manifestations frequently mimic other diseases, such as systemic lupus erythematosus or polyarteritis. Since blood cultures may be sterile in this syndrome, patients have been treated with corticosteroids rather than antibiotics, with disastrous results.

Physical examination usually reveals signs of circulatory congestion with distended neck veins, hypertension, and edema. Other findings which occur in patients with postinfectious glomerulonephritis, such as endocarditis, may include systemic manifestations of immune complex vasculitis, such as skin rash, splenomegaly, and arthritis; and the classic manifestations of intravascular infection, including splinter hemorrhages, Janeway spots, Osler nodes, conjunctival hemorrhages, and Roth spots.

A urinalysis is helpful in establishing the diagnosis. Proteinuria is always present, for example, but is quite variable and, if it is heavy, may indicate a more severe injury. In addition, the urine sediment contains red cells, red cell casts, white cell casts, and granular casts (a so-called "active" sediment). A diagnosis of glomerular disease of acute onset is certain when red cell casts are found in abundance in patients with sudden onset of circulatory congestion, hypertension, as well as renal functional impairment.

Renal function, on the other hand, usually is impaired only mildly to moderately; occasionally a patient may be severely oliguric and require emergency dialysis therapy. Renal functional abnormalities return to normal over a matter of weeks, although proteinuria may be present for six months to a year and microscopic hematuria for several years.

Radiologic evaluation may also be helpful in distinguishing acute disease from an acute exacerbation of chronic disease. In glomerular disease of acute onset, for instance, the kidneys are usually of normal size or slightly enlarged, whereas they may be small in patients with slowly progressive diseases.

Serum complement levels are useful in the evaluation of this syndrome as well, since complement activation is thought to be a major mediator of the damages in immune complex diseases. The third and fourth component of complement and total hemolytic complement activity are diminished during the initial phase of the disease.

Histology

GLOMERULI

LIGHT MICROSCOPY. The glomeruli are diffusely affected, becoming enlarged and hypercellular (Figs. 8-2, 8-5). During the early stage,

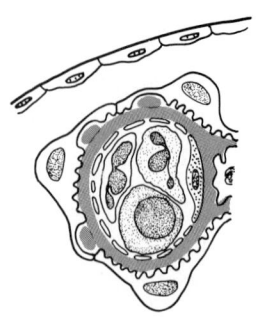

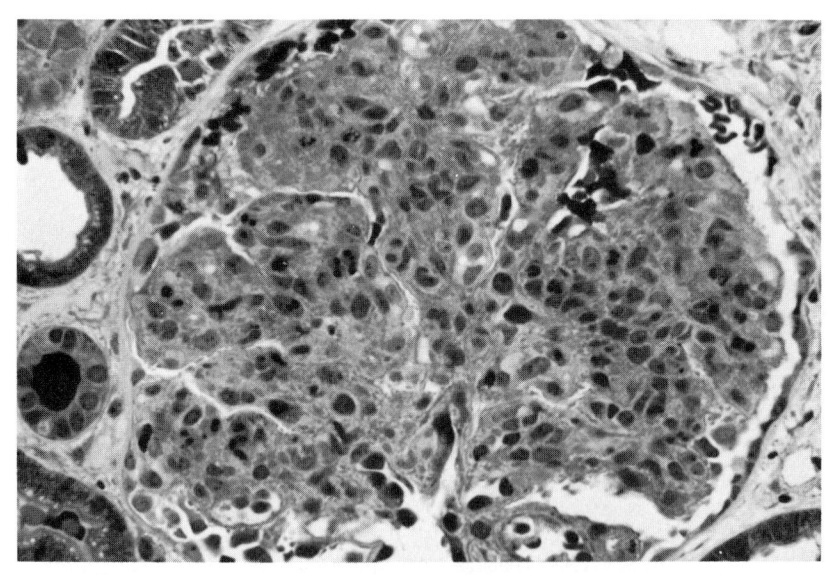

Figure 8-1 Diagrammatic representation of subepithelial deposits and exudation.

Figure 8-2 Light micrograph from a 14-year-old white male with a history of a respiratory infection 10 days prior to admission, and subsequent nausea, vomiting, edema, and focal seizures. On admission his creatinine level was 1.7 mg/100 dl, and the urine contained many cells and casts. Renal function rapidly returned to normal over a one-week period. The glomerulus is diffusely hypercellular and contains many inflammatory cells. (H&E, × 300.)

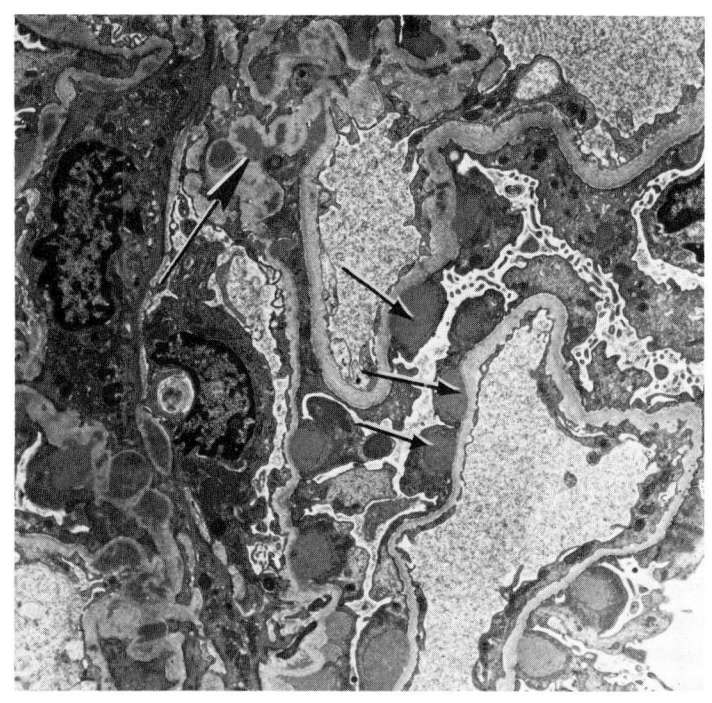

Figure 8-3 Electron micrograph from a 15-year-old patient with severe oliguria and a rising serum creatinine level. The peripheral capillary loops are studded by irregularly distributed deposits (→) on the subepithelial aspect. Deposits may also be seen in the mesangial regions (▶). (×2200.)

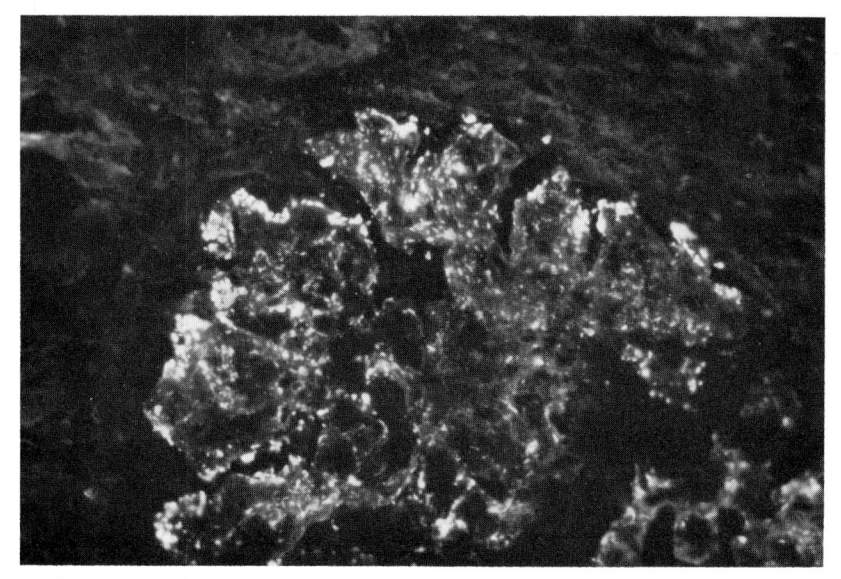

Figure 8-4 Fluorescence micrograph from the same patient as in Figure 8-2. Note that the staining for IgG is irregular in distribution and granular in configuration, and that the peripheral capillary loops are the main sites of deposition. (×300.)

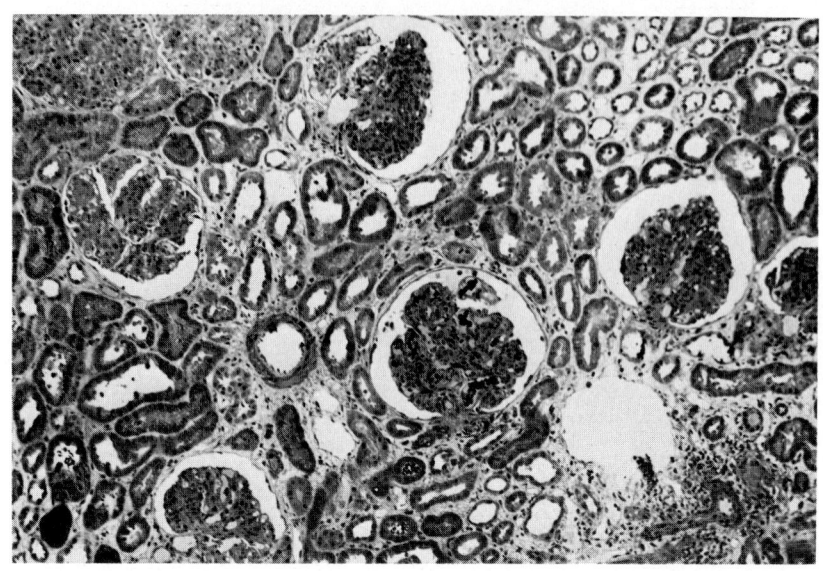

Figure 8-5 Low power photomicrograph of a formalin fixed specimen from a 60-year-old white male who had staphylococcus septicemia and hematuria and proteinuria. The glomeruli are diffusely hypercellular. Formalin fixation causes retraction of the capillary loops within Bowman's space. The interstitium is diffusely edematous and contains a number of inflammatory of cells. (H&E, × 75.)

for example, especially in children, the increase in cells may be due to large numbers of neutrophils, eosinophils, or both. Within a week, the relative number of polymorphonuclear cells decreases and the glomeruli contain large numbers of mononuclear cells, although the time factor is a highly variable feature. At this point it also is difficult to determine whether the cells are mesangial, endothelial, or of circulatory origin.

In addition, within the first few days, epithelial cell hyperplasia is common (Fig. 8-6) and cellular crescents are evident in a few glomeruli. Like the neutrophilic response, however, this appears to be a transient, early feature, since true synechiae rarely form.

Furthermore, the basal lamina of peripheral capillary loops may appear to be thickened on light microscopy, but a thin section demonstrates that this is due to the presence of pedicel effacement (Fig. 8-8) and deposits (Fig. 8-9).

ELECTRON MICROSCOPY. There is also an increase in the number of endothelial cells, many of which have prominent cytoplasmic processes projecting into the capillary lumen (Fig. 8–10). In addition, the usual fenestration of the endothelial cell cytoplasm often is not apparent. In areas where cellularity is marked, it may be impossible to distinguish the exact cell type present, and the capillary spaces may be virtually obliterated by the large number of intraglomerular cells.

The mesangial regions, on the other hand, often are expanded greatly, by either an increased number of cells or edema, or both (Fig. 8–11). Neutrophils often are seen within the confines of the mesangium. When there has been considerable disruption of the mesangial region, however, mesangial cells may be difficult to identify or to distinguish from circulating mononuclear cells. In fact, dead cells and cell debris commonly are found in the mesangial region, raising the question of significant mesangial injury. Deposits of electron-dense material can be found in this region as well, resembling those seen on the peripheral capillary loops. In addition, the peripheral glomerular basal lamina evidences remarkably large numbers of deposits on its subepithelial aspects. The deposits are separated from the lamina densa by the lamina rara externa and from the podocytes by a similar clear area (Fig. 8–3). Deposits within the substance of the glomerular basal lamina are found principally near or over mesangial regions (Fig. 8–11). The structure of the glomerular basal lamina itself, however, is not particularly unusual. Near the mesangial regions, the continuity between the mesangial matrix and the peripheral glomerular basal lamina (the capillary waist) may be disrupted, resulting in coalescence of several capillary loops into one large space.

The epithelial cells are altered considerably. The total number often is increased, and rarely mitotic figures may be seen. Normally epithelial cell cytoplasmic organelles are seen uncommonly in proximity to the glomerular basal lamina, whereas in acute glomerulonephritis, many profiles of rough endosplasmic reticulum, mitochondria, vacuoles, and so forth, may be seen juxtaposed to the glomerular basal lamina (Figs. 8–10, 8–11). There is also an increased number of filaments, which are quite dense in the region adjacent to the deposits. Villous transformation of the epithelial cells is common, although its significance is unknown. The foot processes of the epithelial cells invariably are fused over the deposits.

FLUORESCENCE MICROSCOPY. Deposits of IgG, C3, and properdin are evident, distributed irregularly over the peripheral capillary loops in a subepithelial position (Fig. 8–4). They appear as separate, well-outlined specks of irregular size and shape scattered diffusely over the capillary loops in a random pattern. They also may occur in the mesangial regions. The position of the deposits is shown diagrammatically in Figure 8–1.

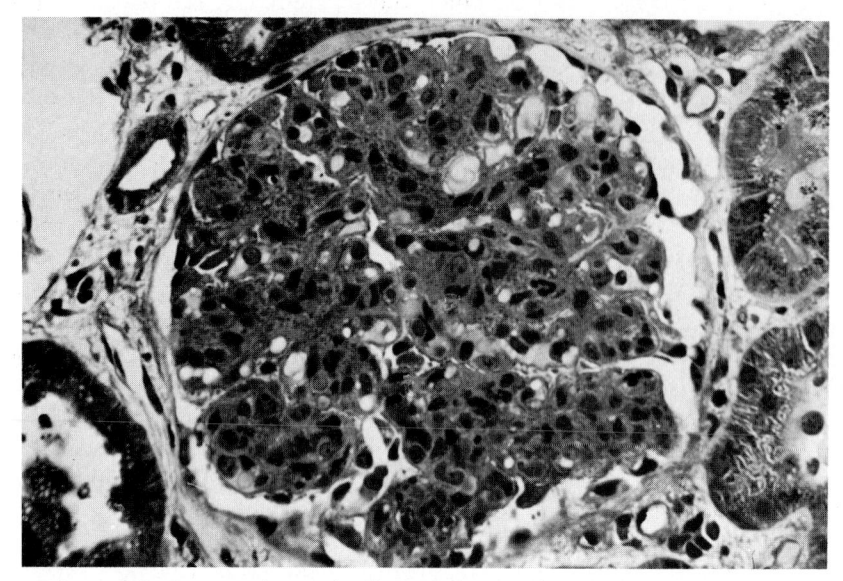

Figure 8-6 Same patient as in Figure 8-2. Note the prominence of the epithelial cells, both parietal and visceral. (H&E, × 300.)

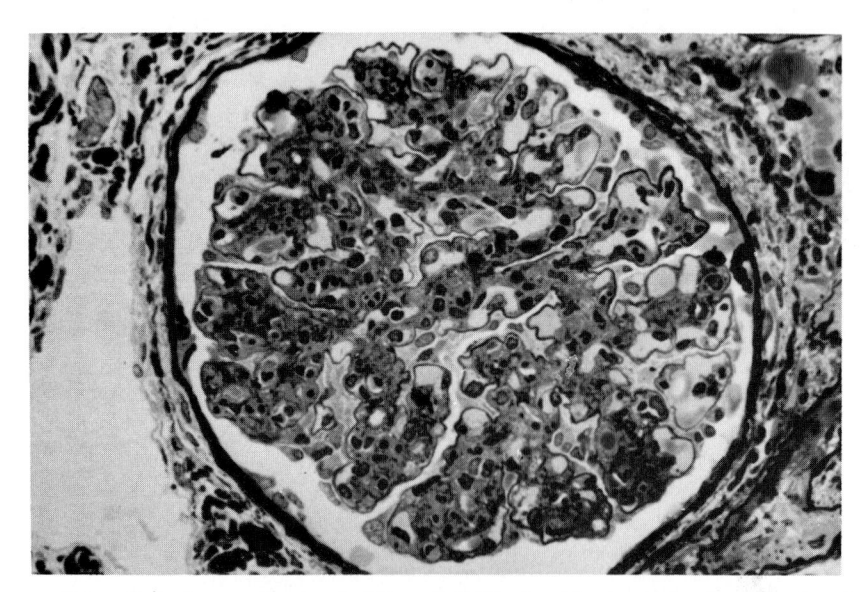

Figure 8-7 Same patient as in Figure 8-2. The basal lamina is clearly outlined, and the majority of proliferating cells and inflammatory cells are seen to lie within the confines of the basal lamina. (Methenamine silver nitrate, × 300.)

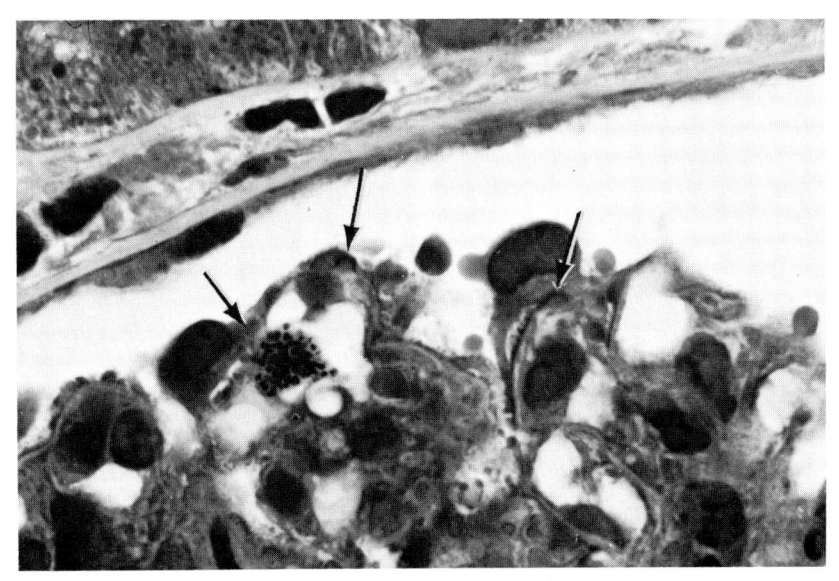

Figure 8-8 High power photomicrograph from same patient as in Figure 8-2, demonstrating effacement of the normal podocyte architecture and the presence of subepithelial deposits (→). In the lumen an eosinophil is clearly defined. (H&E, × 1200.)

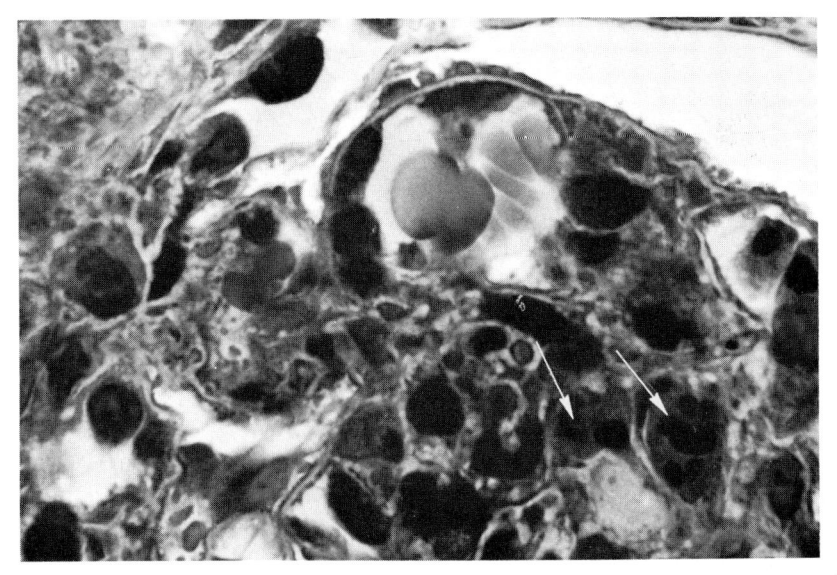

Figure 8-9 Another area similar to that in Figure 8-8. Multiple deposits are noted on the subepithelial aspect of the basal lamina. Multilobulated neutrophils can be seen in the capillary lumen and the mesangial regions (→). (H&E, × 1200.)

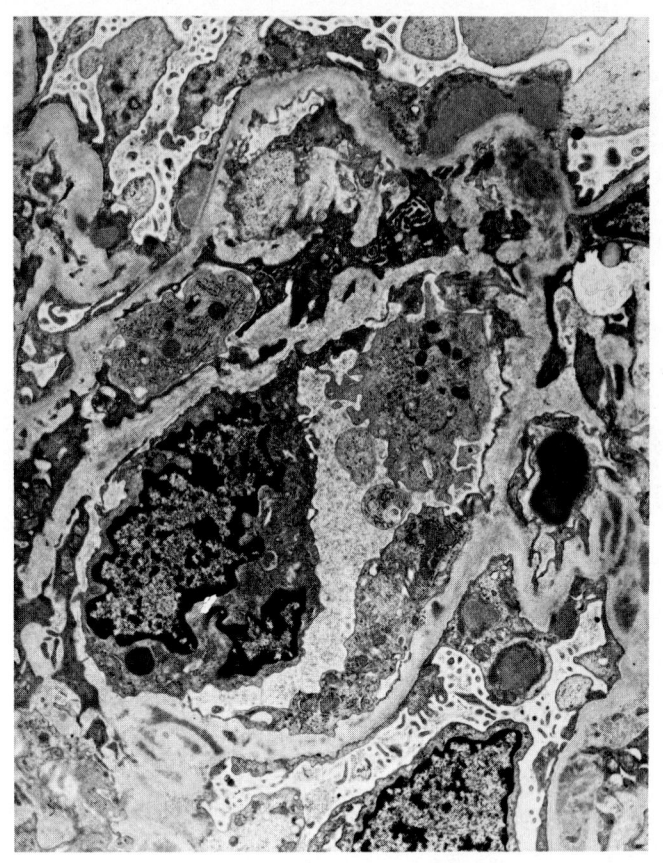

Figure 8–10 Electron micrograph from same patient as in Figure 8–3, demonstrating deposits on the subepithelial aspects of the basal lamina, within the substance of the basal lamina, and in the mesangial matrix. The endothelial cell cytoplasm is quite prominent and thickened in most regions. There is a clear zone (lamina rara externa) between the deposit and the lamina densa. A clear zone is also present between the deposits and the overlying epithelial cell, which has lost the normal pedicellar architecture. ($\times$ 5000.)

TUBULAR CHANGES

LIGHT MICROSCOPY. The most characteristic tubular change is the presence of casts. Red blood cell casts are the most common (Fig. 8–12), but hyaline and granular casts may be recognized. In the absence of interstitial disease, the casts are present only in collecting ducts in medullary rays. Tubular necrosis with formation of granular casts, and dilated, atrophic proximal and distal tubules, or both, may be seen in patients with severe disease and are usually associated with renal failure (see Chapter 6) (Fig. 8–13). Tubular epithelial cell changes commonly are limited to increased numbers of hyaline droplets.

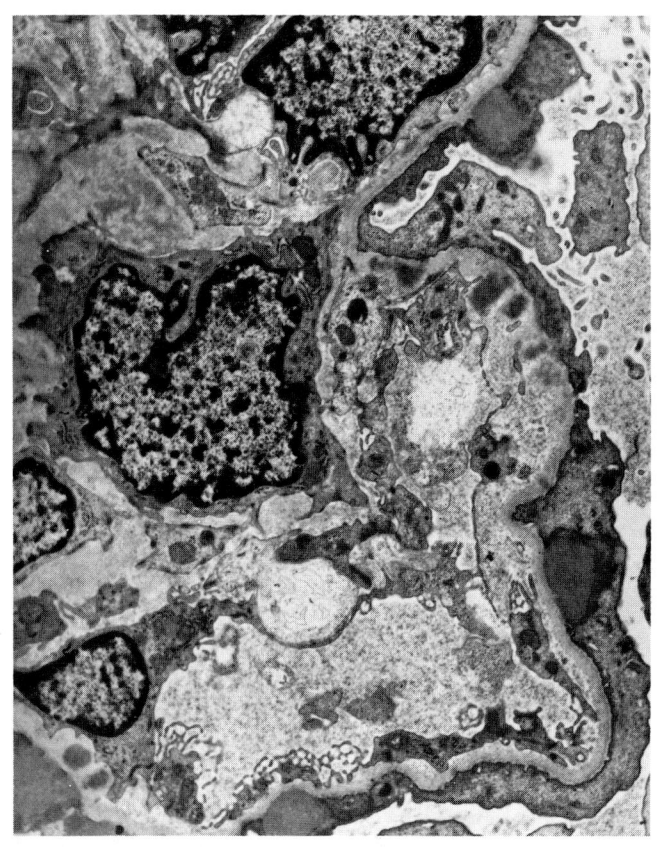

Figure 8-11 Same patient as in Figure 8-10. The mesangial region is expanded and deposits are present within its substance. There is also rarefaction of the mesangial matrix in multiple areas. (× 5000.)

ELECTRON MICROSCOPY. The cells of the proximal tubule are affected only in the most unusual instances. There may be a decreased number of basilar infoldings, lateral interdigitations, and fewer, shorter microvilli. Lysosomes are increased in number as well, but the cell organelles do not appear otherwise altered. The vacuoles noted by light microscopy most often appear to be widened intercellular spaces, although increased numbers of lipid droplets are encountered sporadically (Fig. 8-14).

INTERSTITIUM

In the usual uncomplicated episode of postinfectious glomerulonephritis, the interstitium is unremarkable. As noted in Chapter 6, edema, or infiltrate, or both, in this compartment is reflected by

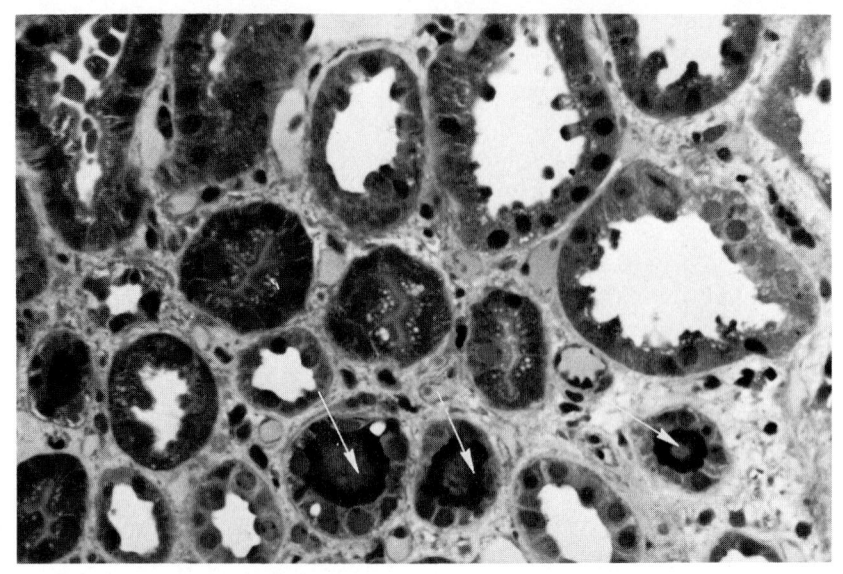

Figure 8–12 Same patient as in Figure 8–2. The interstitium is widened. The capillaries are visible between tubules. Edema and loose connective tissue occupy the majority of this interstitial space. There also appear to be a number of inflammatory cells. Red cells imbedded in a protein matrix are noted in distal tubules and collecting ducts (→). (H&E, × 300.)

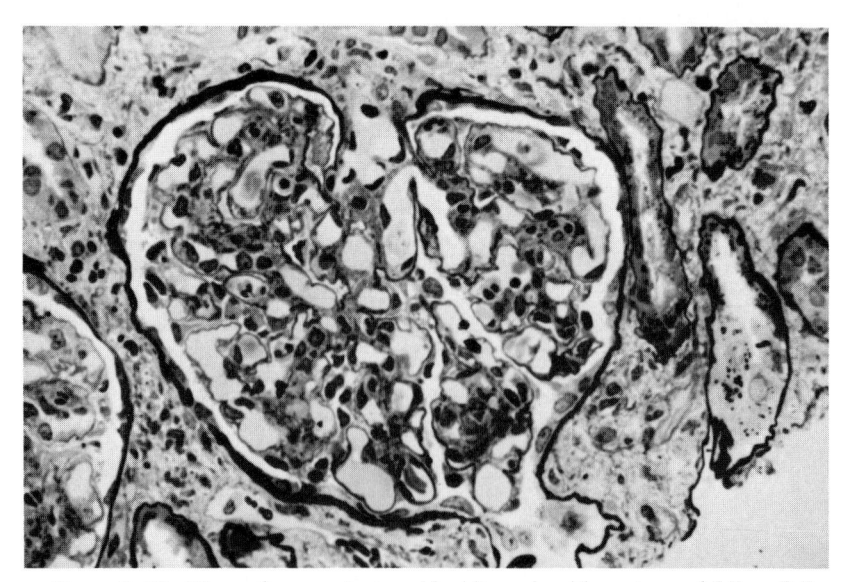

Figure 8–13 Biopsy from an 8-year-old white male with acute renal failure following a streptococcal cellulitis. This patient required dialysis acutely. Note the thickened and wrinkled basal lamina of several proximal tubules to the right of the field. There also is diffuse interstitial edema and infiltrate. (Methenamine silver, × 300.)

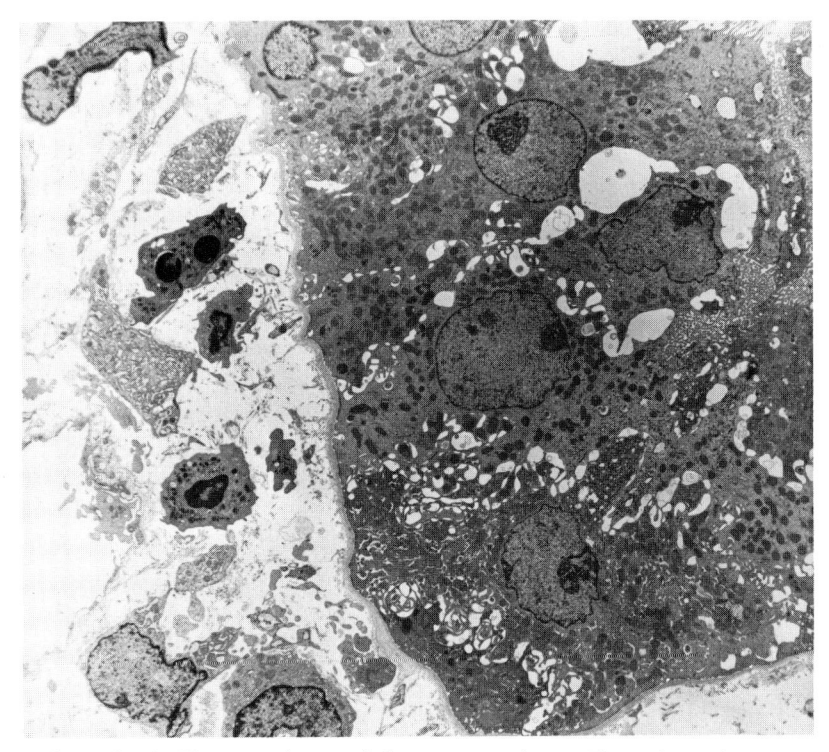

Figure 8-14 Electron micrograph from same patient as Figure 8-3. The proximal tubule has vacuolated intercellular spaces, but otherwise appears normal. The interstitial capillary (lower left) is separated from the basal lamina of the tubule by edema and inflammatory cells. (× 4000.)

changes in renal function. Since generally it is the extraordinary case of postinfectious glomerulonephritis in which renal function is severely affected, there is seldom an abnormality in this compartment. When present the medullary ray or juxtamedullary regions may be the most severely affected (Fig. 8-15). The exact cell type found in the interstices varies, but early in the course neutrophils and eosinophils predominate, with plasma cells and lymphocytes appearing later; however, there is no proliferation of interstitial cells.

Clinical Course and Prognosis

In general, patients with glomerular disease of acute onset secondary to immune complex disease usually have a good prognosis so long as the source of antigen can be removed effectively. In children with poststreptococcal glomerulonephritis, for example, the majority (85 to 95 per cent) regain normal renal function. The original diagnosis should be doubted, however, if progression becomes evident. Although rare, when progression does occur, marked cellular prolifer-

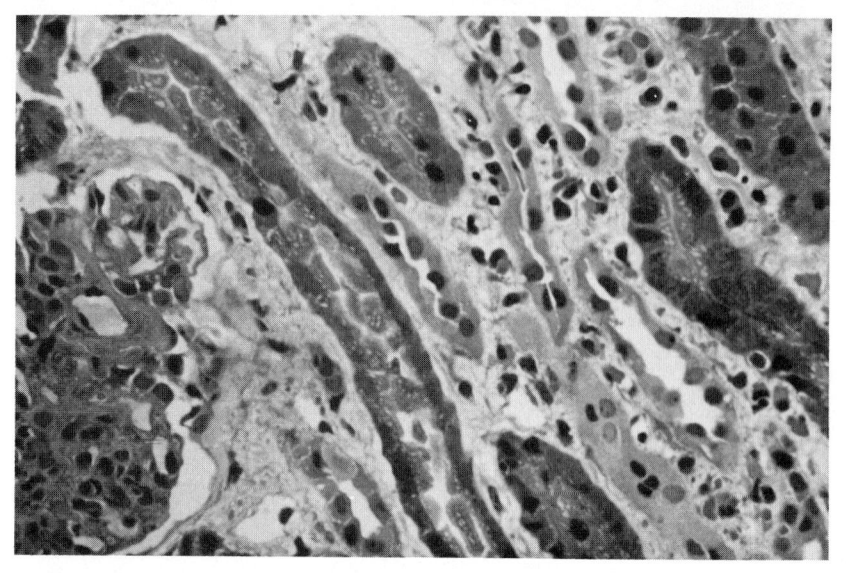

Figure 8-15 Medullary region from same patient as in Figure 8-12. The interstitial space is markedly expanded with the accumulation of edema fluid and large numbers of inflammatory cells. (H&E, × 300.)

ation and necrosis frequently are prominent. It is at this stage that the disparity between age groups becomes apparent.

In addition, the rate and extent of resolution vary in children and adults. In children, the exudation and cellularity may disappear within a period of weeks. There also seems to be a difference even when considering early and late childhood. In a prospective study Dodge and associates (1972) noted that a group of children with a mean age of just over 4½ years, all had healed at rebiopsy; in a second group, however, with a mean age of a little over 9 years, the follow-up biopsy in two years invariably showed some evidence of disease. Whether these changes are significant remains to be seen, but it is clear that resolution occurs by regression of the inflammatory process, the result depending on the patient's age and the degree of injury. In children, the amount of extracellular material laid down and the severity of the inflammatory response vary widely, and complete remodeling occurs frequently, whereas in adults, the healing more often is characterized by scarring.

The general agreement that poststreptococcal glomerulonephritis is a relatively benign condition has been challenged recently by Baldwin and his colleagues (1974). They found that by various clinical measurements 30 to 40 per cent of adults and children have persistent renal disease, whereas histologic abnormalities were present in 70 per cent. Although the degree of functional impairment was rather low (two patients died with uremia), they suggest that 25 to 35 years may be required for its progression from an acute injury to significant renal impairment.

The glomerulonephritis secondary to infected ventriculo-atrial shunts has a good prognosis so long as the infection (usually secondary *Staphylococcus albus*) can be eradicated. This often requires removal of the shunt, together with appropriate antibiotic therapy.

Finally, the nephritis of subacute bacterial endocarditis can present with a wide spectrum of renal involvement. As with most forms of post-infectious nephritis, effective removal of the source of the antigen will result in resolution or stabilization of the renal injury. Quartan malaria is an exception; it apparently initiates an immune response or pattern of injury which causes a high incidence of progression even when the parasite has been eradicated.

References

1. Baldwin, D. S., Gluck, M. D., Schacht, R. C., and Gallo, G.:The long-term course of poststreptococcal glomerulonephritis. Ann. Intern. Med. *80*:342, 1974.
2. Bhorade, M. S., Carag, H. B., Lee, H. J., Potter, E. V., and Dunea, G.: Nephropathy of secondary syphilis. A clinical and pathological spectrum. J.A.M.A. *216*:1159, 1971.
3. Black, J. A., Challacombe, D. N., and Ockenden, B. H.: Nephrotic syndrome associated with bacteremia after shunt operations for hydrocephalus. Lancet *2*:921, 1965.
4. Braunstein, G. D., Lewis, E. J., Galvaneck, E. G., Hamilton, A., Bell, W. R.: The nephrotic syndrome associated with secondary syphilis. Am. J. Med. *48*:643, 1970.
5. Combes, B., Shorey, J., Barrera, A., Stastny, P., Eigenbrodth, E. H., Hull, A. R., and Carter, N. W.: Glomerulonephritis with deposition of Australia antigen-antibody complexes in glomerular basement membrane. Lancet *1*:234, 1971.
6. Dodge, W. F., Spargo, B. H., Traveis, L. B., Srivastava, R. N., Carvajal, H. F., DeBeukelaer, M. M., Longley, M. P., and Menchaca, J. A.: Poststreptococcal glomerulonephritis. A prospective study in children. New Eng. J. Med. *286*:273, 1972.
7. Di Benedetto, B. J., Castronuovo, J., McDonald, H. P., and Friedman, E. A.: Acute renal failure complicating disseminated varicella. N. Y. State J. Med., *70*:298, 1970.
8. Feizi, T., and Gitlin, N.: Immune-complex disease of the kidney associated with chronic hepatitis and cryoglobulinaemia. Lancet *2*:873, 1969.
9. Gutman, R. A., Striker, G. E., Gilliland, B. C., and Cutler, R. E.: The immune complex glomerulonephritis of bacterial endocarditis. Medicine *51*:1, 1972.
10. Hellier, M. D., Webster, A. D. B., and Eisinger, A. J. M. F.: Nephrotic syndrome: A complication of secondary syphilis. Brit. Med. J. *4*:404, 1971.
11. Hendrickse, R. G., Adeniyi, A., Edington, G. M., Glasgow, E. F., White, R. H. R., and Houba, V.: Quartan malarial nephrotic syndrome. Collaborative clinicopathological study in Nigerian children. Lancet *1*:1143, 1972.
12. Levy, R. L., and Hong, R.: The immune nature of subacute bacterial endocarditis (SBE) nephritis. Am. J. Med. *54*:645, 1973.
13. Michael, A. F., Drummond, K. N., Good, R. A., and Vernier, R. L.: Acute poststreptococcal glomerulonephritis: Immune deposit disease. J. Clin. Invest. *45*:237, 1966.
14. More-Maroger, L., Sraer, J., Herreman, G., and Godeau, P.: Kidney in subacute endocarditis. Arch. Pathol. *94*:205, 1972.
15. Rames, L., Wise, B., Goodman, J. R., and Piel, C. F.: Renal disease with *Staphylococcus albus* bacteremia. J.A.M.A. *212*:1671, 1970.
16. Stickler, G. B., Shin, M. H., Burke, E. C., Holley, K. E., Miller, R. H., and Segar, W. E.: Diffuse glomerulonephritis associated with infected ventriculoatrial shunt. New Eng. J. Med. *279*:1077, 1968.
17. Treser, G., Semar, M., Ty, A., et al.: Partial characterization of streptococcal plasma membrane components in acute glomerulonephritis. J. Clin. Invest. *49*:762, 1970.
18. Treser, G., Semar, M., McVicar, M., et al.: Antigenic streptococcal components in acute glomerulonephritis. Science *163*:676, 1969.

Chapter Nine

Glomerular Disease of Acute Onset and Rapid Progression

Introduction

Glomerular disease of acute onset and rapid progression has been described variously as rapidly progressive glomerulonephritis, subacute glomerulonephritis, or extracapillary nephritis. Although it is a relatively uncommon clinical renal syndrome, its fulminant, unremitting course to renal failure is frustrating to the clinician and devastating to the patient.

The syndrome also has varied etiologies (Table 9-1) and occurs as part of a systemic disease in about 40 per cent of the cases (see Section V). This chapter concerns only those of primary renal involvement. Of these a small number appear to be caused by antibody directed against the glomerular basal lamina.

The etiology of antiglomerular basal lamina nephritis has been studied well in experimental animals and man. Masugi produced a model lesion in animals in 1934. The cause of this lesion is postulated to be an autoantibody directed against the glomerular basal lamina. This hypothesis is based on an experiment in which rapidly progressive renal disease is produced by injecting heterologous or homologous glomerular basal lamina into suitable animals. The animals develop antiglomerular basal lamina antibody to the foreign protein, which then cross reacts with native glomerular basal lamina, resulting in severe damage. The antibodies detected in the blood of these animals can be eluted from the kidneys and will cause a similar lesion in syngeneic animals.

Although the initiating events leading to autoimmunity to the glomerular basal lamina in humans are unknown, the end results are the same. Antibodies to the glomerular basal lamina are present in the blood and can be demonstrated by the immunofluorescence technique

TABLE 9-1 Etiologies of Glomerular Disease of
Acute Onset and Rapid Progression

> Primary renal involvement
>   Antiglomerular basal lamina nephritis
>   Immune complex disease
>   Idiopathic
> Systemic syndrome
>   Henoch-Schönlein purpura
>   Polyarteritis nodosa, Wegener's granulomatosis
>   Systemic lupus erythematosus

on the glomerular basal lamina. As with the experimental models, eluates of kidneys removed from these patients contain antibodies against the glomerular basal lamina. On occasion, patients with this syndrome also will have a circulating antibody which cross reacts with pulmonary alveolar basal lamina, leading to a pulmonary-renal complex called Goodpasture's syndrome. Although the disease has proved autoimmunity, the event initiating autoimmunity is unknown. The proportion of cases with anti-GBL antibodies varies among reports, averaging 30 per cent of patients with glomerular disease of acute onset and rapid progression.

As discussed in a previous section, patients with renal disease due to deposition of circulating immune complexes may pursue a course with rapidly deteriorating renal function and irreversible renal failure; however, some patients with circulating antiglomerular basal lamina antibody may have little or no renal injury. The factors which determine a benign rather than progressive course are not understood, but assuredly include the type, distribution, specificity, and amount of antibody or complexes, as well as the host's response to their presence (see Chapter 5).

Clinical Data

In a study of 63 cases with this syndrome at the University of Washington Hospitals, the age distribution spanned a wide range without clear evidence of clustering at any point. Thirty-six patients were men and 27 were women.

The patients presenting with rapidly progressive glomerulonephritis are not too dissimilar from those with acute but nonprogressive disease, but the onset usually is more insidious, with weakness, fatigue, and malaise being the most prominent symptoms. The majority also will have nausea, anorexia, and vomiting. Urinary tract symptoms, including gross hematuria, frequency, or nocturia, are rare.

In addition, half of the patients have a history of an acute febrile illness within one month of the onset of renal failure. The illness is

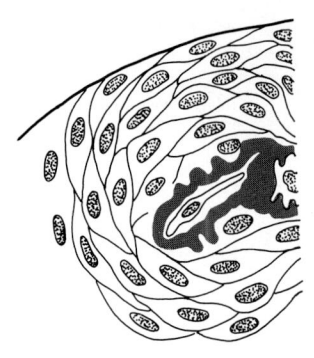

Figure 9-1 Diagrammatic representation of epithelial proliferation and glomerular capillary collapse.

characterized by many as "flu-like" and frequently has abated spontaneously. In many cases this is followed by changes in the urine flow rate or color, which is apparent to the patient.

Fifteen patients in the University of Washington series had been noted to have an episode of "nephritis" in the past, or urinary abnormalities had been recorded (proteinuria, cells, or casts). In all instances these had cleared and no patient had residual impairment of kidney function prior to the onset of the renal syndrome. Hypertension was an

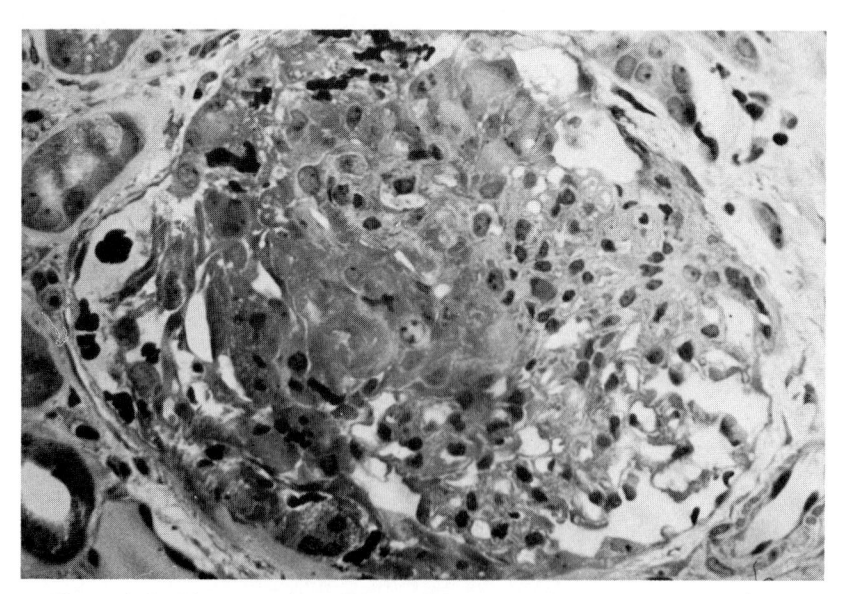

Figure 9-2 Biopsy specimen from a 72-year-old white female with two months' history of progressive renal failure. Serum creatinine level was 12 mg/dl, urine output 400 ml/day. Serum anti-GBL titers were positive. Note the proliferation of epithelial cells in the left portion of the glomerulus. The residual tuft is compressed into the right portion of Bowman's space. (H&E, × 300.)

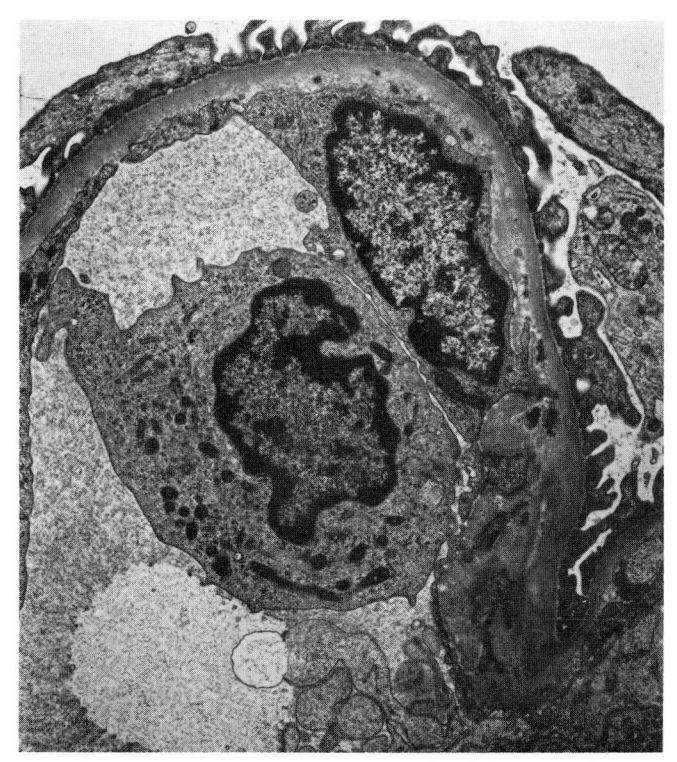

Figure 9-3 Electron micrograph from the same patient as in Figure 9-2. Note that the subendothelial space is expanded and contains a flocculent material. The endothelial cell cytoplasm is swollen in this region. (× 5000.)

uncommon finding at admission. In no case, however, was there severe elevation of the blood pressure. Mild peripheral edema also was present in nearly half the cases.

Nearly all patients were anuric on admission or shortly thereafter. Azotemia also was documented in all cases; in fact, signs and symptoms of uremia precipitated admission in many instances.

Selected laboratory tests can help distinguish an antiglomerular basal lamina antibody nephritis from severe immune complex diseases. For example, elevated antistreptolysin O, antihyaluronidase, or antideoxyribonuclease B levels suggest immune complex disease secondary to a preceding streptococcal infection. Hypocomplementemia is unusual in antiglomerular basal lamina antibody nephritis, although it is common in immune complex disease. A serum assay for circulating antiglomerular basal lamina antibodies is helpful when positive, but may become evident only when the disease is far advanced or following nephrectomy. Unfortunately, the test is available in only a few centers.

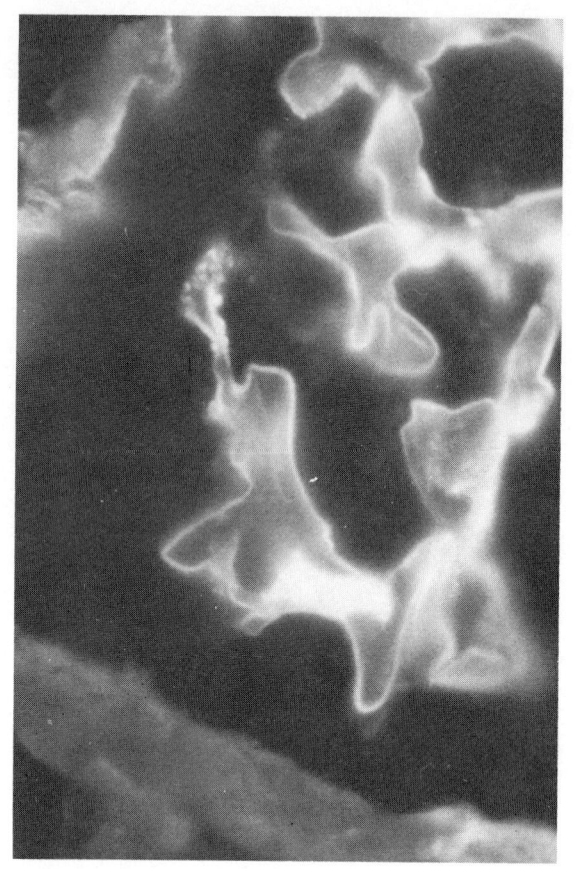

Figure 9–4 Fluorescence micrograph from the same patient as in Figure 9–2. There is a linear, homogeneous deposition of IgG outlining the peripheral GBL. (× 1200.)

Histology

LIGHT MICROSCOPY

GLOMERULI. Rapidly progressive glomerulonephritis typically shows marked proliferation of epithelial cells to form a cellular mass (crescent) that fills the urinary space (Fig. 9–2, 9–5). Nearly all glomeruli are affected. Furthermore, the glomerular tuft is collapsed and usually appears to be hypocellular. Mitotic figures also may be apparent in the crescent, and the proliferative process may extend into the neck of the proximal tubule. It is not known whether the proliferating cells are of parietal or visceral origin. Large numbers of neutrophils also might be evident between epithelial cells. Occasionally, small strands of fibrin may be found in the crescent as well, but this is an inconstant feature. Necrosis within the tuft or involving the crescent

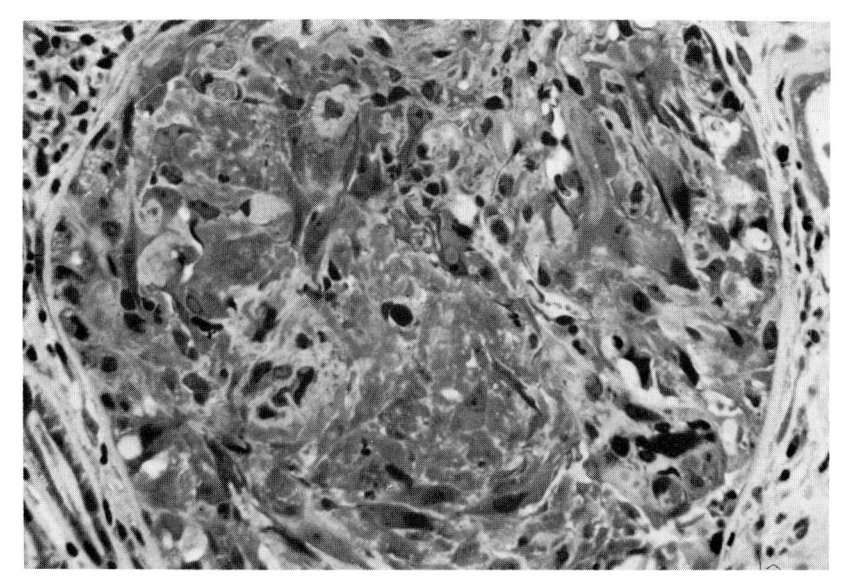

Figure 9-5 Same patient as in Figure 9-2. Note that in this micrograph the glomerular capillary loops are not identifiable within a mass of proliferating cells and extracellular protein. In the 6 to 7 o'clock positions the cellular details are unclear. This appears to be an area of necrosis. (H&E, × 300.)

is not common, but might be a prominent abnormality in individual patients (Fig. 9-5). In such cases, a careful search for a vasculitis is important. The suspicion of vasculitis is heightened when there is variation of involvement among glomeruli and within individual glomeruli (Fig. 9-6).

Proliferation of cells within the tufts can be seen in about one-half of cases (Fig. 9-7). The amount of epithelial cell proliferation, however, often is less severe and less diffuse than in those cases with predominant extracapillary proliferation. The cells include neutrophils as well as presumed endothelial or mesangial cells, or both. The follow-up findings in these patients also suggest that the injury evolves by formation of organized synechiae, increase in mesangial sclerosis, and obsolescence of only the severely affected glomeruli.

INTERSTITIUM. The interstitial edema often is striking early in the clinical course. It usually is diffuse, associated with infiltration of diverse types of inflammatory cells (Fig. 9-8). Later in the course of the disease, the interstitium is diffusely fibrotic, and the number of inflammatory cells decreases. Occasionally the edema and infiltrate, and later the interstitial fibrosis, appear to be concentrated around glomeruli.

TUBULES. Tubular and interstitial changes develop in a parallel manner. The initial alterations include vacuolation and hyaline droplet formation, but red blood cells and hyaline cases in distal tubules are not as prominent as might be expected. Infiltration by mononuclear leukocytes between individual tubular cells also is a feature with extensive in-

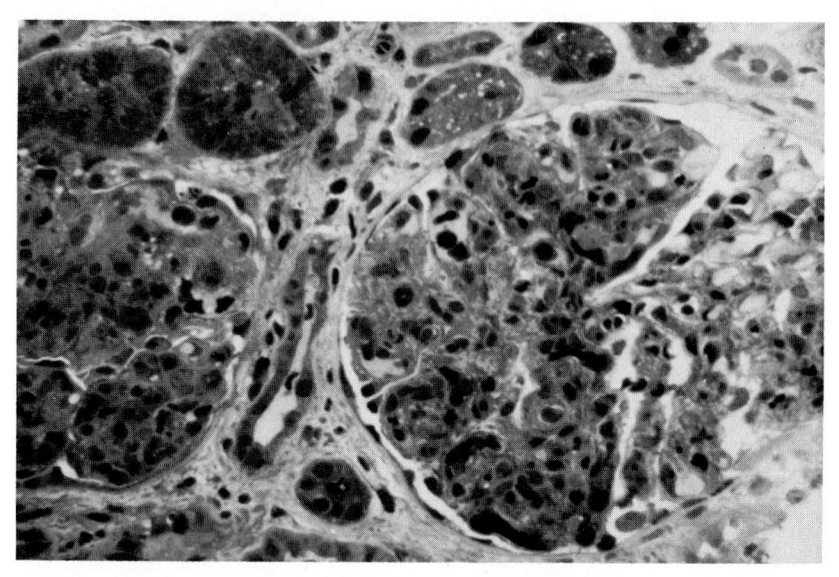

Figure 9-6 Two glomeruli from a 72-year-old white female with a history of migratory pulmonary infiltrates, chest pain, and evanescent neurological findings. The glomerulus on the right is irregularly affected by a proliferative and exudative process. The right segment of this glomerulus appears to be reasonably normal, whereas the left segment contains many cells, including inflammatory cells. There are also diffuse interstitial edema and infiltration. (H&E, × 300.)

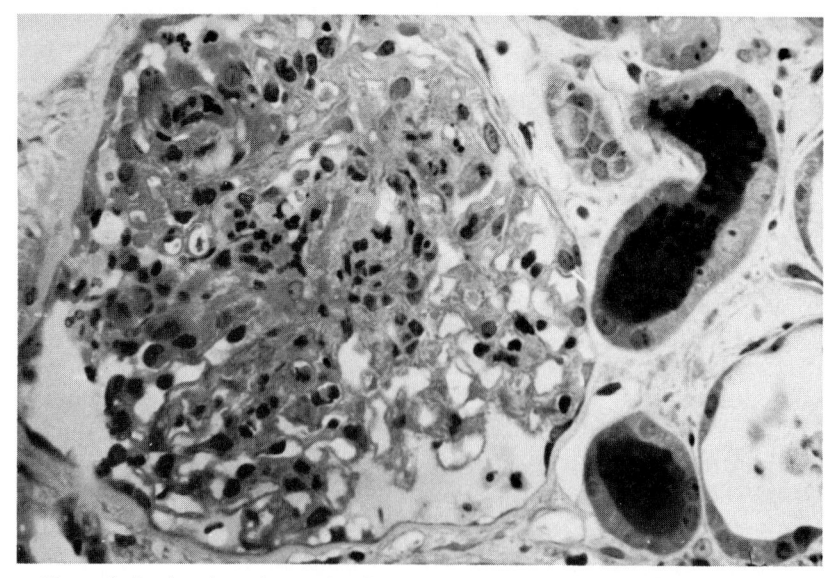

Figure 9-7 Another glomerulus from the same patient as in Figure 9-6. Note that in this glomerulus the primary site of cell proliferation appears to be within the tuft and near the vascular pole. To the right of the micrograph are two distal tubules containing red cells and a protein matrix. (H&E, × 300.)

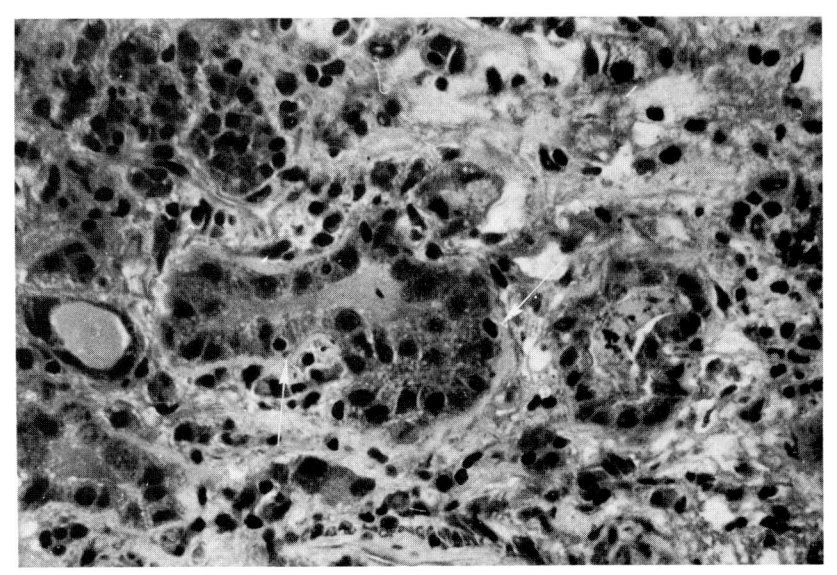

Figure 9-8 Interstitial region from the same patient as in Figure 9-6. Large numbers of inflammatory cells occupy the interstitial space. Mononuclear cells can be seen between tubular epithelial cells (arrows) and in the lumen. (H&E, × 300.)

terstitial involvement (Fig. 9-9). Atrophy and basal lamina thickening accompany the interstitial fibrosis, which develops as the disease progresses.

VESSELS. No specific vascular lesions have been noted. If the underlying etiology is vasculitis, acute inflammatory lesions may be present (see Chapter 18). In those patients who have severe hypertension, however, the vessels may be secondarily affected.

ELECTRON MICROSCOPY

Biopsies characteristically show collapse of glomerular capillary loops and proliferation of epithelial cells, with a lack of identifiable deposits (Fig. 9-3). Light and dark staining epithelial cells also have been described recently (Fig. 9-10). There is widening of the lamina rara interna and endothelial cell swelling (Fig. 9-3). Fibrin may be identifiable in the crescents (Fig. 9-10).

If the biopsy is obtained later in the course of the disease, the cells of the crescent are separated from one another by extracellular material (Fig. 9-11). This consists of both basal lamina and banded collagen fibrils. Since progression of the disease is associated with an increase in connective tissue and decrease in cellularity in the urinary space, the end result is an obsolescent glomerulus.

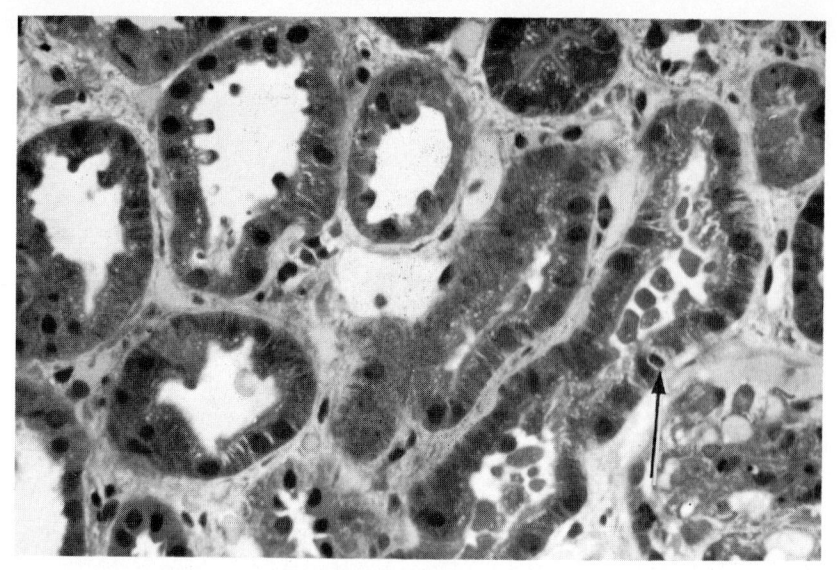

Figure 9-9 Tubular interstitial region from a patient with an area of less prominent infiltration and edema than in Figure 9-8. Note the mononuclear inflammatory cell between proximal tubular epithelial cells (arrow). (H&E, × 300.)

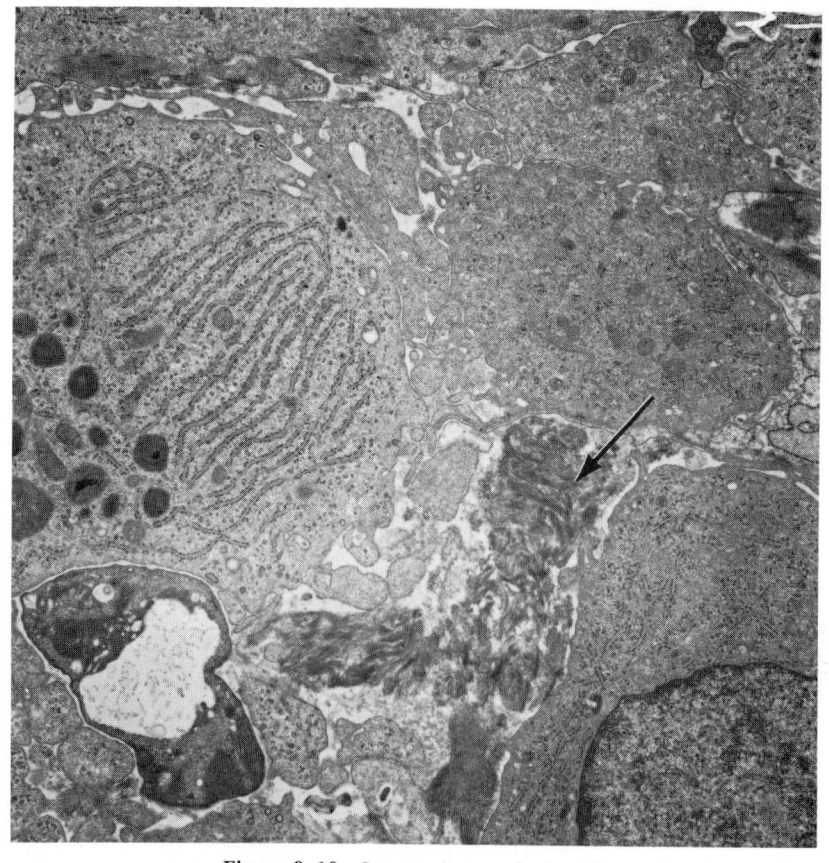

Figure 9-10 *See opposite page for legend.*

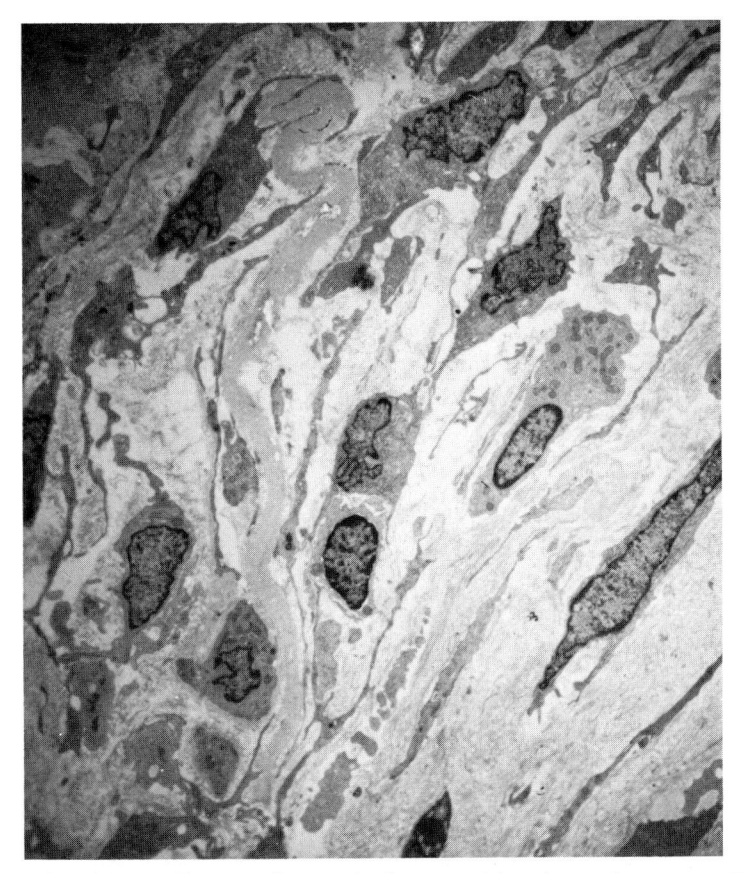

GLOMERULAR DISEASE OF ACUTE ONSET AND RAPID PROGRESSION 113

Figure 9-11 Electron micrograph of an organizing glomerular crescent. There are dense bands of connective tissue and basal lamina-like material lying between lamellae of cells. (× 1500.)

FLUORESCENCE MICROSCOPY

The most often observed abnormality is linear deposition of IgG, usually in association with the C3 component of complement, along the glomerular basal laminae (Figure 9-4). The pattern is seen in those patients having circulating antiglomerular basal lamina antibody, but also has been found in patients with other kidney syndromes that exhibit quite different clinical and histologic findings. Diffuse, irregular deposits of IgG and C3 are found in patients with presumed severe immune

---

Figure 9-10 Electron micrograph of a 77-year-old man with the acute onset of nausea, vomiting, and oliguria. The light microscopic picture resembled that of Figure 9-5. Note the varying cell morphology and the presence of fibrin strands (arrow) between cells. (× 5000.)

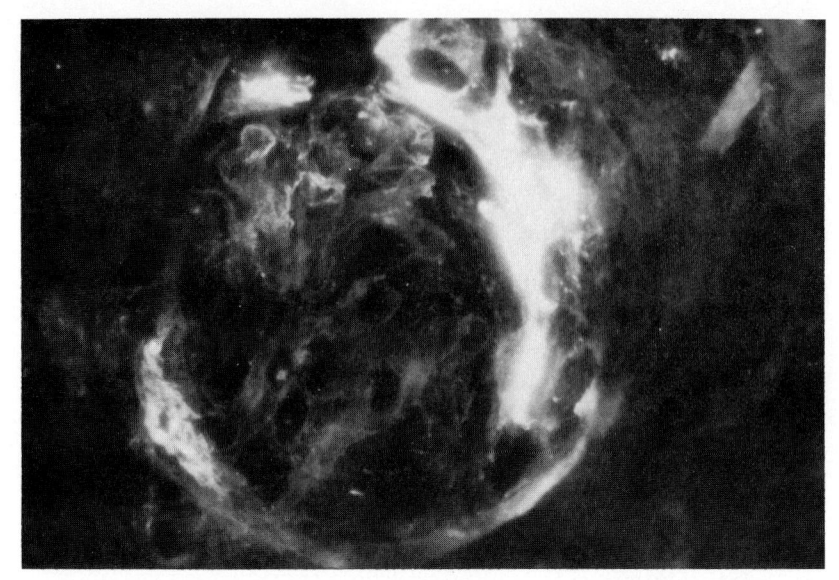

Figure 9-12 Antifibrin fluorescence micrograph on a biopsy from a woman with acute onset of renal failure and an active urine sediment. Marked epithelial cell proliferation was present by light microscopy. The glomerular capillary loops are faintly outlined in the center of the micrograph. The stained material lies within Bowman's space and between proliferating epithelial cells. (× 400.)

complex disease. These cases most often have proliferation of intraglomerular cells as well as crescents. Fibrin is usually present within the crescents (Fig. 9-12).

Clinical Course and Prognosis

The prognosis in this syndrome usually is poor, depending on the etiology, which unfortunately is known in fewer than 50 per cent of cases. Although usually benign, when immune complex disease is severe enough to cause both intra- and extraglomerular proliferation, renal functional impairment can be profound and irreversible.

In the University of Washington study, four of 63 patients ultimately recovered normal renal function. Patients with this renal syndrome in whom a poststreptococcal etiology could be demonstrated had a 60 per cent chance of prolonged satisfactory renal function. Of those in whom a poststreptococcal etiology could not be established, only 5 per cent maintained adequate renal function for more than 1 year.

The histologic changes in the patients with partial recovery of renal function differed from those who remained anuric. In the former group, there were increased numbers of cells within the tuft as well as hyperplasia of glomerular epithelial cells. The major glomerular change in the anuric cases was hyperplasia of only the glomerular epithelial cells.

The amount and type of interstitial disease were of prognostic significance. Those who had interstitial fibrosis involving more than 30 per cent of the tissue were either anuric or had a serum creatinine level greater than 3.5 mg/dl at last follow-up. Those with less interstitial fibrosis as well as reversible glomerular lesions regained renal function.

Patients who also had less than 30 per cent of the interstitium replaced by connective tissue, plus a serum creatinine greater than 3.5 mg/dl at last follow-up, either had advanced or irreversible glomerular changes (obsolescence or necrosis) at the onset. Consequently, early renal biopsy in these cases as a guide to prognosis may be indicated.

Slightly more than half of the patients had a history of an acute "flu-like" illness within one month of the onset of renal failure. The episode was separable temporally from the signs and symptoms of advancing azotemia and uremia in most patients, since changes in urine color or volume occurred at a remote time from the illness. A relationship between viral infections and glomerulonephritis has been noted. For instance, Wilson and Smith (1972) reported on a patient who developed nephritis following an A2 influenza virus infection. The patient had linear deposits of IgG and complement on the glomerular basal lamina. However, the disease was self-limited.

Dodge and co-workers (1972) reported that poststreptococcal nephritis can lead to irreversible or even fatal renal disease when superimposed on preexisting renal disease. In 15 of the University of Washington patients, for instance, there was a history of prior renal disease which had cleared completely. Only one of the patients recovered renal function. It is not known how many of these patients had an antiglomerular basal lamina antibody nephritis.

Although various and at times exceedingly aggressive treatment regimens have been attempted in this renal syndrome, none has proved to be of consistent benefit, since the series is small and it is difficult to rule out spontaneous remission. The presence of fibrin in the crescents and fibrin degradation products in the serum and urine has prompted the use of anticoagulants. The results have been quite variable. Although we recently have studied this phenomenon using kinetic measures of hemostasis, we could not demonstrate significant hemostatic involvement in rapidly progressive glomerulonephritis.

An unresolved problem is whether patients with this disease should receive a renal allograft; the important question is whether there will be a recurrence of the original disease in the graft. Our approach to this problem is to assay the sera of these patients for antiglomerular basal lamina antibodies following binephrectomy in all patients with this syndrome. If antibodies are present, the patient is placed on chronic dialysis until the antibodies disappear. This approach is intuitive and unproved, since patients with circulating antiglomerular basal lamina antibodies have had successful transplantations without evidence of recurrence, while others have recurred.

The exact role of antibody directed against the glomerular basal lamina is in question. Recently, for example, Mathew and colleagues (1975) reported a patient with recurrent pulmonary hemorrhage who had no abnormalities of renal function or urine sediment. Kidney biopsy on several occasions revealed deposition of immunoglobulins in a linear fashion on the glomerular basal lamina, but no other changes. Circulating levels of antiglomerular basal lamina antibody were not reported.

We have followed the case of a similar patient, who initially had a mild decrease in renal function, circulating antiglomerular basal lamina antibodies, and linear fluorescence staining of the glomerular basal lamina. The patient regained normal renal function, and the histologic lesion shows only mild sclerosis.

There are several unresolved issues: Are pulmonary hemosiderosis and Goodpasture's syndrome related? Is the renal lesion in Goodpasture's syndrome (and others) directly related to the presence of the antibody? What is the natural history and therapeutic regimen indicated for this syndrome?

References

1. Bacani, R. A., Velasquez, F., Kanter, A., Pirani, C. L., and Poliak, V. E.: Rapidly progressive (nonstreptococcal) glomerulonephritis. Ann. Int. Med. *73*:703, 1970.
2. Berlyne, G. M., and Baker, S. B.: Acute anuric glomerulonephritis. Quart. J. Med. *33*:105, 1964.
3. Brun, C., Gormsen, H., Hilden, T., Iversen, P., and Raaschou, F.: Kidney biopsy in acute glomerulonephritis. Acta Med. Scand. *160*:155, 1958.
4. Burch, G. E., Chu, K. C., Cololough, H. L., and Sohal, R. S.: Immunofluorescent localization of coxsackievirus B antigen in the kidney observed at routine autopsy. Am. J. Med. *47*:36, 1969.
5. Cameron, J. S.: The natural history of glomerulonephritis. *In* Black, G. (ed.), Renal Disease. Oxford, England, Blackwell Scientific Publications, 1972.
6. Dodge, W. F., Spargo, B. H., Travis, L. B., Srivastava, R. N., Carvajal, H. F., DeBeukelaer, M. M., Longley, M. P., and Menchaca, J. A.: Poststreptococcal glomerulonephritis. A prospective study in children. New Eng. J. Med. *286*:273, 1972.
7. George, C. R. P., Slichter, S. J., Quadracci, L. J., Striker, G. E., and Harker, L. A.: A kinetic evaluation of hemostasis in renal disease. New Eng. J. Med. *291*:1111, 1974.
8. Habib, R.: Classification anatomique des nephropathies glomérulaires. Paediatrische Fortbildungskurze *28*:3, 1970.
9. Harrison, C. V., Loughbridge, L. W., and Milne, M. D.: Acute oliguric renal failure in acute glomerulonephritis and polyarteritis nodosa. Quart. J. Med. *33*:39, 1964.
10. Leonard, C. D., Nagle, R., Striker, G. E., Cutler, R. E., and Scribner, B. H.: Acute glomerulonephritis with prolonged oliguria. Ann. Int. Med. *73*:703, 1970.
11. Lerner, R. A., and Dixon, F. J.: Transfer of ovine experimental allergic glomerulonephritis with serum. J. Exper. Med. *124*:431, 1966.
12. Lerner, R. A., Glassock, R. J., and Dixon, F. J.: The role of antiglomerular basement membrane antibody in the pathogenesis of human glomerulonephritis. J. Exper. Med., *126*:989, 1967.

13. Lewis, E. J., Cavallo, T., Harrington, J. T., and Cotran, R. S.: An immunopathologic study of rapidly progressive glomerulonephritis in the adult. Hum. Pathol. 2:185, 1971.
14. Mathew, T. H., Hobbs, J. B., Kalowski, S., Sutherland, P. W., and Kincaid-Smith, P.: Goodpasture's syndrome: Normal renal diagnostic findings. Ann. Int. Med. 82:215, 1975.
15. Steblay, R. W.: Glomerulonephritis induced in sheep by injections of heterologous glomerular basement membrane and Freund's complete adjuvant. J. Exper. Med. 116:253, 1962.
16. Wilson, C. B., and Smith, R. C.: Goodpasture's syndrome associated with influenza A2 virus infection. Ann. Int. Med. 76:91, 1972.
17. Yuceoglu, A. M., Berkovich, S., and Minkowitz, S.: Acute glomerulonephritis associated with ECHO virus type 9 infection. J. Pediatr. 69:603, 1966.

Chapter Ten

Tubulo-Interstitial Diseases of Acute Onset

Introduction

The most common syndrome associated with severe injury to the tubulo-interstitial compartment is acute renal failure, which is one of the dramatic clinical problems facing physicians who treat critically ill patients. Findings that include a loss of concentrating capacity and a rapid, steadily increasing azotemia, with or without oliguria (less than 500 ml daily) establish the diagnosis of acute renal failure. Although this syndrome frequently is associated with specific clinical problems to be described, the exact pathogenesis of suppression of renal function often is obscure.

It has been useful clinically to divide the major causes of acute renal failure into three diagnostic categories: prerenal, postrenal, and renal (Table 10–1). This classification stresses the fact that prerenal and postrenal causes are rapidly reversible and, therefore, should be diagnosed and treated early. Some of the causes of primary renal injury also are treatable, such as acute interstitial nephritis from pyelonephritis or drug reactions, and metabolic disorders such as hypercalcemia and hyperuricemia.

ACUTE TUBULO-INTERSTITIAL INJURY

Although the pathogenesis of oliguria associated with acute tubulo-interstitial injury is still being debated, micropuncture studies have suggested that at least three factors are involved. Alterations due to acute circulatory or toxic damage produce changes in glomerular capillary pressure, permeability, and blood flow leading directly to a reduction in filtration and urine formation. At the same time, intratubular

TABLE 10-1 Major Causes of Acute Renal Failure

I. Prerenal (diminished renal perfusion)
   A. Fluid and electrolyte depletion
   B. Hemorrhage
   C. Septicemia

II. Postrenal (obstruction)
   A. Prostatism
   B. Bladder or other pelvic or retroperitoneal tumors
   C. Renal calculi
   D. Ureteral blockage after surgery or instrumentation

III. Primary renal injury
   A. Acute tubular injury
      1. "Ischemic" (consequent to circulatory inadequacy, obstetric complications)
      2. Toxins (carbon tetrachloride, heavy metals, methanol, ethylene glycol, etc.)
      3. Hemoglobinuria (mismatched transfusions, malaria, etc.)
      4. Myoglobinuria (crush injuries, exercise rhabdomyolysis)
      5. Burns (combination of 1, 3, 4)
   B. Acute glomerulonephritis (Chapters 8 and 9)
   C. Arterial or venous obstruction (Chapter 11)
   D. Acute diffuse interstitial nephritis
   E. Intrarenal precipitation (hypercalcemia, sulfonamides, urates, myeloma protein, etc.)

obstruction occurs, retarding the flow of filtrate and promoting backleakage across damaged epithelium. These factors are not mutually exclusive, nor are all necessarily present in any patient; moreover, they probably vary in importance among different patients and from time to time in the same patient. All the foregoing factors emphasize the inaccuracy of the term "acute tubular necrosis" as a description of the basic abnormality. In reality, the tubular lesions are variable, but edema and inflammation of the interstitial tissue are always present. The only constant sign is the apparent integrity of the glomeruli and vessels.

Clinical Data

The clinical manifestations of renal failure secondary to acute tubular injury can be divided into four phases: (1) prodromal, (2) anuric or oliguric, (3) diuretic, and (4) recovery. The prodromal phase varies in duration, depending upon causative factors, such as the dosage of toxin ingested or the length and severity of hypotension. The anuric or oliguric phase is defined by the loss of nephron function, as exhibited by a suppression of urine volume, a concentrating defect (urine-to-plasma osmolarity ratio of 0.9 to 1.1), and a rapidly rising serum creatinine level. Although frequently oliguria is the earliest sign, it never occurs in approximately 20 per cent of the patients. On

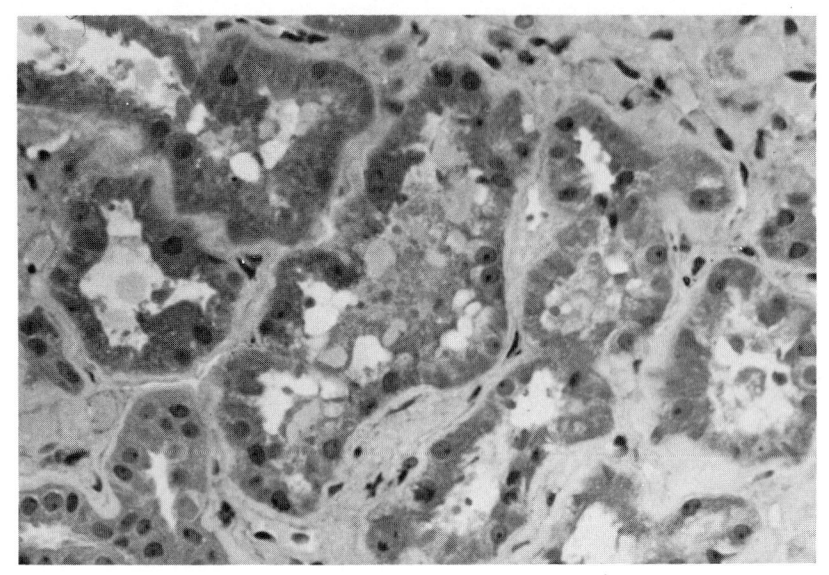

Figure 10-1 Specimen from a 68-year-old female with rheumatoid arthritis who was admitted with pneumonia, sepsis and hypotension. The proximal tubular epithelial cell cytoplasm is swollen and vacuolated. (H&E, × 300.)

the other hand, a concentrating defect and progressive azotemia are always present. The management of such cases, however, is easier than their oliguric counterparts.

The urinary sediment gives valuable clues to diagnosis. In prerenal failure, moderate numbers of hyaline and finely granular casts are evident. The sediment of acute tubulo-interstitial injury characteristically contains numerous renal tubular cells, tubular cell casts, and coarse granular casts. Red cells, hemoglobin casts, and red cell casts may be seen as well if hemoglobinuria or glomerulonephritis are present. Urine with scanty sediment that contains only rare white cells, as well as red cell, hyaline, and granular casts, suggests that obstruction may be the etiology.

The chemical urinalysis usually reveals some proteinuria and a urine sodium concentration which is less than 15 mEq/liter in prerenal disease, but usually greater than 20 mEq/liter with primary renal injury or obstruction. A plain film of the abdomen also may help in diagnosis by demonstrating a stone or by establishing kidney size (which would be normal or large in acute renal failure, for instance). If the clinical picture suggests obstruction, retrograde ureteral catheterization should be performed.

Histology

GLOMERULI. No lesions are noted in the glomeruli.
TUBULES. Quite often no histologic abnormalities or only minor

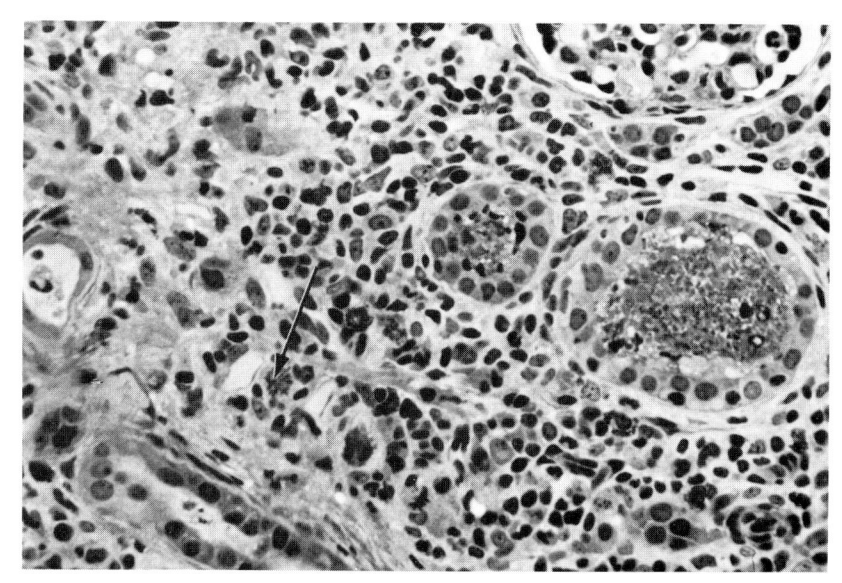

Figure 10-2 Same patient as in Figure 10-1. Here the interstitial infiltration is marked and the tubular epithelium is infiltrated by inflammatory cells. At the lower right portion of the micrograph there appears to be karyorrhexis and karyolysis of the epithelial cells. Mitotic figures are noted in the interstitium (arrow). (H&E, × 300.)

cell swelling is seen in the tubules (Fig. 10-1). However, they may show varying degrees of necrosis, infiltration with acute inflammatory cells, or both, depending on the severity of the initial injury (Fig. 10-2). In severe injury the tubular basal laminae may be disrupted (Fig. 10-3). In these instances, restoration of the normal tubular achitecture is impaired, and permanent damage results.

INTERSTITIUM. The interstitium is not involved in mild cases, but may show varying degrees of edema. The characteristic lesion of severe injury is a diffuse infiltration of all interstitial spaces with inflammatory cells consisting of large numbers of neutrophils and mononuclear cells. With time, this lesion is replaced by broad bands of fibrosis (Fig. 10-4).

VESSELS. No distinctive vessel changes, either arteriolar or venous, are evident.

Clinical Course and Prognosis

It is crucial to rule out prerenal and postrenal causes of acute renal failure in patients with this syndrome. In the former, oliguria responds to correction of the disorder producing a reduction in renal blood flow. On the other hand, postrenal causes usually require prompt urologic intervention to prevent irreversible renal damage. If oliguria occurs in the presence of certain "high risk" conditions (shock, sepsis, nephro-

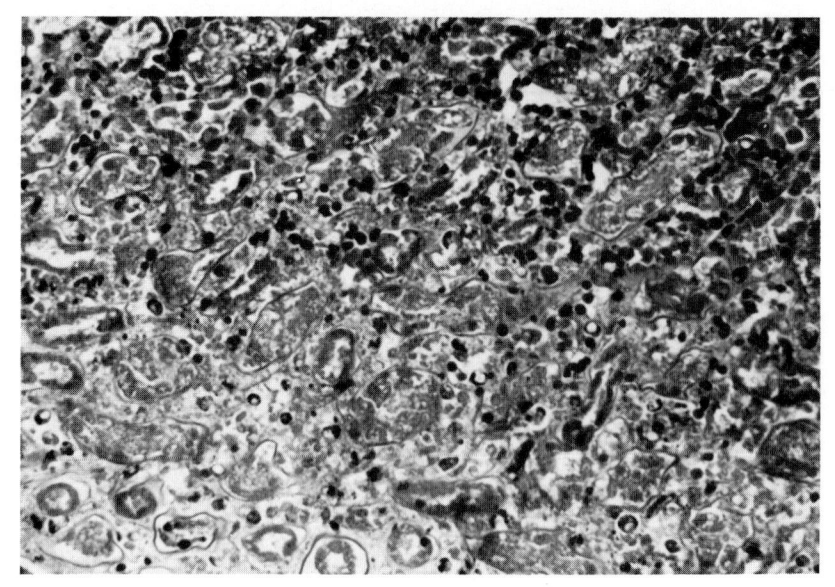

Figure 10-3 Renal biopsy from a renal transplant patient with arterial obstruction. The tubular basal laminae are disrupted and frayed. The cellular architecture is severely altered. (H&E, × 300.)

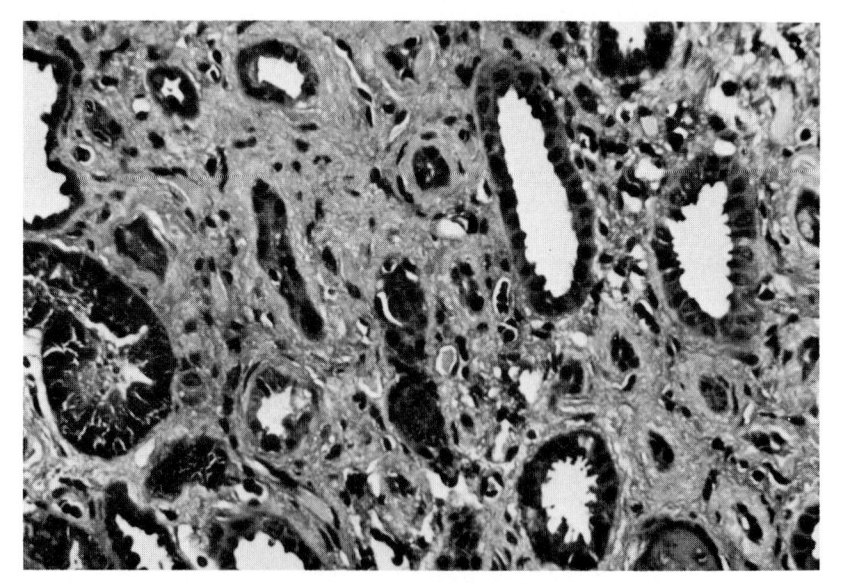

Figure 10-4 Renal biopsy from a 63-year-old man three months after ingestion of ethylene glycol and a prolonged period of renal failure. The interstitial space is prominent. Dense connective tissue and a small number of inflammatory cells lie in this region. Atrophied tubules with thick basal laminae are prominent in the central portions of the micrograph. (H&E, × 300.)

toxins, cardiopulmonary bypass), acute tubulo-interstitial injury should be suspected. In these situations, support of the circulation along with the induction of a solute diuresis in the prodromal or early oliguric phase may prevent or modify the development of oliguria. In the past this had been attempted with furosemide (2 to 3 mg/kg intravenously), mannitol (0.5 to 1 g/kg intravenously), or both. The lack of response to furosemide creates no problems, but an inability to excrete mannitol does expand the extracellular volume and may precipitate pulmonary edema in susceptible patients. Recent clinical and laboratory experience suggests that dopamine (3 to 5 μg/kg/min intravenously) along with furosemide (10 to 15 μg/kg/min intravenously) may be even more effective in reversing oliguria. Such therapy may prevent the decrease in glomerular filtration and intratubular obstruction which usually occur in acute tubulo-interstitial injury but may have no effect on other factors. Many cases treated in this manner appear to be converted from oliguric to non-oliguric acute renal failure. However, even this modification may be useful as clinical management of the non-oliguric patient is usually simpler.

The oliguric phase may last from hours to weeks, depending on the cause and extent of injury. If it had not been done previously, a renal biopsy often is performed if this phase is prolonged over 20 to 30 days to determine the potential reversibility of the lesion. The management of established renal failure consists of proper fluid and electrolyte control, adequate nutrition, early and frequent dialysis, and control of infections.

The diuretic phase is important because mismanagement could cause death. During this period, urine flow begins again, but a continued impairment of tubular transport prevents normal renal function. The urine is similar to an ultrafiltrate of plasma, so large quantities of electrolytes and water may be lost. Although the urine volume might be high, the excretion of urea and creatinine is so low that their plasma levels continue to rise, or fall very slowly. The duration of this phase is variable, but usually lasts 5 to 7 days.

Finally, the recovery phase is characterized by a return to a more normal tubular function and glomerular filtration rate, with electrolyte and water conservation, which results in a fall in urine volume, as well as decreasing azotemia. Although renal function may not return entirely to normal in every patient, a slow improvement continues for several months after the onset of diuresis.

Fortunately, long-term clinical and histologic studies indicate that complete recovery is the rule, even in the presence of prolonged renal failure and diffuse tubular injury. Therefore, barring frank cortical necrosis, it appears that acute tubular damage usually is completely reversible.

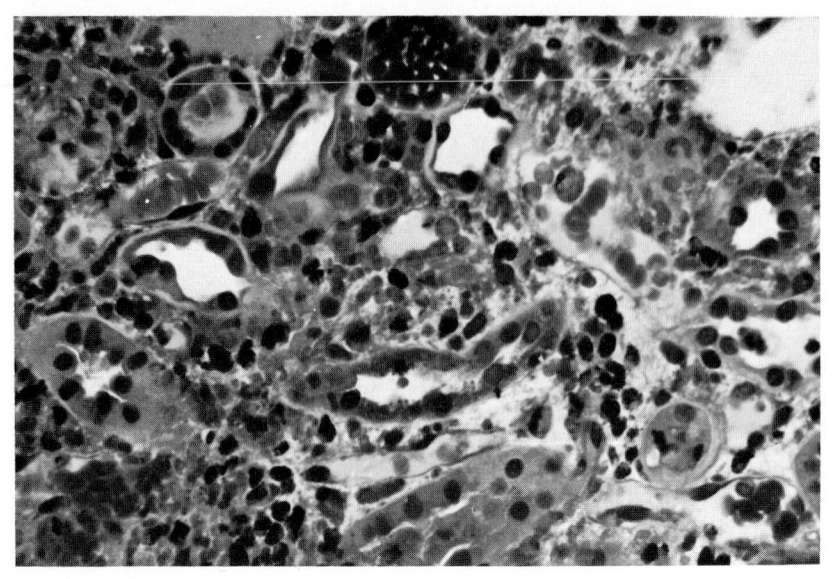

Figure 10-5 A 60-year-old man with low back pain and fever treated with methicillin. A penicillin allergy was subsequently documented. The tubulo-interstitial region is markedly widened by an intense inflammatory infiltration consisting predominantly of eosinophils. (H&E, × 300.)

ACUTE DIFFUSE INTERSTITIAL NEPHRITIS

Acute diffuse interstitial nephritis is an uncommon disorder, but one which must be considered among the important causes of acute oliguric renal failure. Councilman, for example, reviewed the literature in 1898 and reported 42 cases. At that time and during the four succeeding decades it was recognized as a lesion that occurred largely in children with acute febrile infections, particularly streptococcal infections or diphtheria. With the control and decline of these infections, the dominant cause of acute diffuse interstitial nephritis became drug reactions, particularly to sulfonamides, penicillin, and methicillin. A few cases also have been reported following colistimethate sodium, phenindione, and nitrofurantoin administration.

Clinical Data

The initial clinical presentation of acute diffuse interstitial nephritis is rapid renal failure. There are no typical features which would distinguish this syndrome from other forms of oliguric renal failure, but the following clinical clues are helpful in suggesting its existence: (1) exposure to drugs, and (2) presence of symptoms and signs suggesting a hypersensitivity state such as rash or eosinophilia.

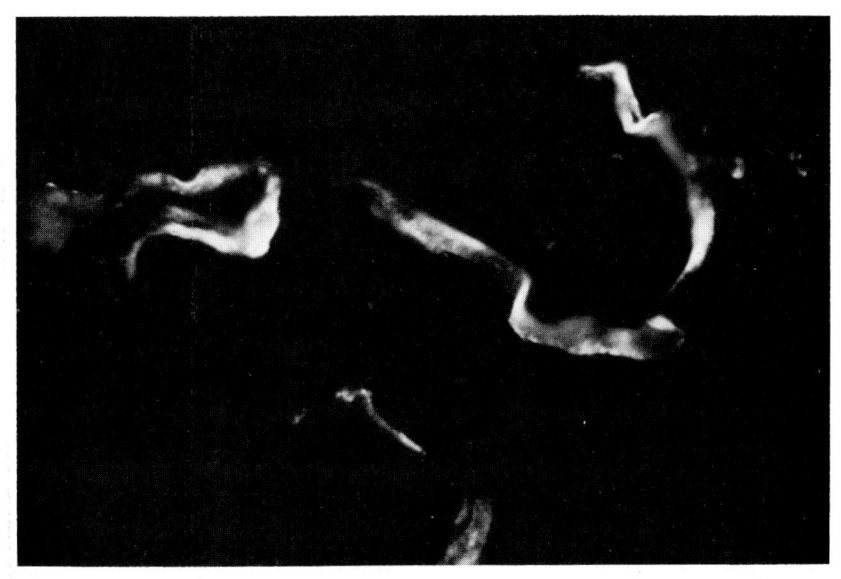

Figure 10-6 Fluorescence micrograph with anti-IgG antibody. The tubular basal lamina is irregularly outlined. This is a biopsy specimen from the same patient as in Figure 10-5. (× 300.)

Histology

LIGHT MICROSCOPY. Dense interstitial infiltration with inflammatory cells and pronounced edema is evident (Fig. 10-5); the inflammatory cells vary, but often are primarily neutrophils or eosinophils. There does not appear to be a predilection for a particular anatomical site, but the medulla frequently is affected. Glomerular, tubular, and vascular lesions seldom occur.

IMMUNOFLUORESCENCE MICROSCOPY. In the majority of cases, the immunofluorescent staining is nonspecific. Occasionally, linear staining of tubular basal lamina with IgG and complement has been reported in patients with penicillin or methicillin hypersensitivity (Fig. 10-6).

Clinical Course and Prognosis

According to Rich (1960), four types of renal involvement are associated with drug hypersensitivity: (1) periarteritis nodosa, (2) acute proliferative glomerulonephritis, (3) focal necrotizing glomerulonephritis, and (4) acute interstitial nephritis. In our experience, the fourth type is most commonly associated with drug administration, whereas the other three are seen only rarely. Rich also outlines a spectrum of changes ranging from focal areas of interstitial inflammation with no clinically detectable functional abnormality, to diffuse interstitial inflammation involving both kidneys and leading to necrosis of tubular epithelium. Anuria and uremia leading to death have been reported with extensive involvement.

The long-term results in patients with acute diffuse interstitial nephritis, however, look encouraging. The evidence available suggests that progressive renal disease will not occur, although the patient may be left with some residual renal dysfunction.

Recently there also has been increasing confirmation of the immunologic nature of this disorder when associated with methicillin. Border and his colleagues, for example, found antitubular basal lamina antibodies in the serum of a patient in whom severe renal failure developed while receiving methicillin. A renal biopsy showed a severe mononuclear interstitial infiltrate with focal areas of tubular degeneration. IgG, complement, and a methicillin antigen assumed to be dimethoxyphenylpenicilloyl were present in a linear pattern along the tubular basal lamina, but not on the glomerular basal lamina. The dimethoxyphenylpenicilloyl-tubular basal lamina "hapten protein conjugate" apparently led to an immune response with antitubular basal lamina antibodies being involved in the immunopathogenesis of the patient's interstitial nephritis.

References

1. Andres, G. A., and McCluskey, R. T.: Tubular and interstitial renal disease due to immunologic mechanisms. Kidney Int. 7:271, 1975.
2. Bailey, R. R., Natale, R., Turnbull, D. I., and Linton, A. L.: Protective effect of frusemide in acute tubular necrosis and acute renal failure. Clin. Sci. Mol. Med. 45:1, 1973.
3. Border, W. A., Lehman, D. H., Egan, J. D., Sass, H. J., Glode, J. E., and Wilson, C. B.: Antitubular basement-membrane antibodies in methicillin-associated interstitial nephritis. New Eng. J. Med. 291:381, 1974.
4. Briggs, J. D., Kennedy, A. C., Young, L. N., Luke, R. G., and Gray, M.: Renal function after acute tubular necrosis. Brit. Med. J. 3:513, 1967.
5. Bull, G. M., Joekes, A. N., and Lowe, K. G.: Renal function studies in acute tubular necrosis. Clin. Sci. 9:379, 1950.
6. Councilman, W. T.: Acute interstitial nephritis. J. Exp. Med. 3:393, 1898.
7. Finn, W. F., Arendshorst, W. J., and Gottschalk, C. W.: Pathogenesis of oliguria in acute renal failure. Circ. Res. 36:675, 1975.
8. Flamenbaum, W.: Pathophysiology of acute renal failure. Arch. Intern. Med. 131:911, 1973.
9. Luke, R. G., Linton, A. L., Briggs, J. D., and Kennedy, A. C.: Mannitol therapy in acute renal failure. Lancet 2:980, 1965.
10. Rich, A. R.: Visceral hazards of hypersensitivity to drugs. Trans. Amer. Clin. Climat. Assn. 72:46, 1960.

Chapter Eleven

Vascular Diseases of Acute Onset (Except Vasculitis)

Introduction

Excluding vasculitis (Section V), there are five types of changes which occur in the kidney related to vascular disease of acute onset: (1) malignant nephrosclerosis, (2) infarction from arterial occlusion, (3) renal cortical necrosis, (4) renal vein thrombosis, and (5) atheromatous embolization. Because clinical presentation and pathologic changes differ, each type of disorder will be discussed separately.

MALIGNANT NEPHROSCLEROSIS

Introduction

Although there is disagreement concerning a precise definition of malignant hypertension, the diagnosis is based clinically upon the findings of persistent diastolic blood pressure greater than 120 mm Hg and neuroretinopathy (hemorrhages, exudates, and papilledema). If the blood pressure is not reduced, the disease invariably is fatal within one year, with death usually resulting from either cardiac or renal failure, stroke, or a combination of these. Most cases of malignant nephrosclerosis appear in the course of benign, essential hypertension. Recent studies suggest that nearly 1 per cent of the patients with essential hypertension develop this complication.

Arteriolar nephrosclerosis is the most common background for the development of malignant nephrosclerosis. However, malignant nephrosclerosis may be associated with a variety of other renal syn-

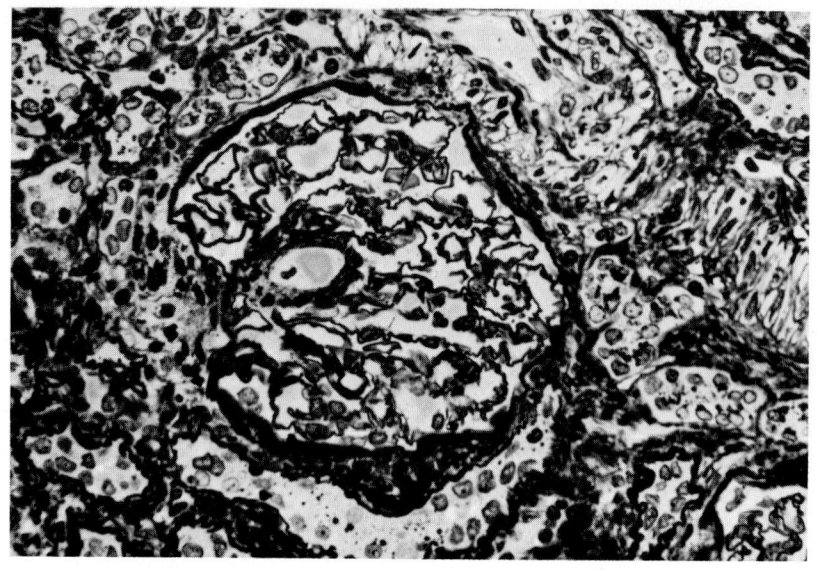

Figure 11-1 Silver stain from a 47-year-old female with a 2 month history of rising blood pressure, elevated serum creatinine levels, and increasing cardiac failure. The glomerular basal lamina is wrinkled and irregular. The number of cells is normal or slightly decreased. (Methenamine silver, × 300.)

dromes, including glomerulonephritis, chronic interstitial nephritis, polyarteritis nodosa, renal vascular disease, radiation nephritis, hydronephrosis, scleroderma, and polycystic disease. Malignant nephrosclerosis also may develop *de novo* without prior history of hypertension.

Clinical Data

The peak incidence of this disease occurs in the fourth and fifth decades in women and about 10 years later in men. Patients usually have severe headaches and blurring of vision, which may or may not be associated with papilledema. Because many patients present with significant neurologic symptoms and findings, it may be difficult to differentiate malignant hypertension from brain tumor.

In addition, the diastolic blood pressure is frequently in excess of 120 mm Hg, and the heart is enlarged, revealing electrocardiographic evidence of left ventricular hypertrophy. Congestive heart failure also may be present. Grade IV hypertensive retinopathy, as described by Keith and his associates (1939), is evident as well, which includes papilledema, retinal hemorrhages, and exudates. Neurologic findings also vary from slight obtundation to deep coma.

Laboratory data may show varying degrees of renal insufficiency, urinary findings including proteinuria that occasionally may be in the nephrotic range, and hematuria, which may be microscopic or gross.

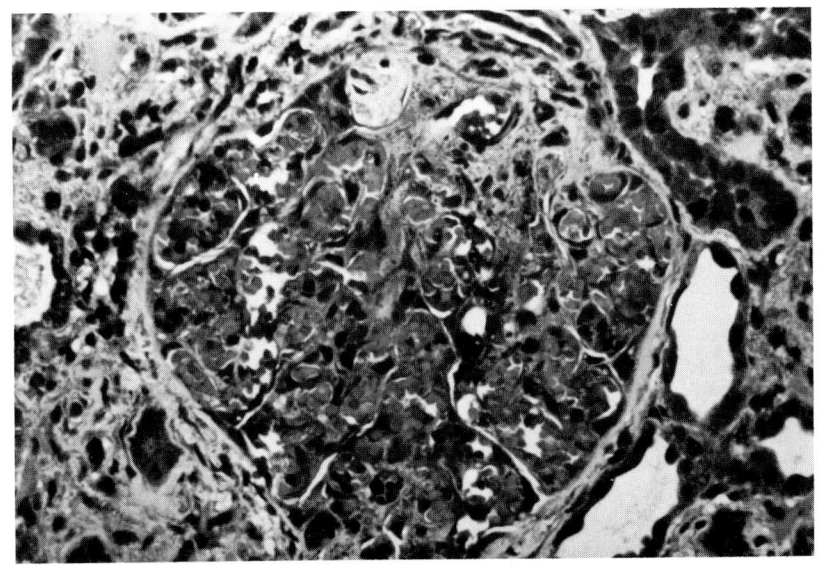

Figure 11-2 Glomeruli from the same patient as in Figure 11-1. The capillary spaces are distended with blood cells and amorphous masses of serum protein. (H&E, × 300.)

Except in those renal syndromes that are associated with glomerulonephritis, only occasional red cell casts are present.

Histology

GLOMERULI. The glomerular lesions are characterized by ischemia, hemorrhage, and thrombosis (Fig. 11-1). The ischemia, in contrast to that seen in milder forms of hypertension, is associated with a wrinkled, thickened, and contracted basal lamina (Fig. 11-2 and 11-3). Very striking when present is the finding of necrosis with deposition of fibrin and large numbers of red cells within vascular channels leaking into extravascular spaces (Fig. 11-4). In such lesions, there is a loss of cellular detail, with karyorrhexis and karyolysis. This change usually affects a relatively small number of glomeruli (5 to 20 per cent), and therefore may not be present in a renal biopsy specimen.

Changes in Bowman's basal lamina also have been stressed by several authors, the alterations variously described as duplication of the basal lamina or a nodular increase in the amount of extracellular material in this region, beginning at the vascular pole and spreading circumferentially (Fig. 11-2).

TUBULES. There is considerable disruption of the normal tubular architecture, as well as atrophy, thickened basal lamina, and a total

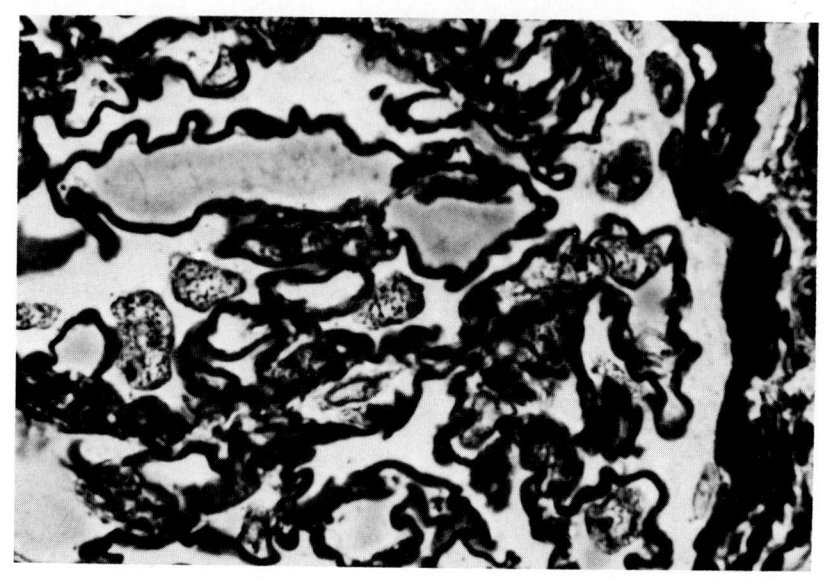

Figure 11-3 High power photomicrograph of the same patient as in Figure 11-1 to illustrate the irregular, wrinkled glomerular basal lamina surrounding collapsed capillary lumina. Note that the Bowman's basal lamina is duplicated and thickened. This is even more prominent in Figure 11-4. (Methenamine silver, × 1200.)

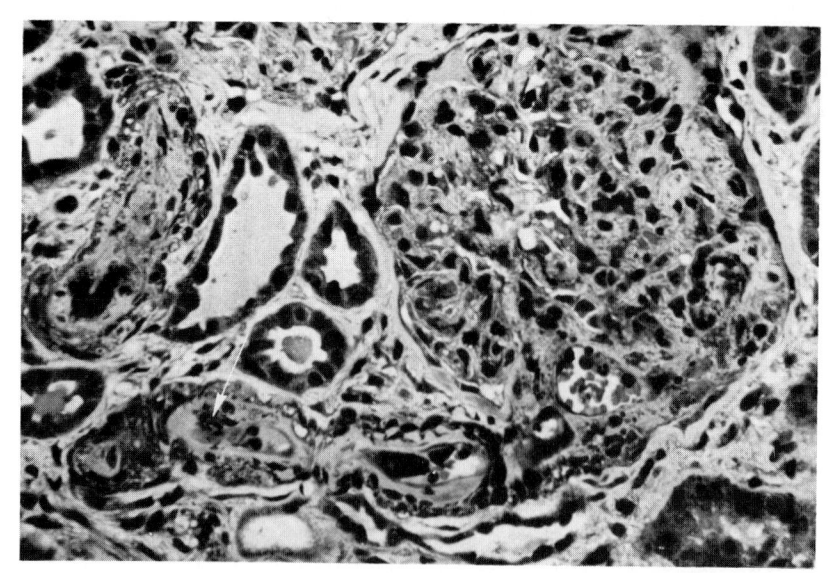

Figure 11-4 Photomicrograph of the same patient as in Figure 11-1. The subendothelial space is markedly expanded in the efferent arterial space and in some areas there is nuclear debris within these spaces (arrow). (H&E, × 300.)

decrease in the number of tubular profiles (Fig. 11-4). In the remaining atrophic tubules, casts and sloughed cells often are present.

INTERSTITIUM. The interstitium is increased in amount owing to edema and a diffuse increase in the amount of interstitial connective tissue, with a loss of interstitial capillary structures. Although broad bands of scar, characteristic of primary interstitial and primary glomerular lesions, are not common, this may be a prominent feature in patients who have long-standing hypertension.

VESSELS. The arteriolar lesion also is prominent, replacing the normal structures in the wall, or in a segment of the wall, with an eosinophilic homogeneous acellular mass of material which contains fibrin and many other serum proteins (Fig. 11-5). This usually is associated with marked decrease in the size of the vascular lumen, and often nearly complete disruption of the normal architecture of the vessel, as well as the loss of cellular detail. This is an irregular lesion, however, affecting fewer than half of the identifiable afferent arterioles in an individual biopsy.

The injuries to the larger vessels are characterized either by a localized process similar to that seen in the arteriole, or by a concentric lamellar thickening of the space between the internal elastic lamella and the intima (Fig. 11-6, 11-7, and 11-8). This enlarged space contains myoendothelial cells and fibroelastic connective tissue. The latter change is frequently seen in patients who have had essential hypertension.

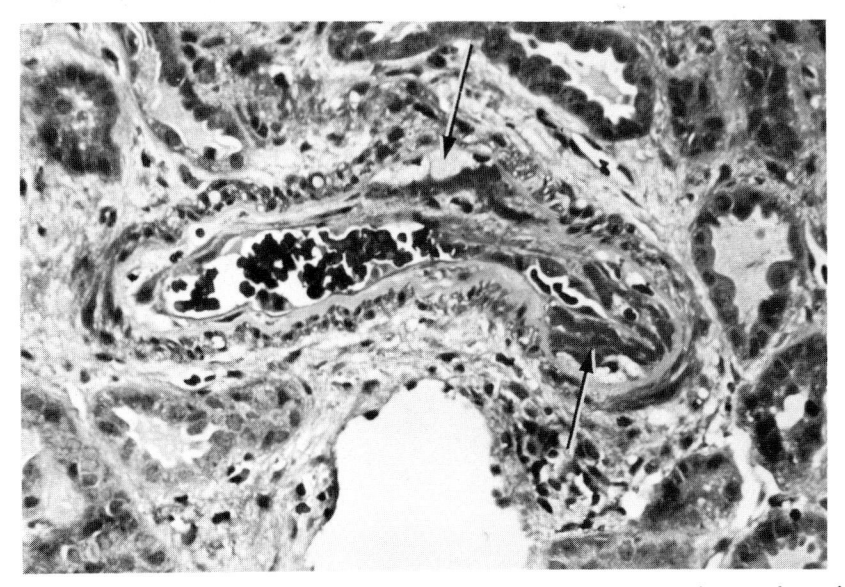

Figure 11-5 Same patient as in Figure 11-1. Note the serum protein vacuoles and fibrin lying within the subendothelial space (arrows). (Trichrome, ×   .)

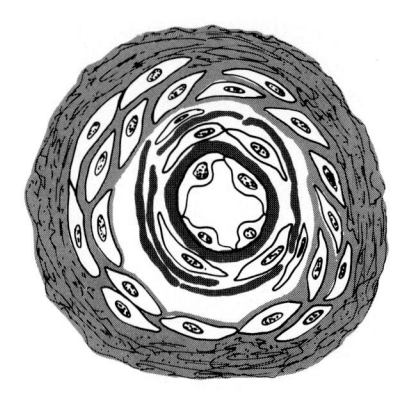

Figure 11-6 Diagrammatic representation of a vessel showing intimal hyperplasia with reduplication of the elastic lamina.

Clinical Course and Prognosis

Untreated patients with malignant nephrosclerosis die in a relatively short period of time, approximately half of them by 6 months and most of the remainder within 1 year. Sixty to 70 per cent of the patients die as a result of uremia with or without accompanying heart failure; 20 per cent die from cerebrovascular accidents.

Aggressive lowering of blood pressure can significantly reduce the mortality and morbidity associated with malignant nephrosclerosis. Pa-

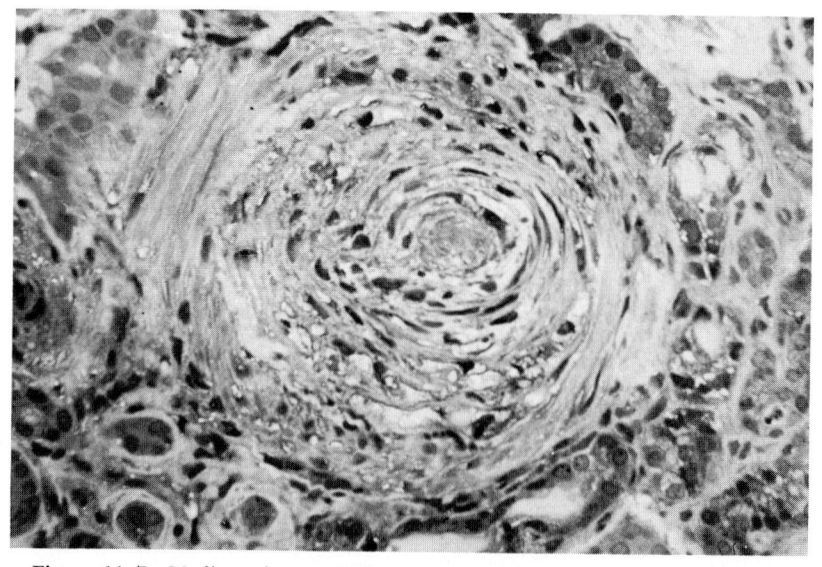

Figure 11-7 Medium size artery from a 28-year-old female with an acute onset of hypertension, oliguria, and malaise. Blood pressure was markedly elevated, and she required hemodialysis. The media appear to be intact. The lumen is separated, however, by multiple layers of elongated cells resembling smooth muscle cells. The lumen is tiny and appears to be filled with coagulated protein. (H&E, × 300.)

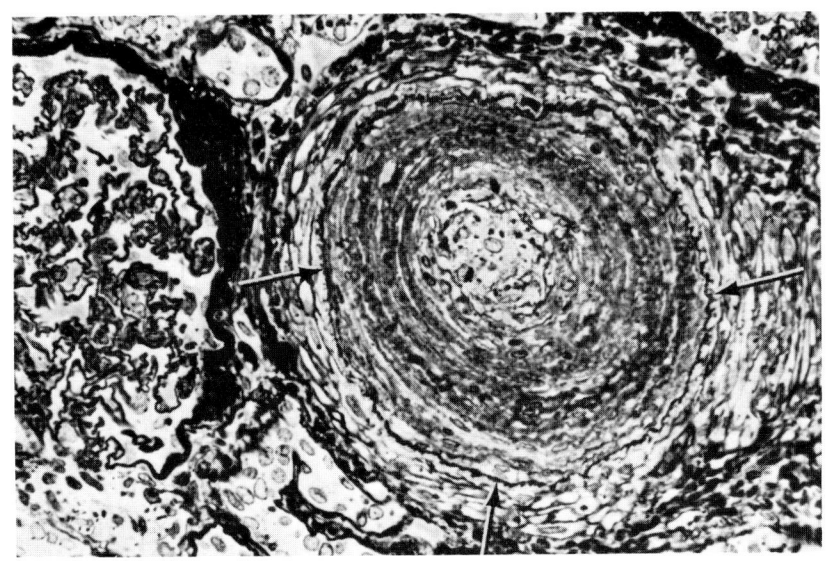

Figure 11-8 Silver stain of same vessel as in Figure 11-2. The internal elastic lamina (arrows) is adjacent to the relatively normal media. Centrad to this are multiple layers of basal lamina which separate cells. The lumen is barely distinguishable in the central region. Note the wrinkled, thickened basal lamina in the adjacent glomerulus. (Methenamine silver, × 300.)

tients without significant renal failure have the best prognosis, and if hypertension can be reduced satisfactorily, most of them are alive after 3 to 5 years. Previous research had also suggested that treatment of patients with renal failure (glomerular filtration rate less than 50 ml/min) led to further reduction of glomerular filtration rate as the arterial pressure was lowered, but the studies were carried out at a time when dialysis and transplantation therapy were not readily available. Recent observations indicate that patients who are aggressively treated despite this period of decreased function show a subsequent improvement in renal function. The blood pressure of patients with malignant hypertension and renal failure should be dealt with vigorously, and meticulous attention should also be given to the management of their renal status.

RENAL INFARCTION

Research is scant on the frequency of renal infarction, although the condition has been discussed in medical literature since Traube's description in 1856. Most studies have been autopsy reviews, which largely predate the antibiotic era, and consequently the majority of cases in the past were associated with bacterial endocarditis secondary to embolic occlusive disease of the renal artery or its branches. With current laboratory tests, however, based on awareness that the diag-

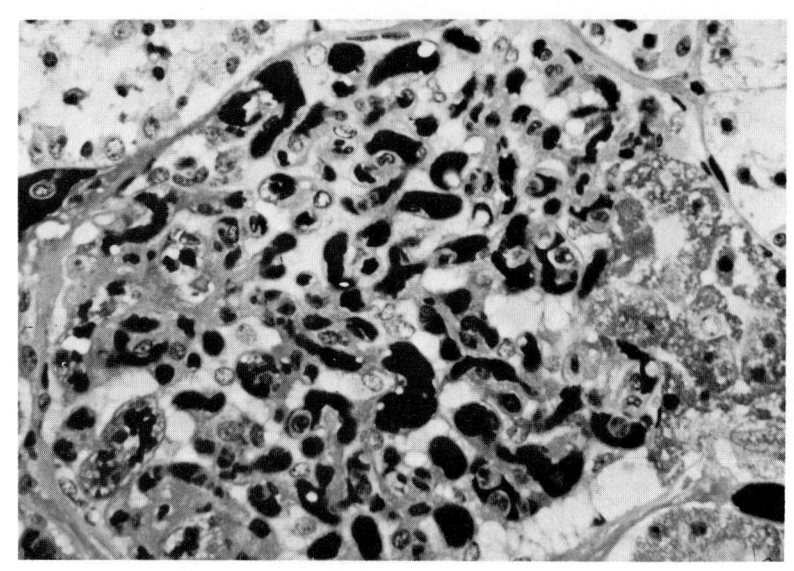

Figure 11-9 Biopsy of renal transplant with acute occlusion of the renal artery. The glomerular capillary loops are stuffed with red blood cells. The cellular architecture is obscured by karyorrhexis and karyolysis. At the right hand corner of the micrograph the cells of the proximal tubule are noted to be herniating into Bowman's space. (H&E, ×300.)

nosis is possible, early recognition is taking place with increasing frequency.

The causes of renal infarction may be divided broadly into those due to occlusion of the renal artery or its branches, and those due to renal vein thrombosis. Currently, occlusion of the renal artery is caused most frequently by embolism, arteriosclerotic narrowing, and trauma. In addition, a special form of arterial infarction (cortical necrosis) has bilateral involvement, presenting as acute renal failure. Renal infarction due to thrombosis of the renal veins is restricted largely to infants in whom severe extracellular depletion has occurred.

Clinical Data

Urinary or systemic findings are present in fewer than 50 per cent of patients with renal infarction. When the diagnosis is recognized, it is usually because pain, fever, proteinuria, and microscopic hematuria are evident. Typically, steady, aching abdominal pain develops, which may localize in the flank or become more generalized. Fever, nausea, and vomiting also may appear. The patient rarely notices a change in the urine, although some decrease in urine volume usually occurs. When the patient is examined, fever and tenderness of the region of the in-

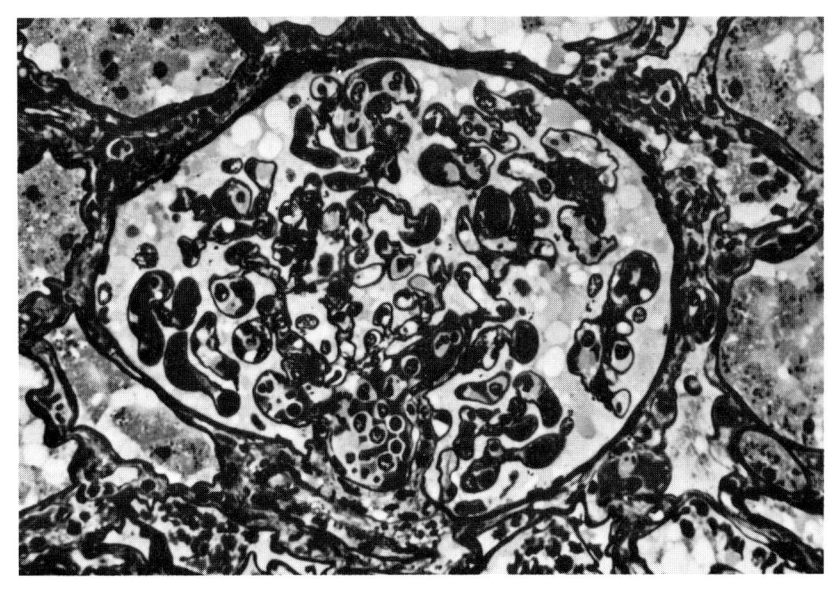

Figure 11-10 Silver stain of same specimen as in Figure 11-9. The basal lamina is intact in both the glomeruli and the adjacent tubules. (Methenamine silver, × 300.)

volved kidney may be found. When infarction is a result of arterial occlusion, the kidney is small and not palpable. With thrombosis of the renal veins, however, the kidney usually is tender and enlarged enough to be palpated readily.

In addition, there is usually a leukocytosis. The urinalysis typically shows proteinuria and microscopic hematuria; gross hematuria is rare. If the diagnosis is considered early, serum and urine levels of enzymes such as lactic dehydrogenase, alkaline phosphatase, and glutamic oxalacetic transaminase frequently are elevated. Hypertension also occurs frequently and begins a few days after the infarction. It may remain elevated for several weeks, but usually it subsides.

Histology

Renal infarction is characterized histologically by complete loss of cellular detail, extravasation of red blood cells into extracellular spaces, and relative preservation of the extracellular (basal lamina) components of the kidney (Figs. 11-9 and 11-10). When this process is focal or irregular, the margins are characterized by hyperemia, infiltration of the marginal zone by leukocytes, and proliferation of cells contained in the adjacent tubules and glomeruli, which still maintain their blood supply (Fig. 11-11).

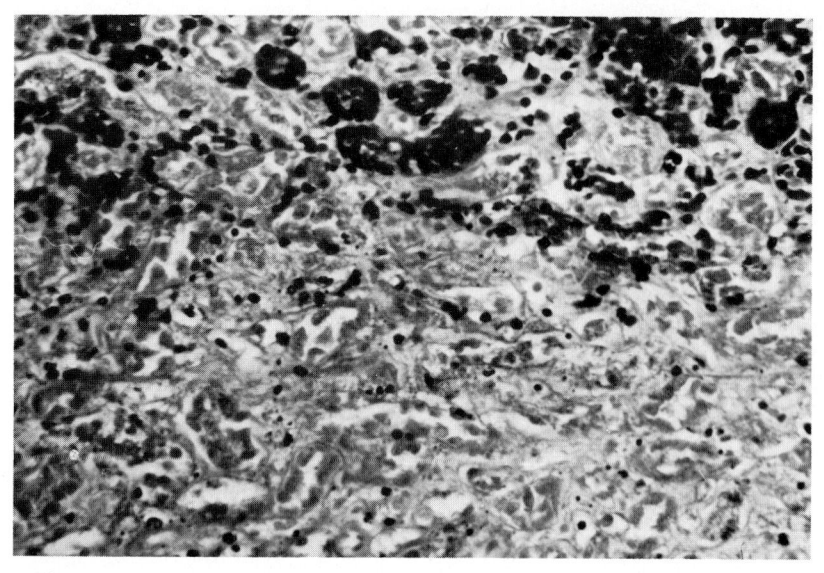

Figure 11-11 Interstitium of a biopsy specimen from a patient with renal vein thrombosis, demonstrating marked engorgement of interstitial capillaries and loss of cellular detail. (H&E, × 300.)

Clinical Course and Prognosis

When renal infarction is suspected, excretory urography should be performed. An absence or marked diminution in excretion of the contrast media or radionuclide on the involved side during the first two weeks is noted.

Areas of infarction large enough to produce sustained hypertension occasionally have been associated with normal or only minimally abnormal excretory urograms or scans. Impaired excretion also could be due to obstruction of the ureter, and if ureteral filling cannot be demonstrated, retrograde pyelograms are frequently the next diagnostic step. In infarction without other renal abnormalities, this procedure will reveal a normal-appearing, nondilated pelvis and collecting system. With renal thrombosis, however, there may be wide separation of the calyces due to interstitial edema, resembling polycystic kidneys.

The combination of history, signs and symptoms, virtual absence of excretory function on the involved side, and a normal collecting system strongly indicate renal infarction. If this diagnosis seems likely and an attempt to relieve the obstruction is to be considered, then arteriography should be performed promptly. In addition, the diagnosis of infarction due to arterial occlusion could be corroborated by radiologic evidence of diminution in renal size, which might be observable as early as 2 weeks after infarction. Calcium deposits also may be viewed radiographically within months following the event. Finally, the major indications for surgical removal of all or part of an infarcted kidney are the development of infection in the damaged tissue and the appearance of hypertension which cannot be controlled by drug therapy.

With increased awareness of renal infarction, however, and early diagnosis by arteriography, reports show successful surgical relief of obstruction, often followed by recovery of normal renal function. Subsequent tests and morphologic investigations indicate no detectable functional abnormality.

RENAL CORTICAL NECROSIS

Renal cortical necrosis fortunately is rare; it is characterized by necrosis of cortical tissue with sparing of the medulla. It usually is not difficult to distinguish this syndrome from infarction or other acute renal failure syndromes. Although the diagnosis may be suspected clinically at the outset, it can be confirmed only from the typical pathologic findings obtained by renal biopsy or postmortem examination. This disease has been recognized for almost a century, but its etiology and pathogenesis are still debated.

It is clear, however, that cortical necrosis results from ischemia and is associated with arteriolar thrombosis, although it is not evident why, under similar clinical circumstances, one patient develops curable acute renal failure with tubulo-interstitial changes, whereas another develops irreversible cortical necrosis. Renal cortical necrosis can occur at any age; approximately 10 per cent of the cases have occurred in infancy and childhood. After maturity, most of the patients are women, who develop the disease in association with pregnancy. Other predisposing causes include infection, circulatory insufficiency, intravascular coagulation, or nephrotoxins.

Clinical Data

Renal cortical necrosis presents as anuric acute renal failure. The onset of anuria usually is associated with an event of circulatory insufficiency. Most cases occur during pregnancy, related to some complication, such as toxemia, premature separation of the placenta, septic abortion, or postpartum hemorrhage. Except in those cases associated with infection, the patient usually is afebrile, feels well, and is mentally alert. Abnormal physical findings are minimal.

The urine volume is low, however, and may be absent in the first few days. In some cases the urine flow has risen to 300 to 500 ml daily after the fourth or fifth day, but it is rarely greater than this. Urinalysis results, when available, show marked proteinuria and either gross or

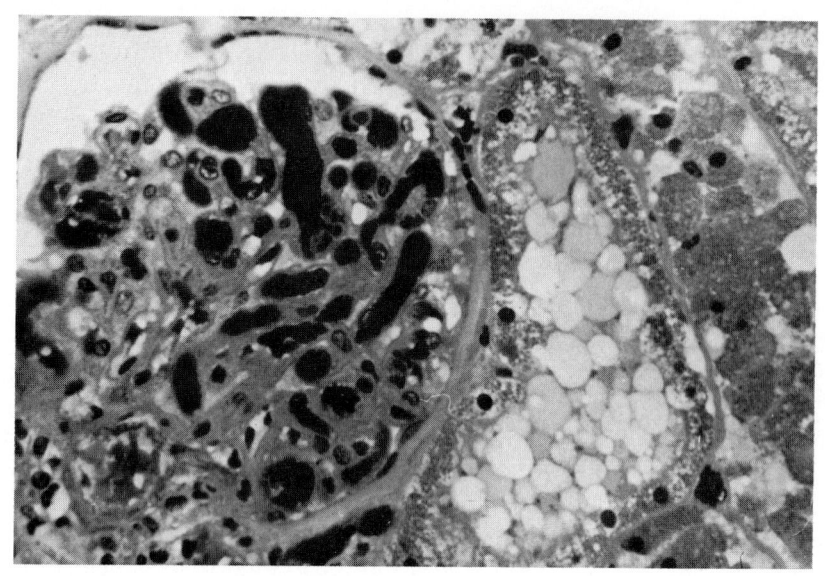

Figure 11-12 Biopsy specimen from a patient with acute renal failure and no perfusion of the cortex found by renal arteriography. The glomerular capillary loops are filled with red blood cells and protein. Note that the efferent arteriole also is packed with similar material. (H&E, × 300.)

microscopic hematuria; leukocytes are present in variable numbers, but casts of any type are infrequent.

Serial radiograms initially show enlarged kidneys, as in any form of acute renal failure. The renal size then diminishes and may be reduced to about half the normal size in 6 to 8 weeks. At this state, calcification (often linear) appears, especially marked at the corticomedullary junction.

Histology

The anatomic features include necrosis of cells and thrombosis of the vascular structures (Figs. 11-12 and 11-13). The process may not involve all of the cortex, and consequently there may be areas of surviving parenchyma, usually in a subcapsular position. In most cases the intact parenchyma is insufficient to maintain adequate renal function.

Clinical Course and Prognosis

Because of the severity of the injury in cortical necrosis, reversal of the renal failure rarely occurs. In general, patients with histologic con-

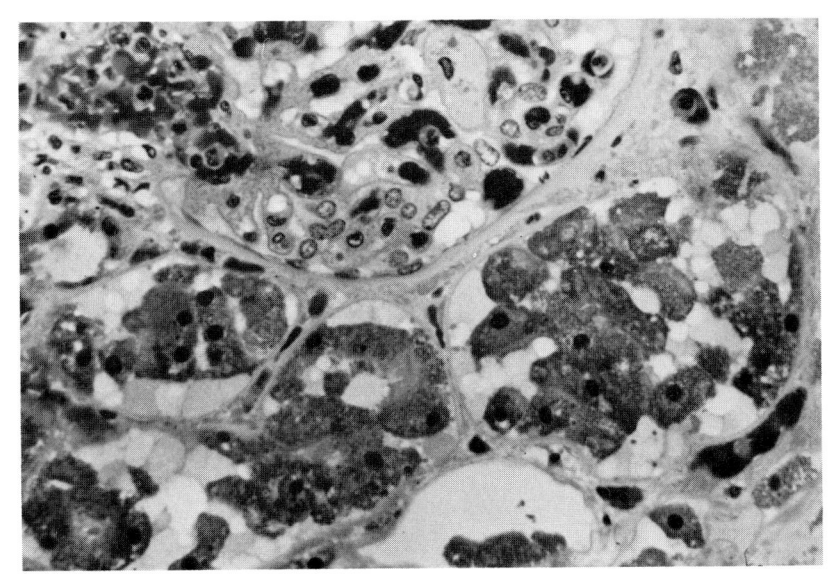

Figure 11-13 A different area from the same specimen as in Figure 11-12. Here the tubular epithelial cells can be seen to detach from the tubular basal lamina. The efferent arterial of the adjacent glomerulus is filled with red blood cells, inflammatory cells, and protein. Here again the glomerular capillaries are filled with red blood cells. (H&E, × 300.)

firmation of cortical necrosis require definitive long-term treatment of uremia by dialysis or transplantation.

RENAL VEIN THROMBOSIS

In 1840, Rayer was the first to describe renal vein thrombosis. This condition is rare, difficult to diagnose, and usually considered seriously only when the nephrotic syndrome is present. Thrombosis of the renal veins also may be secondary to disease of the renal parenchyma. Amyloidosis is the most frequent primary diagnosis, but it also has been associated with membranous glomerulonephritis and diabetic glomerulosclerosis. In addition, thrombosis has been associated with perirenal disease, trauma to the renal veins, hypernephroma and thrombophlebitis of the lower extremities and inferior vena cava. In infants, it commonly develops as a consequence of severe extracellular volume depletion following gastroenteritis.

Clinical Data

Clinically, renal vein thrombosis presents two different pictures. In children, it is associated with loin pain, fever, hematuria, edema, leukocytosis, and renal failure. In adults, it is more insidious, presenting with the onset of proteinuria, or an increase in preexisting proteinuria, and deterioration to renal function.

Consequently, the diagnosis of renal vein thrombosis is difficult and often missed. Radiographic examination may show an enlarged, nonfunctioning kidney. The definitive procedure, phlebography, will reveal thrombosis manifested by filling defects in the major renal veins or filling of collateral veins. Varicosities of renal veins may be associated with hematuria, and sometimes are evident through urography, displaying irregularly shaped filling defects in the kidney pelvis.

Histology

GLOMERULI. The changes present in renal vein thrombosis depend on the rapidity of the occlusion. If acute and complete, renal infarction may ensue. The process is commonly one of more gradual onset. In this case, the changes cover the spectrum of renal morphology from minimal lesions to sclerosing lesions, which may be indistinguishable from the typical membranous lesion (see page 000). There is little concrete evidence to support the concept that renal vein thrombosis leads to the development of the membranous lesion.

TUBULES AND INTERSTITIUM. No characteristic changes in the tubules and interstitium are present, although one should be suspicious of this lesion in patients with glomerular injury and interstitial infiltrate with patchy edema.

VESSELS. No lesions occur in the vessels.

Clinical Course and Prognosis

The current therapeutic approach to renal vein thrombosis is unsatisfactory. Surgical methods usually are not successful because the thrombosis is often bilateral, and it is rarely limited to the trunk of the vein, usually extending for a variable distance into the smaller tributaries and even into the renal parenchyma. Furthermore, nephrectomy is frequently required because of uncontrolled bleeding or transection of collateral veins as one nears the kidney.

Moreover, improvement following medical therapy is often limited; heparin and oral anticoagulation treatment have been used and apparently are of benefit, but spontaneous recovery has also been recorded. Recently, thrombolytic therapy with streptokinase or urokinase has been tried and may be beneficial.

ATHEROMATOUS EMBOLIZATION

Atheroemboli to the kidney can produce a clinical syndrome involving either rapid deterioration of renal function or a more slowly progressive renal failure, depending on the amount of atheromatous material obstructing the renal arteries. It may occur spontaneously in patients with advanced arteriosclerosis, subsequent to vascular surgery or following arteriography.

Clinical Data

Atheromatous embolization to the kidneys occurs most commonly in elderly patients and increases in incidence with age. It should be suspected in patients with renal failure of unknown etiology over the age of 60 years, especially if they have signs of advanced arteriosclerosis. Suspicion should be heightened if the renal insufficiency follows aortography or major vascular surgery. A history of hypertension is common in patients with spontaneous embolization.

Signs of peripheral embolization are helpful but are not often present. When embolization is widespread, however, this syndrome has been confused with polyarteritis because of the multiplicity of organ involvement. Embolization to the retina can cause sudden blindness, and the bright yellow crystalline plaques can be seen lodged at bifurcations of arterioles on funduscopic examination.

There are no distinctive laboratory or urinary sediment abnormalities in this syndrome. The diagnosis can only be confirmed by careful examination of a renal biopsy specimen.

Histology

Atheromatous embolization to the kidneys causes an irregular injury to the kidney from occlusion of small blood vessels with atheromatous material.

There are no distinctive abnormalities of the glomeruli except in the rare case in which the atheromatous material can be seen lodged in the afferent arterioles. Those glomeruli in the involved segment of the kidney show various degrees of ischemia, as discussed earlier in this chapter.

Tubular injury varies from mild ischemia to focal areas of necrosis, depending on the degree of vascular occlusion. Specific changes are limited to the blood vessels. If the biopsy is obtained early in the course, needle-shaped inclusions representing cholesterol crystals together with amorphous eosinophilic material can be seen occluding

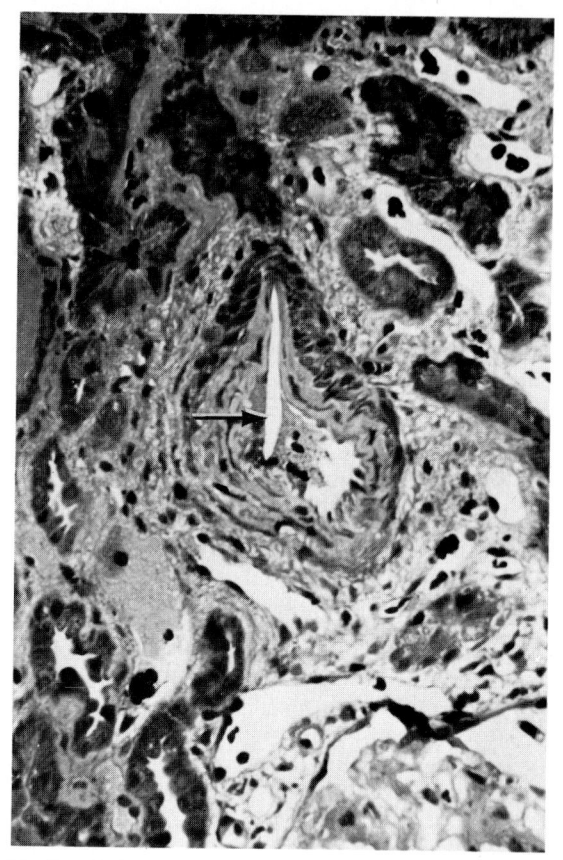

Figure 11–14 Renal biopsy from a 72-year-old male with severe arteriosclerosis who had the spontaneous onset of renal failure. Note the cholesterol crystal and amorphous material partially occluding the lumen of the vessel (arrow). (H&E, × 300.)

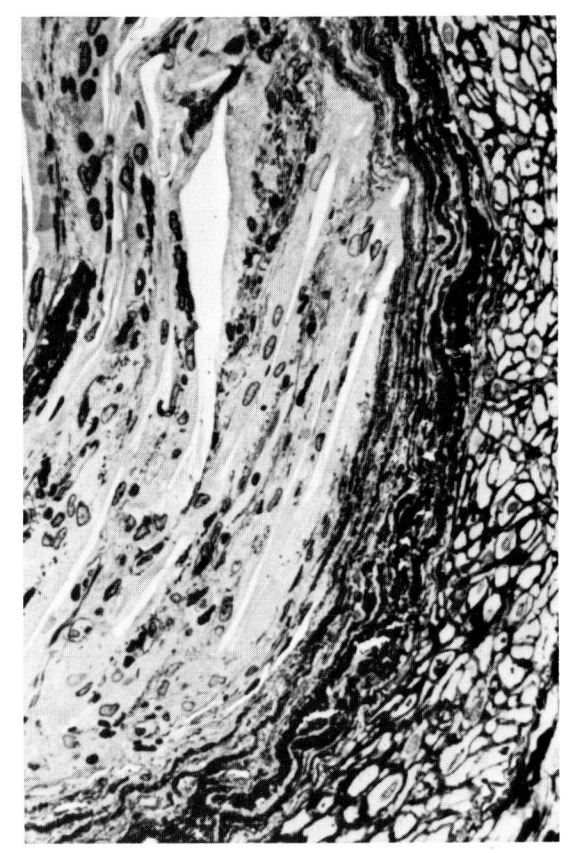

Figure 11–15 Same patient as in Figure 11–14. Larger vessel with multiple crystals surrounded by cells and amorphous material. Also present are multinucleated giant cells. (Methenamine silver, × 300.)

the arteriole (Fig. 11–14). Later changes consist of concentric sclerosis around the emboli and the formation of multinucleated giant cells surrounding the crystals (Fig. 11–15).

Clinical Course and Prognosis

Massive atheromatous embolization to the kidney produces rapid deterioration of renal function, which for the most part is irreversible. Although rarely it occurs spontaneously, this syndrome is most commonly seen following aortic surgery or aortography.

Spontaneous embolization has a more insidious onset, and the patients are often azotemic when they first come to the physician's attention. Progressive renal failure, usually occurring in a matter of weeks, is common.

References

1. Abeshouse, B. S.: Thrombosis and thrombophlebitis of the renal veins. Urol. Cutan. Rev. *49*:661, 1945.
2. Bechgaard, O.: The natural history of benign hypertension. *In* Bock, K. D., and Cottier, P. T. (eds.), *Essential Hypertension: An International Symposium.* Berlin, Springer-Verlag, 1960.
3. Duggan, M. O.: Acute renal infarction. J. Urol. *90*:669, 1963.
4. Gwyn, W. B.: Biopsies and the completion of certain surgical procedures. Can. Med. Assoc. J. *13*:1217, 1923.
5. Hamburger, J., Richet, G., Crosnier, J., Funck-Bretano, J. L., Antoine, B., Ducrot, H., Mery, J. P., and Montera, H.: Nephrology (translated by Anthony Walsh). Philadelphia, W. B. Saunders Co., 1968.
6. Heptinstall, R. H.: Malignant hypertension: A study of 51 cases. J. Path. Bact. *65*:423, 1953.
7. Hoxie, H. J., and Coggin, C. B.: Renal infarction: Statistical study of two hundred and five cases and detailed reports of an unusual case. Arch. Intern. Med. *65*:587, 1940.
8. Kassirer, J. P.: Atheroembolic renal disease. New Eng. J. Med. *280*:812, 1969.
9. Keith, N. M., Wagener, H. P., and Barker, N. W.: Some different types of essential hypertension: Their course and prognosis. Amer. J. Med. Sci. *197*:332, 1939.
10. Kincaid-Smith, P., McMichael, J., and Murphy, E. A.: The clinical course and pathology of hypertension with papilledema (malignant hypertension). Quart. J. Med. *27*:117, 1958.
11. Llach, F., Arieff, A. I., and Massry, S. G.: Renal vein thrombosis and nephrotic syndrome. Ann. Intern. Med. *83*:8, 1975.
12. Loomis, L., Ocker, J. M., Jr., and Hodges, C. B.: Dynamic treatment of renal artery embolism: A case report and review of the literature. J. Urol. *96*:131, 1966.
13. Rayer, P. F. O.: Traie des maladies des reins et des alterations de la secretion urinaire. Vol. 2. Paris, J.-B. Balliére, 1840.
14. Riff, D. P., Wilson, D. M., Dunea, G., Schwartz, F. D., and Kark, R. M.: Renocortical necrosis. Partial recovery after 49 days of oliguria. Arch. Intern. Med. *119*:518, 1967.
15. Schottstaedt, M. P., and Sokolow, M.: The natural history and course of hypertension with papilledema (malignant hypertension). Amer. Heart J. *45*:331, 1953.
16. Sheehan, H. L., and Moore, H. C.: Renal Cortical Necrosis and the Kidney of Concealed Accidental Hemorrhage. Springfield, Ill., Charles C Thomas, 1953.
17. Traube, L.: Uber ben Zusammenhang von Herz—und Nieren—Krankheiten. Berlin, Verlag von August Hisschwald, 1856.
18. Wells, J. D., Margolin, E. G., and Gall, E. A.: Renal cortical necrosis. Clinical and pathologic features in 21 cases. Amer. J. Med. *29*:257, 1960.
19. Whelan, J. G., Jr., Ling, J. T., and Davis, L. A.: Antemortem roentgen manifestations of bilateral renal cortical necrosis. Radiology *89*:682, 1967.
20. Woods, J. W., and Blythe, W. B.: Management of malignant hypertension complicated by renal insufficiency. New Eng. J. Med. *277*:57, 1967.

Section III

SLOWLY PROGRESSIVE RENAL DISEASES

Chapter Twelve

Slowly Progressive Glomerular Disease

Introduction

Slowly progressing glomerular disease presents a clinical enigma. Among patients with chronic uremia this is the most common syndrome, yet its true incidence in the general population is unknown. Because of the disease's slowly progressive nature, a patient may be asymptomatic for years, the disease becoming evident only when the renal injury is advanced. Consequently, the majority of patients in this group escape the attention of physicians unless routine screening urinalyses are performed.

This condition raises a number of questions: What is the etiology of persistent progressive glomerulonephritis? Could this syndrome represent the end stage of a progressive form of an acute glomerular disease such as poststreptococcal glomerulonephritis? The answers to these questions are complex, but it is uncommon to obtain a history of previous acute glomerular disease in such patients, and serologic studies implicating prior streptococcal infections are unconvincing. However, Baldwin et al. (1974) reported an increased incidence of proteinuria and hypertension following poststreptococcal glomerulonephritis, and some patients had progressive renal failure. Does this syndrome also have an immune, infectious, or metabolic etiology? Although immunoglobulins and complement can be histologically demonstrated in the glomeruli of some patients, they provide only indirect evidence of immune etiology, and immunity to renal antigens measured in some patients with this syndrome may be the consequence rather than the cause of injury. Searches for an infectious or metabolic etiology have been fruitless.

Intrarenal coagulation has been implicated in the pathogenesis of many renal syndromes, including this one. Evidence to support this assumption is based on the findings of coagulation by-products in the urine, in the blood, and occasionally in the renal parenchyma. As with the presence of immunoglobulins, however, it is difficult to determine whether their localization is the cause of or secondary to the injury. For example, in research recently completed at this institution, the hemostatic system could be implicated in some patients whose primary histologic lesion was progressive sclerosis. These studies suggest a role for the hemostatic system in the pathogenesis of glomerulonephritis. Finally, because slowly progressive glomerular disease represents a conglomeration of chronic diseases of diverse etiologies which share the eventual common pathway of slowly progressing sclerosis, this category should shrink and ultimately disappear as our understanding of renal disease increases.

Benign recurrent hematuria (page 157) and hereditary nephritis (page 160) also will be discussed in this chapter in order to contrast these diseases with slowly progressive glomerular disease syndromes, since both may present similar clinical findings. Membranous, focal sclerosing, and membranoproliferative glomerulonephritides are slowly progressive glomerular diseases commonly associated with nephrotic syndrome and will be discussed in Chapter 16.

Clinical Data

The insidious nature of slowly progressive glomerular disease makes it difficult to date the onset of the illness accurately. Hematuria is rarely obvious to the patient. Occasionally the illness is evidenced by recurrent episodes of gross hematuria and proteinuria, which may represent either flare-ups of a slowly progressive illness or separate, unrelated episodes of acute glomerulonephritis. The patient often is unaware of the illness until objective signs are noted on routine medical examinations or symptoms of severe renal failure or hypertension lead to medical evaluation.

During the early phase of slowly progressive glomerular diseases, laboratory findings are limited to signs of a persistent but mild inflammatory process. Hematuria and proteinura, which are the most common findings, may, for instance, be very inconspicuous, so that they are apparent only by careful examination of the urine. The presence of cellular and protein casts depends on the stage and extent of the injury. Waxy and broad casts appear only when there is significant interstitial scarring, tubular atrophy, and tubular dilatation late in the disease.

Histology

GENERAL. In this group of diseases the spectrum of changes is enormous, varying from a barely detectable lesion to a completely sclerotic kidney. Furthermore, progression of the lesion varies, depending on the presence and type of associated cellular proliferation and/or deposits. It is, therefore, essential that the changes be interpreted and quantitated carefully and reported accurately.

LIGHT MICROSCOPY. A characteristic of this group of diseases is an increase in the amount of extracellular material, often in the mesangial matrix, with or without significant hypercellularity. The early changes, then, may be very difficult to detect (Figs. 12–1 and 12–2). Silver methenamine stains of more advanced lesions (see Fig. 12–5) and electron microscopy reveal that the increase frequently is a result of collapsed capillary loops, in addition to a well-defined expansion of mesangial extracellular material (Fig. 12–3). Organized synechiae in a significant number of glomeruli often are present as well, possibly involving up to half of the glomerular architecture (Fig. 12–6). Synechiae characteristically are associated with duplication of Bowman's basal lamina and a direct continuity between this basal lamina and that of the glomerulus (Figs. 12–7 and 12–8).

The sclerosing process is characterized by a slow decrease in cellularity and increase in the amount of extracellular material, which expands to efface capillaries, and enlarging synechiae, both of which lead to obliteration of Bowman's space (Figs. 12–9 and 12–10). The end result is an enlarged but completely sclerotic glomerulus (Fig. 12–11). The changes are reasonably uniform among glomeruli. As a result, the glomeruli all tend to reach the stage of complete sclerosis within a relatively short period of time, giving the false impression that the glomerular disease is "rapidly progressive," when, in fact, it is the end stage of a prolonged process.

In contrast to these findings, patients who have a rapidly advancing glomerular disease may have few recognizable glomeruli when the process has reached the point at which the kidney is small and shrunken. Similarly, patients who have a primary vascular or tubulointerstitial disease with secondary glomerular ischemia will at the end stages have many small obsolescent glomeruli.

Depending on the stage of the disease, the interstitium is variably affected, often appearing to be involved early and extensively by interstitial infiltration of chronic inflammatory cells and fibrosis (Fig. 12–12). There does not seem to be a predilection for a specific area of the cortex, although thickening of Bowman's capsule and fibrosis in the immediately adjacent area are the earliest changes recognizable. Tubular atrophy occurs in areas of interstitial fibrosis and infiltration. The vascular lesion is nonspecific and resembles that seen in slowly progressive vascular disease, possibly as a result of hypertension (Fig. 12–13).

Text continued on page 156

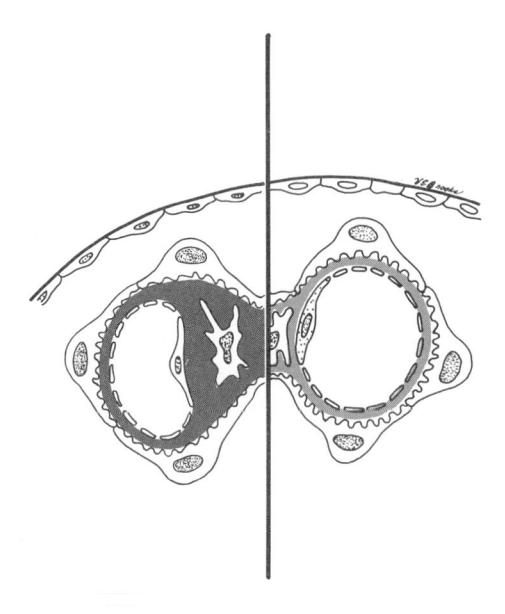

Figure 12–1 Diagram of a glomerulus, showing an increase in mesangial matrix.

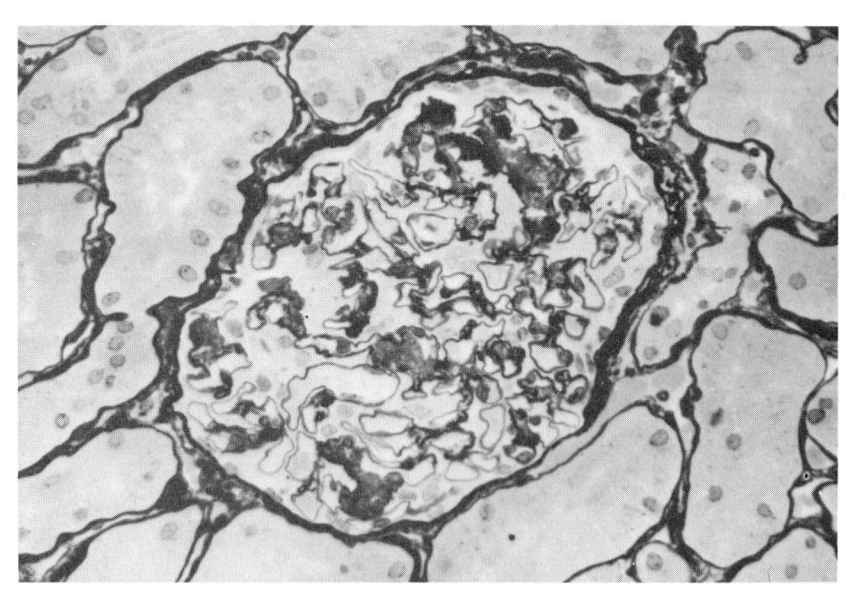

Figure 12–2 Renal biopsy from a 65 year old man with proteinuria and hyperlipidemia. All glomeruli are affected in a similar manner. The mesangial regions are expanded by silver-positive material, but there is no increase in the number of cells. Although the peripheral glomerular basal lamina is normal, Bowman's membrane is thickened. (Silver methenamine, ×300.)

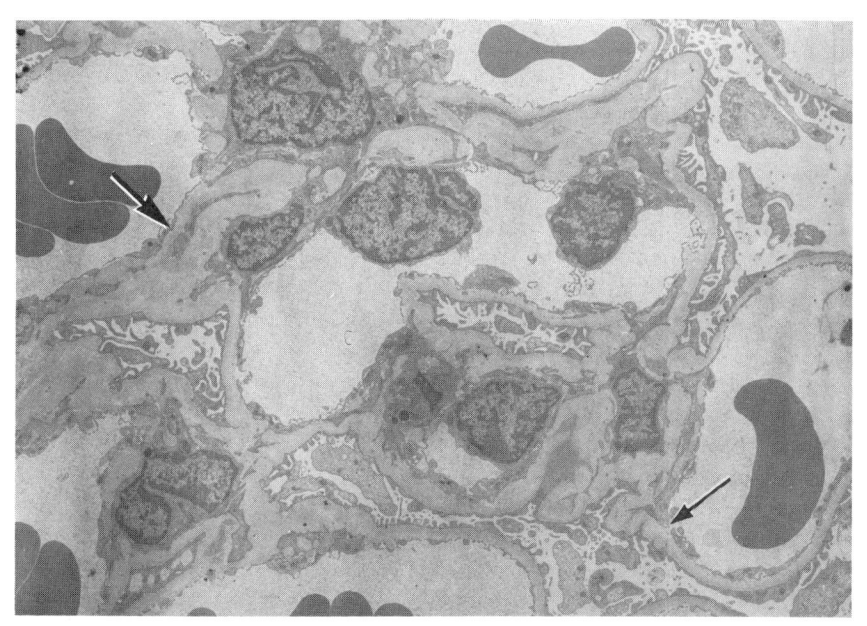

Figure 12-3 Electron micrograph from the same patient as in Figure 12-2. The epithelial cell foot processes are generally intact, although small areas of effacement can be seen. The peripheral basal lamina is unremarkable except near the mesangial regions, where it is wrinkled (light arrow). The endothelial and mesangial cells are unremarkable. The major change is in the mesangial regions, where there is a diffuse, although modest, increase in the amount of extracellular material (heavy arrow) (×2200.)

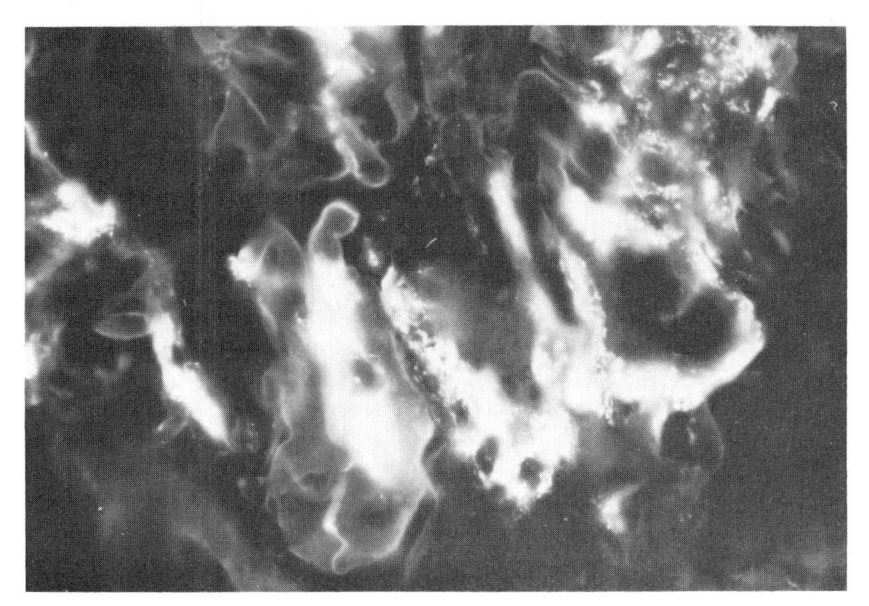

Figure 12-4 Fluorescent micrograph using a fluoresceinated anti-IgG. There is prominent staining in the mesangial region in a granular pattern. The peripheral basal lamina shows irregular and very much lighter staining. The latter is a nonspecific finding in patients who have slowly progressive glomerular disease. (×1200.)

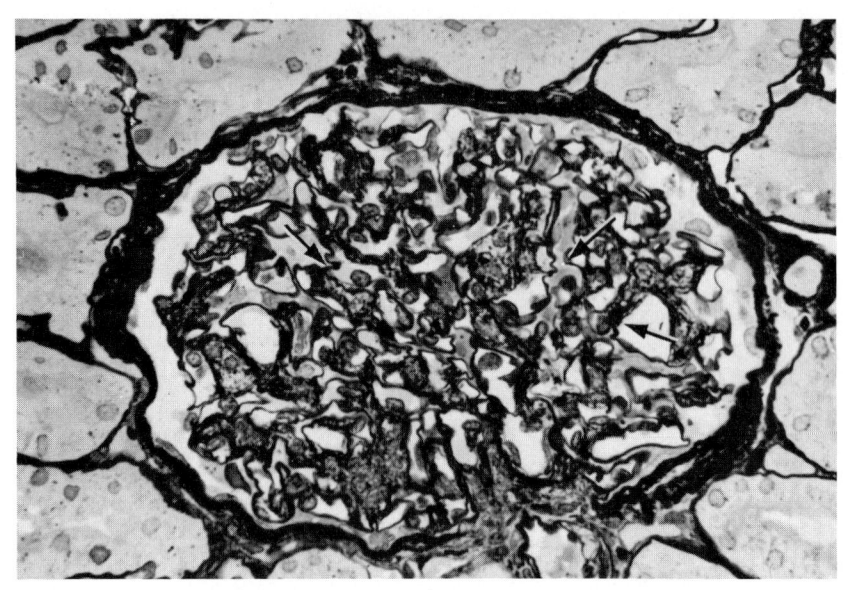

Figure 12-5 This biopsy specimen from a 31 year old man demonstrates somewhat more diffuse sclerosis in the mesangial regions and more prominent wrinkling of the basal lamina near the mesangial regions (arrows). (Silver methenamine, ×300.)

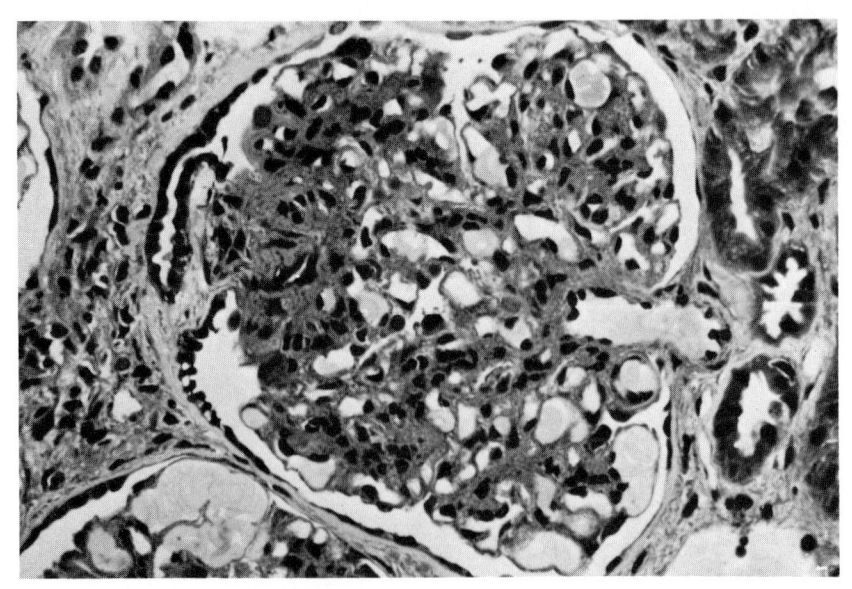

Figure 12-6 Six weeks prior to biopsy this 15 year old male had a grossly red urine of acute onset. His creatinine clearance was normal and 24 hour protein excretion was 0.33 g. Two of 54 glomeruli were obsolescent; the rest showed diffused intraglomerular cell proliferation and mesangial cell sclerosis. Synechiae similar to those seen here were present in 18 of 54 glomeruli. Note that there is a connection between the extracellular material of Bowman's capsule and the glomerulus. (H&E, ×300.)

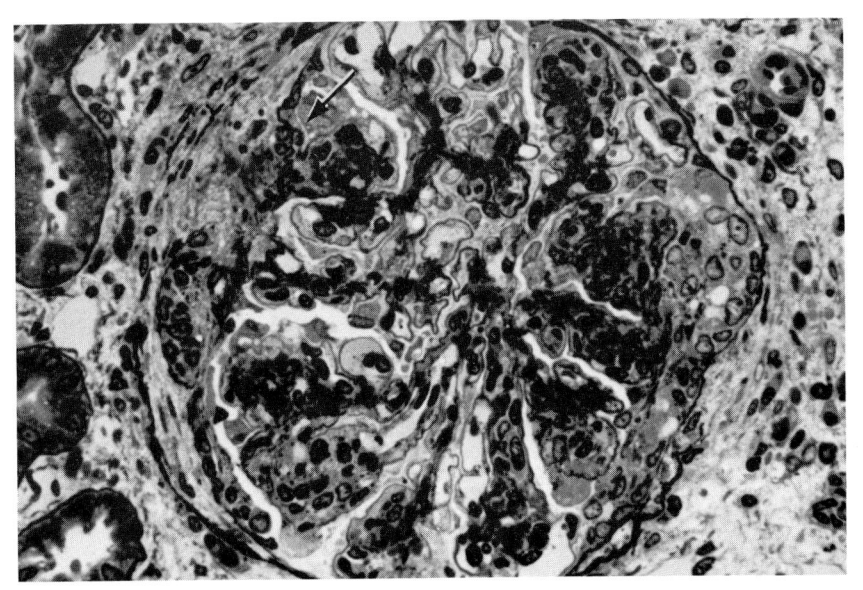

Figure 12-7 In this biopsy specimen from a 26 year old woman, the normal thin line representing Bowman's basal lamina is seen to be frayed and split in the area of the synechia (arrow). (Silver methenamine, ×300.)

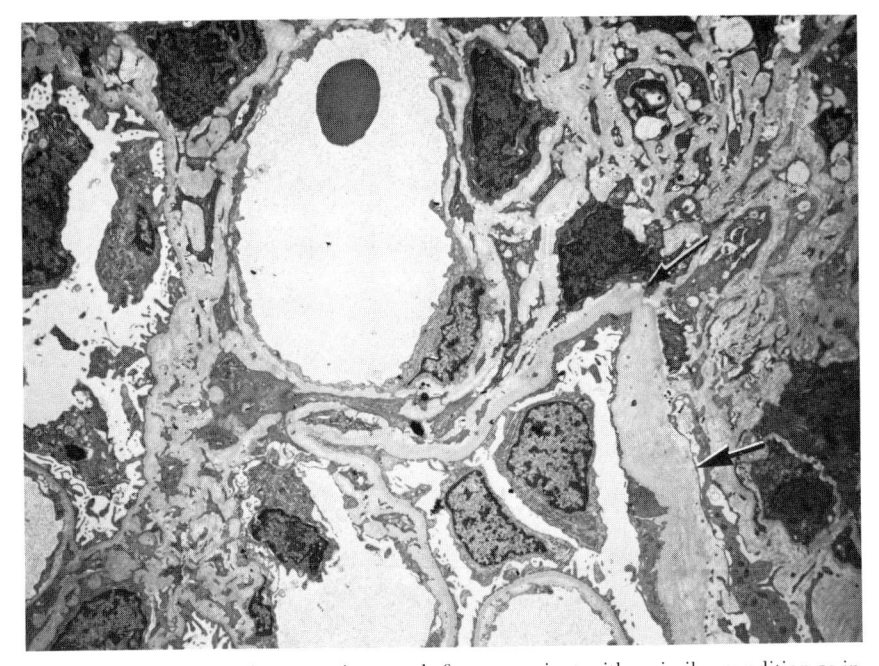

Figure 12-8 An electron micrograph from a patient with a similar condition as in Figures 12-6 and 12-7. Bowman's capsule is directly continuous with that of the peripheral basal lamina (light arrow). Note that Bowman's membrane is thickened and duplicated in this region, and that there is an increase in the amount of extracellular material (heavy arrow) (×2200.)

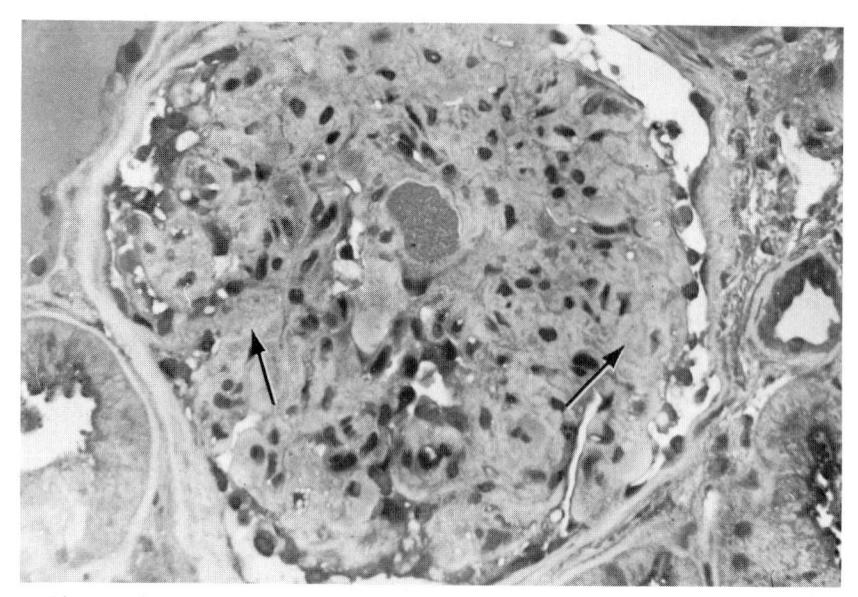

Figure 12-9 This 44 year old woman has had known proteinuria for 26 years. Renal function has recently deteriorated. The capillary spaces are nearly obliterated by a marked increase in the amount of poorly staining extracellular material (arrows). Note that the number of cells is not increased, and that the glomerulus maintains nearly normal size. (H&E, × 300.)

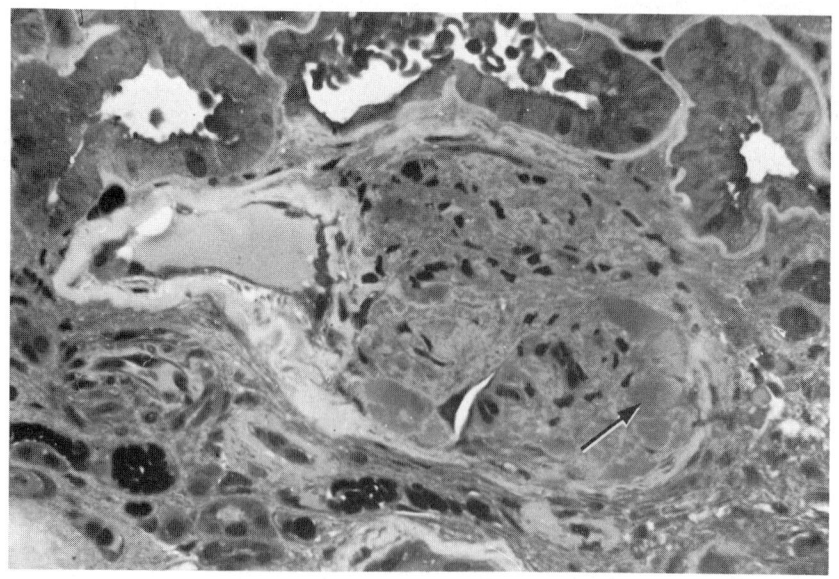

Figure 12-10 A glomerulus from the same patient as in Figure 12-9. Seven of 10 glomeruli had this appearance. The glomerular architecture is almost totally replaced by pale-staining extracellular material in which are embedded a small number of cells. There are several "lakes" of serum protein, presumably occupying spaces which previously were vascular channels (arrows). (H&E, × 300.)

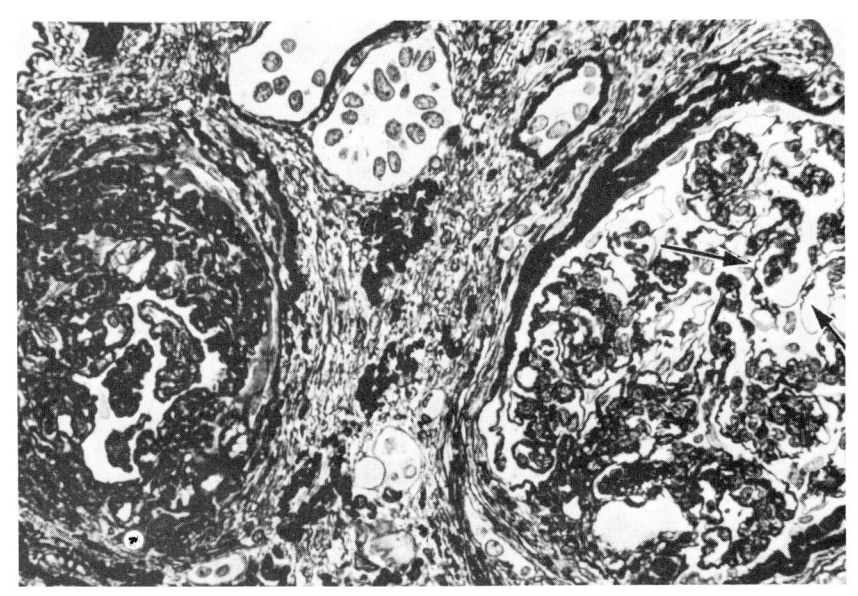

Figure 12-11 Silver-stained preparation of glomeruli from the same patient. In addition to the mesangial sclerosis, there also is wrinkling of the peripheral basal lamina near the mesangial regions (arrows). The glomerulus on the left is obsolescent. Note, however, that it maintains a nearly normal size, which is characteristic of patients who have a slowly progressing sclerosing process in their glomeruli. (Silver methenamine, × 300.)

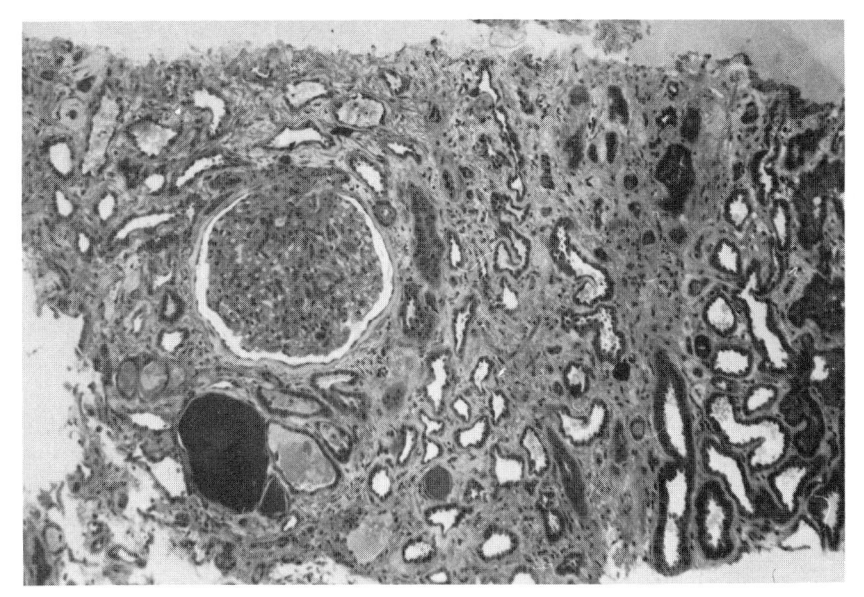

Figure 12-12 Specimen from a 28 year old man who had an episode of acute nephritis at 2 years of age, which was complicated by the nephrotic syndrome. Sixteen years later he was again noted to have proteinuria with normal renal function. At present he has hypertension, serum creatinine clearance is 2.3 mg per 100 ml, 24 hour protein excretion is 12 g. As noted previously, the glomerular size remains normal or large, even though the surrounding tubules and interstitium are atrophied and fibrotic. Scattered throughout the interstitium are large numbers of lymphocytes and plasma cells. Casts are noted in the dilated tubules. (H&E, × 75.)

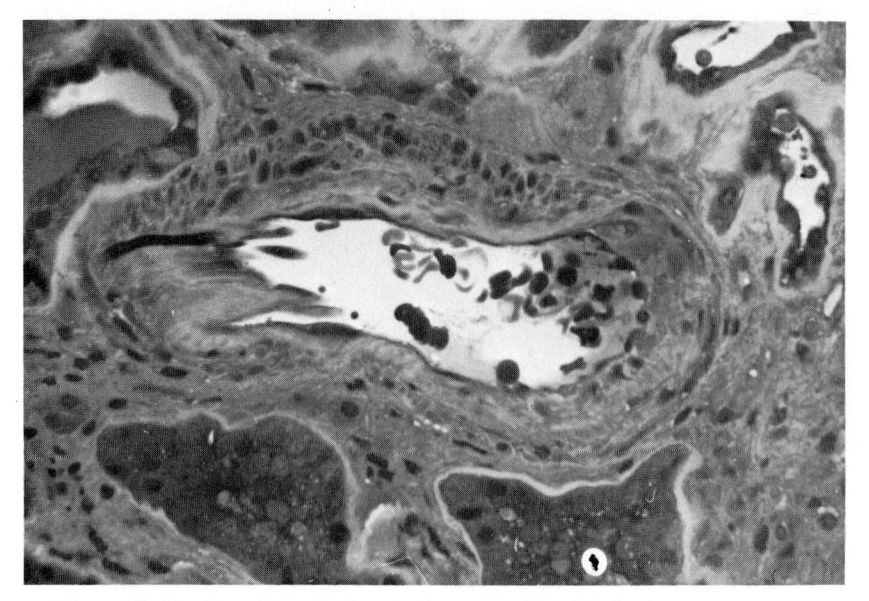

Figure 12–13 A medium-sized artery from a patient with slowly progressive glomerular disease (same patient as in Figures 12–9 through 12–11). There is an increased amount of extracellular material between individual cells of the media as well as below the internal lamina. (H&E, × 300.)

ELECTRON MICROSCOPY. As previously noted, the increase in extracellular material involves the glomerular basal lamina and mesangial regions. Early in the disease process the increase may be quite subtle and electron microscopy is very helpful. Deposits of protein and hyalin frequently are present in the areas of expanded extracellular material.

FLUORESCENCE MICROSCOPY. Deposits of immunoglobulins are inconsistent in glomeruli and may be absent (Fig. 12–4). It may be possible to identify certain specific forms, such as the membranous or membranoproliferative type (see Chapter 16).

In summary, the histologic lesions evidenced by light and electron microscopy that suggest the presence of irreversible and progressive renal disease are those of fairly severe and diffuse glomerular sclerosis, synechiae in a large number of glomeruli, substantial interstitial disease, and an accumulation of extracellular material over a defined period of time.

Clinical Course and Prognosis

Discussion of the clinical course and prognosis of this group of diseases is made difficult by the marked variability from patient to patient. Some may show an apparent rapid course leading to renal failure, whereas the majority have slow progression of the disease over

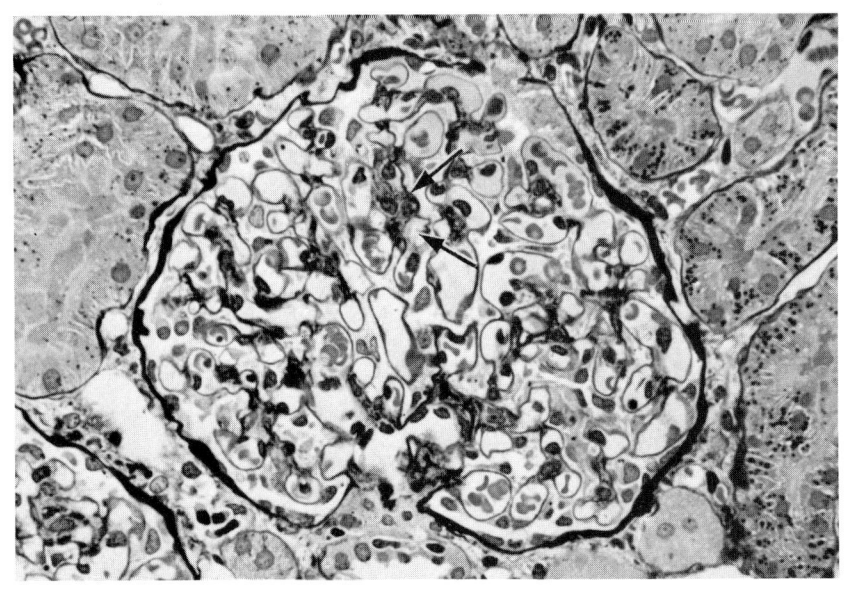

Figure 12-14 Renal biopsy from a 15 year old male with normal renal function and no proteinuria, but an 8 month history of episodic hematuria. Of 18 glomeruli, six were noted to have a modest increase in the number of mesangial cells in localized areas (arrows). (Silver methenamine, × 300.)

many years. The degree of activity on renal biopsy is helpful in predicting the rate of progression, but it is only a rough estimate. The best means of determining progression is by observing the patient carefully at different points of time with renal function studies, careful urinalysis, and, if doubt remains about the underlying lesion's activity, a repeat renal biopsy. With these parameters, the clinical course can be estimated with reasonable reliability.

Although many forms of therapy have been attempted in this syndrome, none has conclusively been proved effective in preventing progression. The nature of the disease process makes controlled, thorough investigation extremely difficult for treatment protocols, since observation must be continued over a period of years. Furthermore, no study fulfilling these requirements has substantiated a beneficial effect from any form of therapy other than blood pressure control.

BENIGN RECURRENT HEMATURIA (IgA DISEASE)

Clinical Data

Benign recurrent hematuria is characterized by recurrent episodes of macroscopic hematuria in both children and young adults, without evidence of significant renal disease. The syndrome is described most often as occurring one to two days after an episode of a viral syndrome. Boys are affected twice as frequently as girls, and there is no evidence of a systemic disease. Proteinuria is present in approximately half the patients. A urine sediment examination confirms the presence of hematuria, although red cell casts are noted relatively infrequently. As previously noted, 24 hour urine protein excretion usually is less than 1 g, and most often less than 100 mg. Glomerular filtration rate and serum creatinine and serum complement levels are normal, and hypertension is not evident in this syndrome.

Most researchers agree that the clinical course is benign. Bodian and colleagues (1965) first noted immunoglobulins deposited in the mesangial regions. Berger (1969) then fully developed this as a separate clinical entity when he described the presence of diffusely distributed mesangial deposits containing IgA, IgG, and C3 fraction of complement in patients with recurrent episodes of hematuria without progression to renal failure.

Histology

LIGHT MICROSCOPY. The morphologic features may range from normal to a mild generalized proliferative glomerulonephritis. The majority, however, show proliferation involving localized areas within glomeruli, frequently in the mesangial regions (Fig. 12–14). The proliferation may vary within each glomerulus and among glomeruli, the majority being uninvolved. The presence of glomerular sclerosis and synechiae differs somewhat among series, but generally this is not a prominent characteristic.

ELECTRON MICROSCOPY. The peripheral capillary loops, including the cells and extracellular material, are usually normal. The major findings are limited to the mesangial regions, where a focal increase in mesangial matrix and mesangial cells is found, as well as areas of electron-dense "deposits" within the increased mesangial matrix (Fig. 12–15). Similar deposits also have been reported in Bowman's capsule.

IMMUNOFLUORESCENCE MICROSCOPY. With immunofluorescence microscopy, in contrast to the irregular, local, and focal distribution of cellularity previously noted, there is a diffuse mesangial deposition and localization of IgA, IgG, and occasionally C3 component of complement; the amounts of IgA noted are in excess of IgG (Fig. 12–16). There is only occasional peripheral basal lamina localization of immunoglobulins. In one study, properdin also was noted in a distribution similar to that of C3.

Clinical Course and Prognosis

The course of the disease appears to be remarkably slow in most reported series. Berger's initial report (1969) stated that renal function

SLOWLY PROGRESSIVE GLOMERULAR DISEASE 159

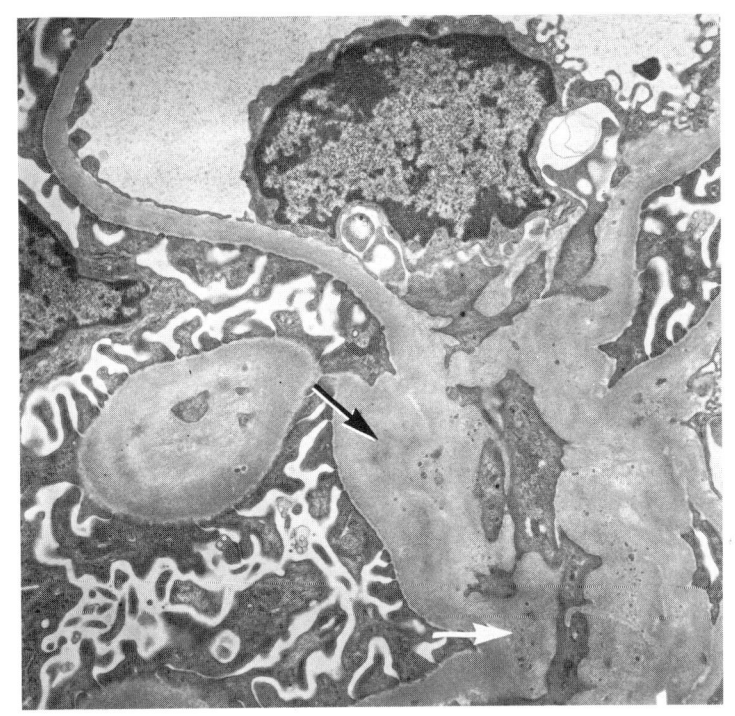

Figure 12-15 Electron micrograph from the same patient as in Figure 12-14. In a few of the mesangial regions there is an increase in the amount of extracellular material and cell debris (light arrow). There also is a small amount of more darkly staining material presumed to be deposits (dark arrow). ($\times 2200$.)

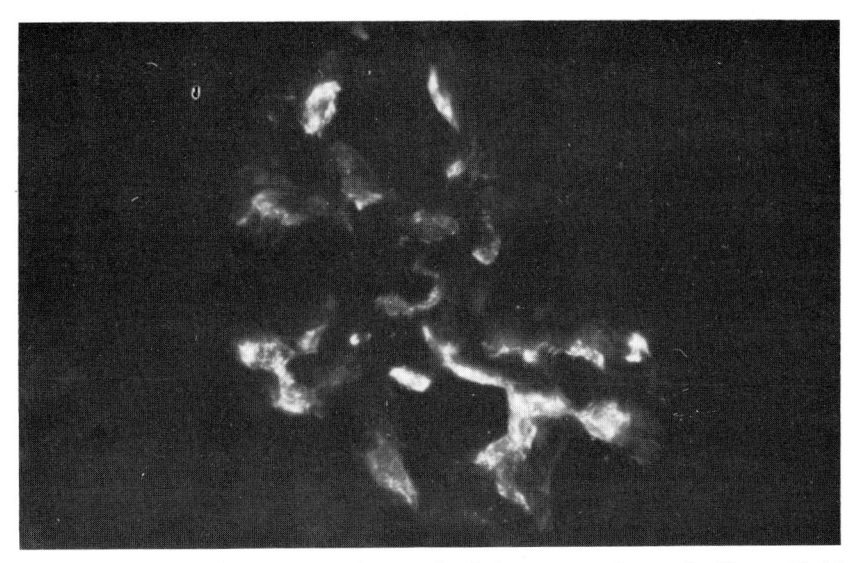

Figure 12-16 Fluorescence micrograph of the same patient as in Figure 12-14. utilizing fluoresceinated anti-IgA. Deposits of IgA are prominent in the mesangial regions and were present in all of the glomeruli examined. No other immunoglobulins were seen in this patient. ($\times 300$.)

remained normal in all but three of 55 children. A subsequent study by Roy and associates (1973) of 16 children suggested that those with segmental glomerular sclerosis may have a more ominous prognosis, since four of these developed renal functional impairment. Additionally, in a study of 20 patients by McCoy and his colleagues (1974), renal functional deterioration was noted in only one patient, who also was found to have mild hypertension. Thus, it appears that this is a relatively benign syndrome, characterized by intermittent or persistent hematuria, which becomes accentuated after even modest viral illnesses. Many of the reports indicate that it is difficult to separate this syndrome from others without the aid of renal biopsy. Since the prognosis is so different in benign recurrent hematuria than in other conditions, biopsy would be a particularly useful technique in the early diagnosis in this syndrome.

HEREDITARY NEPHRITIS

Introduction

Hereditary nephritis was first described by Guthrie in 1902. Alport in 1927 reported its association with deafness, and this syndrome now bears his name. From recent reports, hereditary nephritis (Alport's syndrome) appears to be a disease of abnormal basal lamina production involving both glomeruli and tubules. Although Alport's syndrome is the most well-recognized form of hereditary nephritis, as renal diseases are being more closely examined from a genetic standpoint, other types with varying clinical expression are being discovered. This section, however, will deal only with Alport's syndrome.

Clinical Data

In most kindreds, renal involvement appears to be associated with the X chromosome, with males being affected predominantly. In families in which the females are involved, the syndrome is usually milder than in the affected males. Recurrent hematuria in childhood is a common initial manifestation. Persistent proteinuria is common, but it rarely occurs in the nephrotic range. Microscopic urinalysis shows the same characteristics as are found in any type of chronic glomerulonephritis, with occasional red blood cell casts, granular casts, and, depending on the degree of tubulo-interstitial disease, broad and waxy casts.

Approximately 30 to 50 per cent of patients will have neural sensory deafness, which often may be subclinical and determined only by audiometry.

Hereditary nephritis also has been associated with various ocular abnormalities, as well as megathrombocytopenia.

Other renal diseases of a hereditary nature, such as medullary cystic disease, polycystic disease, nail-patella syndrome, and Fabry's disease, may be confused with Alport's syndrome. Careful clinical evaluation and renal biopsy are helpful in establishing the diagnosis and prognosis in the individual case, and may be useful in genetic counseling.

Histology

The anatomic descriptions of renal biopsies in the literature vary considerably, reflecting in large part the various times in the course of the disease at which the patient is examined. Generally, early in the course the changes appear mainly in glomeruli, whereas in advanced injury, the tubules and interstitium are prominently affected.

GLOMERULI. Mesangial hypercellularity involving a small number of glomeruli is the most consistent early light microscopic change (Fig. 12–17). At this time, the basal lamina is normal on light microscopy but can be seen to be multilaminated or frayed by electron microscopy (Fig. 12–18). At later times, the basal lamina is prominently thickened, and the hypercellularity is less prominent. In one early series complement components were found deposited in mesangial regions and peripheral capillary loops, and in another hypocomplementemia was found in two of five patients studied. However, in our experience and that of most others, immunoglobulins or other protein deposits are not features at either the fluorescence or electron microscopic levels of observation.

TUBULES. Few changes are present early in the disease process save for the presence of red blood cells and occasionally red blood cell casts in the lumen. Later, there is tubular atrophy in areas of associated interstitial fibrosis. On electron microscopy, a change similar to that seen in the glomeruli (multilayering and fraying of the basal lamina) is apparent. The epithelial cells often contain lipid, but this is an inconstant feature. Tubular basal lamina thickening parallels the increasing tubular atrophy and interstitial fibrosis.

INTERSTITIUM. Changes are not seen in the interstitium early in the disease. It has been suggested that the interstitial foam cells often present in an otherwise normal interstitium and seen primarily at the corticomedullary junction are characteristic of Alport's syndrome (Fig. 12–19). However, these cells are seen in so many patients with other renal syndromes that it is difficult to assign to them a diagnostic function.

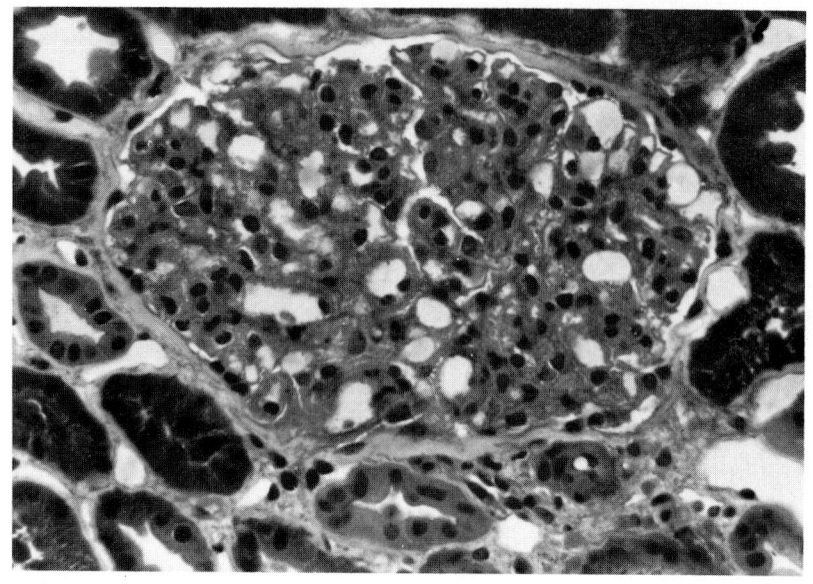

Figure 12-17 Biopsy specimen from a 17 year old male with persistent hematuria and mild proteinuria. A younger sibling has similar urinary abnormalities and a maternal uncle has renal failure. The only apparent abnormality is a mild increase in the number of mesangial cells. (H&E, × 300.)

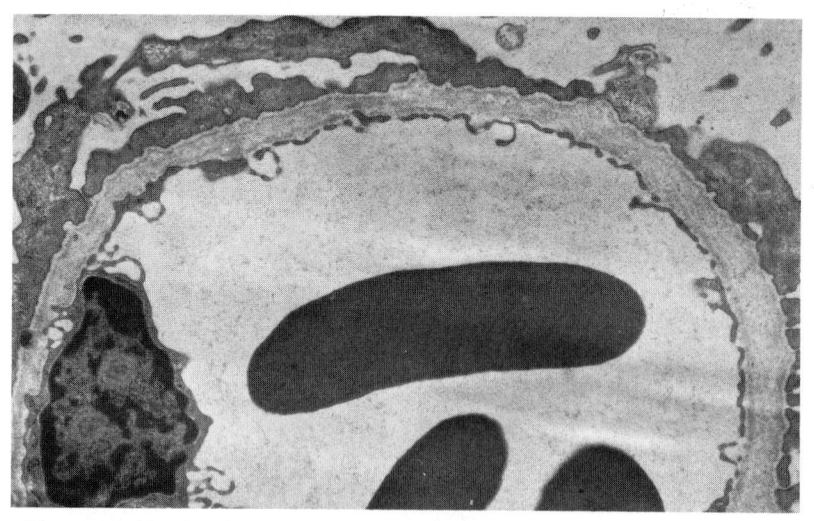

Figure 12-18 An electron micrograph from the same biopsy as in Figure 12-17. Note the multilayering and fragmentation of the basal lamina. This abnormal basal lamina stains poorly if at all with silver methenamine. (× 4000.)

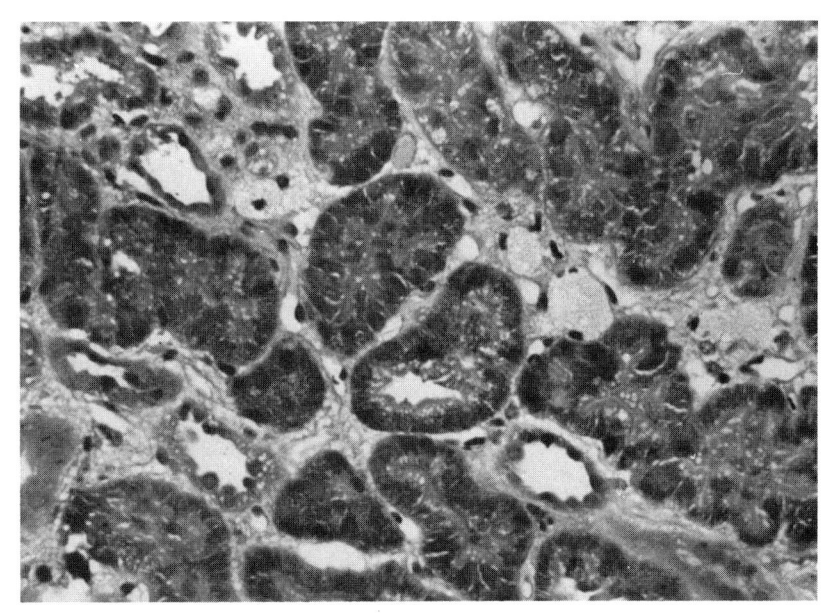

Figure 12-19 Same biopsy as in Figure 12-17. There is a mild, generalized increase in interstitial connective tissue. Also present are interstitial foam cells. (H&E, ×300.)

VESSELS. No vascular lesions have been described in Alport's syndrome.

Clinical Course and Prognosis

The clinical course is not different from other forms of slowly progressive renal diseases. Renal failure ensues after a long course of proteinuria and hematuria. Hypertension may occur with progressive azotemia but is not a distinctive feature of this syndrome. The development of the nephrotic syndrome is rare.

References

Slowly Progressive Glomerular Disease
1. Baldwin, D. S., Gluck, M. C., Schacht, R. G., and Gallo, G.: The long-term course of poststreptococcal glomerulonephritis. Ann. Int. Med. *80*:342, 1974.
2. Bodian, M., Black, J. A., Kobayashi, N., Lake, B. D., and Shuler, S. F.: Recurrent hematuria in childhood. Quart. J. Med. *34*:359, 1965.
3. Heptinstall, R. H.: Pathology of end-stage renal disease. Am. J. Med. *44*:656, 1958.

4. Rakowski, T. A., Argy, W. P., Curtis, J. J., and Schreiner, G. F.: Percutaneous renal biopsy in end-stage renal failure. Clin. Res. *23*:37A, 1975.

Benign Recurrent Hematuria
1. Berger, J.: IgA glomerular deposits in renal disease. Transpl. Proc. *1*:939, 1969.
2. Levy, M., Beaufils, H., Gubler, M. C., and Habib, R.: Idiopathic recurrent macroscopic hematuria and mesangial IgA–IgB deposits in children (Berger's disease). Clin. Nephr. *1*:63, 1973.
3. McCoy, R. C., Abramowsky, C. R., and Tisher, C. C.: IgA nephropathy. Am. J. Path. *75*:123, 1974.
4. Roy, L. P., Fish, A. F., Vernier, R. L., and Michael, A. F.: Recurrent macroscopic hematuria, focal nephritis, and mesangial deposition of immunoglobulin and complement. J. Pediatr. *82*:767, 1973.

Hereditary Nephritis
1. Alport, S. C.: Hereditary familial congenital hemorrhagic nephritis. Brit. Med. J. *1*:504, 1927.
2. Epstein, C. J., Sahud, M. A,. Piel, C. F., Goodman, J. R., Bernfield, M. R., Kushner, J. H., and Ablin, A R.: Hereditary macrothrombocytopathia, nephritis and deafness. Am. J. Med. *52*:299, 1972.
3. Purriel, P., Drets, M., Pascale, E., Cestau, R. S., Borras, A., Ferreira, W. A., De Lucca, A., and Fernandez, L.: Familial hereditary nephropathy (Alport's syndrome). Am. J. Med. *49*:753, 1970.
4. Sherman, R. L., Churg, J., and Yudis, M.: Hereditary nephritis with a characteristic renal lesion. Am. J. Med. *56*:44, 1974.
5. Spear, G. S., Whitworth, J. M., and Konigsmark, B. W.: Hereditary nephritis with nerve deafness. Am. J. Med. *49*:52, 1970.
6. Spear, G. S., and Slusser, R. J.: Alport's syndrome. Emphasizing electron microscopic studies of the glomerulus. Am. J. Path. *69*:213, 1972.

Chapter Thirteen

Slowly Progressive Tubulo-Interstitial Diseases

Introduction

The primary anatomic manifestations of slowly progressive tubulo-interstitial diseases reflect the generalized or localized changes in the tubulo-interstitial area, including tubular atrophy, interstitial fibrosis, and infiltration by chronic inflammatory cells (Figs. 13–1 and 13–2). Until appropriate diagnostic techniques are developed, this designation represents a convenient way to group renal diseases of unknown etiology which produce principally tubulo-interstitial changes, much as the title slowly progressive glomerulonephritis is used for many renal diseases of unknown causes in which the alterations are mostly glomerular (Table 13–1). Unlike the slowly progressive glomerulopathies, however, tubulo-interstitial disease may be patchy in its distribution, diseased areas alternating with healthy or less diseased sections.

Tubulo-interstitial changes are associated with most renal diseases, however, and determining whether the tubulo-interstitial lesion is the

TABLE 13–1 Conditions Associated With Chronic Tubulo-Interstitial Nephropathy

1. Urinary tract obstruction
2. Parenchymal infection (pyelonephritis)
3. Transplant rejection (Section VI)
4. Nephrotoxins
5. Metabolic disease
6. Hereditary disease
7. Malignancy
8. Balkan nephropathy
9. Idiopathic
10. Radiation Nephritis

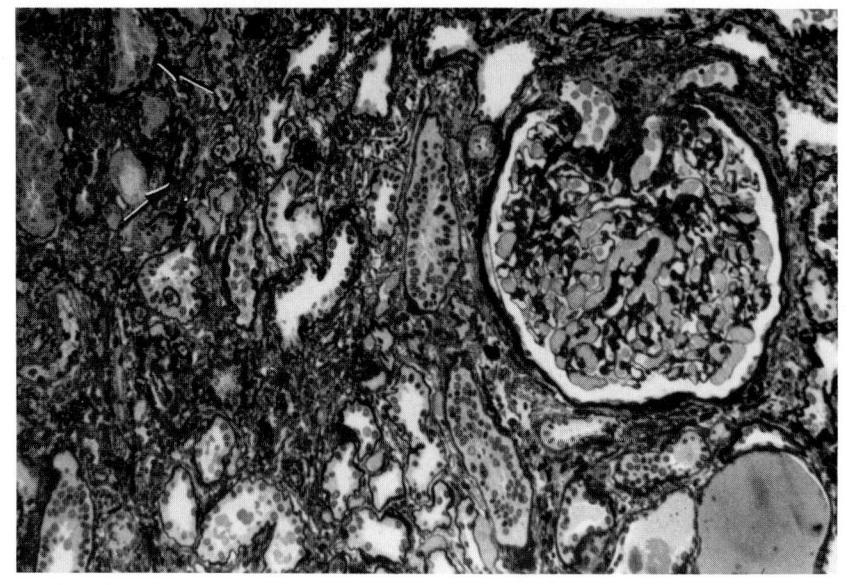

Figure 13-1 This 28 year old male had long-standing obstructive uropathy. The glomerulus appears normal, while the surrounding interstitium is densely fibrotic. The encased tubules are quite abnormal; some are dilated and contain casts and others are small and atrophic and have thickened basal lamina (arrows). (Silver methenamine, ×75.)

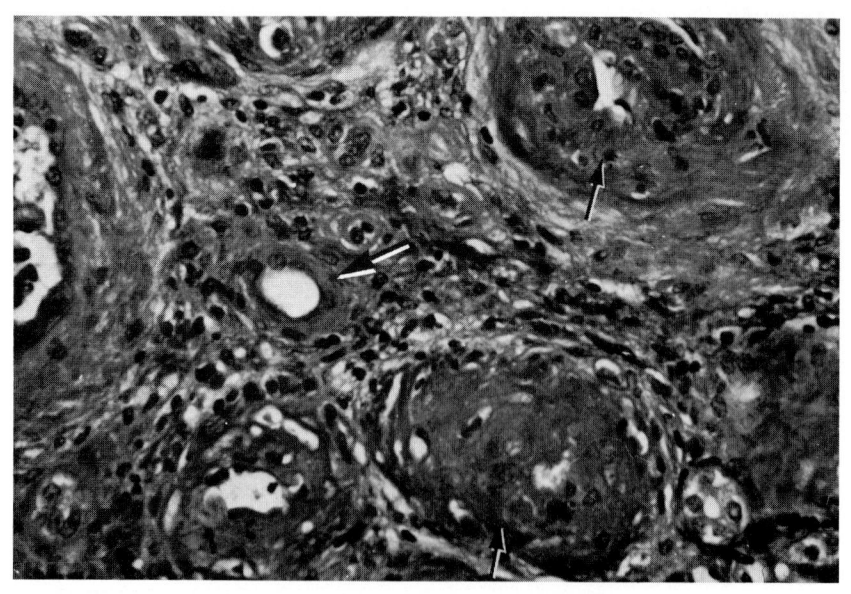

Figure 13-2 Biopsy from a 46 year old woman with chronic obstructive renal disease. The biopsy consists mainly of obsolescent glomeruli (light arrows). Only a few tubules are recognizable, and these are atrophic (heavy arrow). The interstitium is filled with connective tissue and a large number of mononuclear inflammatory cells. (H&E, ×300.)

dominant one is often difficult. The diagnosis is clear only when the tubulo-interstitial area is the single compartment affected.

Tubulo-interstitial nephropathy causes few common clinical features. Symptoms indicating the presence or progression of renal disease generally are absent until late in the course of the disease. Patients therefore frequently present with signs of end stage renal disease or are discovered to have significant abnormalities when examined for other medical problems. There may also be signs and symptoms of a variety of primary illnesses which could underlie interstitial nephritis (Table 13–1). The benchmarks of renal disease, however, such as edema, excessive proteinuria, or macroscopic hematuria, are not associated with this syndrome in the early stages.

Although they are not specific to tubulo-interstitial nephropathy, the following three findings often represent the initial clinical manifestations in patients with this disease: (1) polyuria, (2) renal tubular acidosis, and (3) inability to conserve sodium. These abnormalities are caused by the loss of normal tubulo-interstitial functions, indirectly affecting renal blood flow and glomerular filtration. These changes in tubular function are more frequent in tubulo-interstitial disease than in glomerulonephritis, and although they suggest the site of involvement, they are not helpful in determining the etiology of the syndrome.

CHRONIC INFECTIOUS PYELONEPHRITIS

Clinical Data

Chronic pyelonephritis is a common variety of tubulo-interstitial nephritis. Unfortunately, this has produced the impression that chronic tubulo-interstitial nephritis and infectious pyelonephritis are synonymous, leading to the use of the term pyelonephritis for all tubulo-interstitial nephropathies, irrespective of the existence of a urinary tract infection. Most patients with true chronic pyelonephritis have obstruction in the urinary tract. When bacterial infection is present there generally is no pain or disturbance of voiding apart from some increase in nocturnal frequency. The radiologic findings indicate asymmetry and irregular renal atrophy, with distortion of the renal pelvis. Frequently chronic pyelonephritis occurs in the absence of a history of acute pyelonephritis. The diagnosis of chronic pyelonephritis in the absence of obstruction now is made less frequently because of better understanding of the pathologic processes and the development of better radiologic and urologic techniques.

Histology

Renal biopsy is not useful in evaluating this condition, since the changes are irregular in distribution and the papilla usually is not accessible to the biopsy needle. In addition, other, less invasive techniques allow better quantification of the injury (see Chapter 6).

Clinical Course and Prognosis

Although the course of chronic pyelonephritis is variable, it is typical for the disease to progress very slowly. Hamburger and associates (1968) have suggested that there are four factors which influence the outcome of the disorder: (1) the microorganism involved, (2) the presence of hypertension, (3) recurrent episodes of pyelonephritis, and (4) the presence and type of urinary tract obstruction.

It is clear that the last three factors are of critical importance in the rapidity in which progression occurs in humans, but the first factor, although well established in laboratory animals, may not apply in humans. Animal studies have suggested, for example, that infections with *Escherichia coli* are less damaging to renal structure than are those with strains of Proteus, Pseudomonas, and Enterococci. The associated vascular damage seen with uncontrolled blood pressure has been demonstrated to accelerate renal damage regardless of the primary nephropathy. Frequent exacerbations of acute pyelonephritis may also produce changes in renal structure and deterioration of function.

Finally, continued urinary tract obstruction acts both by predisposing the kidney to infection or perpetuating the existing renal infection, and by increasing the pelvic pressure, which directly damages the kidney. Functional disorders, however, such as vesicoureteral reflux, are less harmful than mechanical obstruction. The operative correction of reflux, important as a preventive measure, is of little value when chronic pyelonephritis is advanced.

TOXIC TUBULO-INTERSTITIAL NEPHROPATHY

The kidney is particularly susceptible to toxins and drugs which gain access to the circulation. It receives a very high proportion of the cardiac output in relation to its weight, has a large vascular surface area, and is a metabolically active organ. Furthermore, the reabsorption of salt and water in the tubules serves to concentrate nonreabsorbable solutes within the lumen. Their concentration at this site, therefore, may be several times that in the plasma and thus may reach toxic concentrations. Finally, the epithelial cells are exposed to large amounts of ingested heavy metals as a consequence of their function of transporting ions into and from the tubular fluid. Thus, these cells may have increased likelihood of suffering heavy metal poisoning.

In the medulla, the interstitial fluid is hyperosmotic as the result of the operation of the countercurrent concentration mechanism. Thus, drugs entering the medullary interstitial fluid may be concentrated to levels far beyond those encountered in the bloodstream, lymph, or other body fluids. Few drugs have been studied for such effects except for N-acetyl-p-aminophenol, a metabolite of phenacetin which appears in higher concentrations in the medulla than in the plasma.

Analgesic Abuse

Prior to 1950, few cases of analgesic nephropathy were described. The recognized toxic tubulo-interstitial nephropathies, such as those due to the sulfonamides, were associated with acute disease and were thought to be the result of a hypersensitivity reaction. However, beginning in 1953 with the report of Spühler and Zollinger, attention was drawn to the increasing number of patients with chronic tubulo-interstitial nephropathy associated with few symptoms until end stage renal disease occurred. They ascribed these changes to abuse of analgesics, especially those containing phenacetin. The study of Bengtsson (1962) demonstrated clearly the increased frequency of papillary necrosis in women with tubular-interstitial nephritis and urinary tract infection associated with analgesic abuse, compared to those patients with interstitial nephritis and urinary infection alone.

Subsequent studies also demonstrated the secondary nature of bacterial infection in the production of renal damage by these agents. Although many questions remain concerning the nature of the agent(s) and the mechanisms involved, there is a causative relationship between analgesics and tubulo-interstitial nephritis.

CLINICAL DATA

There is nothing distinctive about the clinical features of analgesic nephropathy. In reported series, however, the syndrome is more frequent in women than in men. The diagnosis often is based on a strong clinical suspicion and persistent interrogation of the patient. A history of analgesic abuse rarely is volunteered and the ingenuity of the physician may be taxed in obtaining an accurate history. Analgesic abuse should be suspected, however, in any patient with renal disease or recurrent urinary tract infection when associated with pyelonephritis.

The patient generally is unaware of the progressive nature of the renal disease prior to the development of uremic symptoms, as is common with most types of chronic renal disease. The appearance of papillary necrosis, however, may cause fulminating illness resembling a very severe attack of acute pyelonephritis, or occasionally patients may give a history of repeated attacks of lumbar pain, hematuria, and perhaps renal colic. Suspicion of papillary necrosis may be confirmed

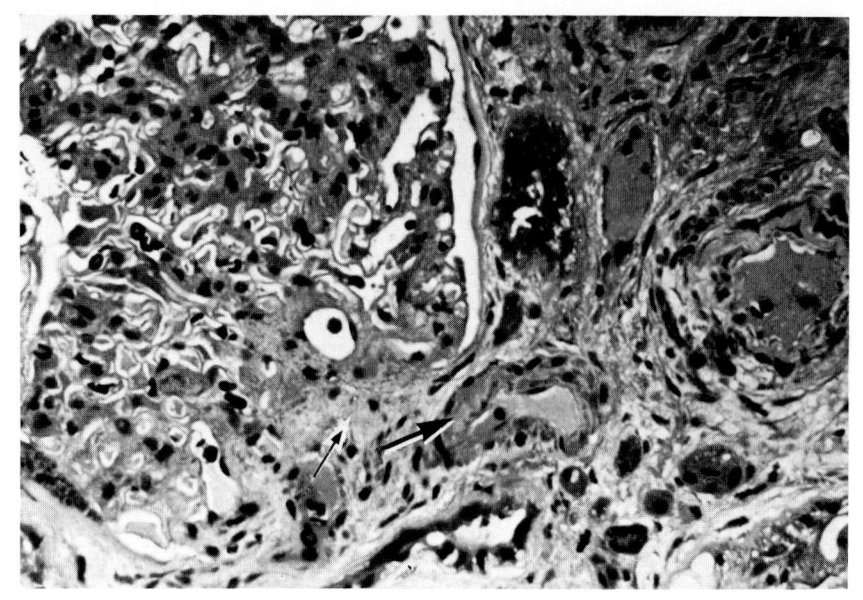

Figure 13-3 Biopsy from 46 year old woman who had a long history of analgesic ingestion. The glomeruli appear relatively normal save for sclerosis near the vascular pole (small arrows). The interstitium contains a large amount of connective tissue, as well as a number of mononuclear inflammatory cells. The associated vessels have "hyaline" in their walls (large arrow). (H&E, ×300.)

by finding fragments of the necrosed papilla in the urine or by radiologic examination.

HISTOLOGY

Renal biopsy is not often used in patients with chronic renal failure and would be useful only in differentiating acute from chronic changes and in determining the potential reversibility of the lesion.

Little is known about the early histologic changes in this disease, for cortical changes occur late; when such changes are present, medullary rays are most severely affected, and the proximal tubules tend to be spared. The late changes consist of diffuse interstitial fibrosis, tubular atrophy, and interstitial infiltration with lymphocytes (Fig. 13-3). The glomeruli are normal, and vessel changes, when present, reflect the degree of interstitial change.

CLINICAL COURSE AND PROGNOSIS

The importance of accurately assessing a patient's intake of analgesic mixtures cannot be overemphasized. There is evidence that regression, or at least stabilization, of the renal lesion may be possible if the patient stops ingesting the responsible analgesic.

Heavy Metal Nephropathy

The association between renal disease, hypertension, and arteriosclerosis was noted in lead workers over 100 years ago. Henderson provided evidence incriminating lead poisoning as a cause of chronic tubulo-interstitial nephritis in children. Many other heavy metals are associated with chronic progressive disease in humans as well, including cadmium, mercury, gold, uranium, copper, bismuth, thallium, arsenic, and iron.

Clinically the features are similar to those of other slowly progressive tubulo-interstitial diseases: slow progression of disease, small amounts of protein in the urine, and impairment of renal concentrating capacity in the early stages of disease.

Lead nephropathy is associated with a history of poisoning in the patient or a sibling, gout, impairment of intellect, euphoria or psychiatric disorders, and neuropathy. Gout has been noted in over 50 per cent of patients, and is a frequent presenting symptom of the disease.

HISTOLOGY

The histologic changes of acute intoxication with heavy metals are those of proximal tubular injury. Specific intranuclear or cytoplasmic inclusions are present in lead poisoning. These inclusions are eosinophilic and acid fast, and have been shown not to contain lead. Chronic heavy metal intoxication, however, presents the histologic picture of interstitial fibrosis, tubular atrophy, and normal glomeruli and vessels.

Gold nephropathy has recently received renewed interest, and studies indicate that there are a number of patients who develop subepithelial deposits in their glomeruli (Fig. 13–4) and lysosomal crystalloids in their proximal tubules (Fig. 13–5). A glomerular lesion also has been reported in chronic mercury intoxication resembling membranous nephropathy.

CLINICAL COURSE AND PROGNOSIS

Older studies emphasized the relationship between lead exposure and chronic renal disease. Perhaps the best study, however, is that of Henderson (1958), who followed 401 children who had lead poisoning. Of these, 165 died from 6 to 34 years later. Chronic nephritis or hypertension occurred in 108 who died. Of the remaining 187 traced, three had hypertension, and 17 had proteinuria and hypertension. Consequently, the study provides highly suggestive evidence of a relationship between early lead intoxication and subsequent renal failure. The chronic effects of other heavy metal intoxication have not been as well described.

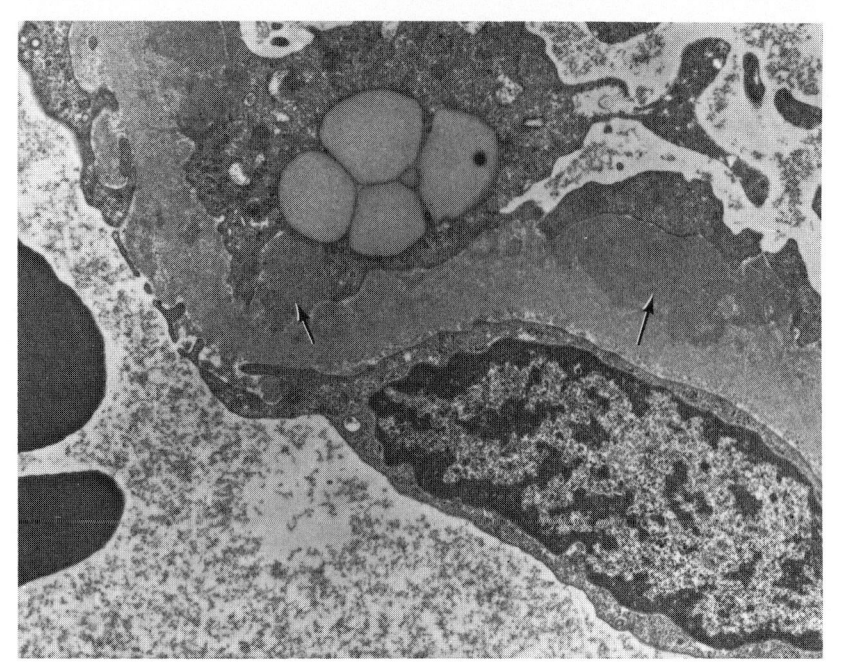

Figure 13-4 A biopsy from a 46 year old female with a 10 year history of rheumatoid arthritis. Following the institution of gold therapy 1 year ago, she developed persistent proteinuria of less than 1 g/24 hr. The most obvious abnormalities are irregular deposits of electron-dense material on the epithelial aspect of the glomerular basal lamina (arrows). The epithelial foot processes in these areas are effaced. ($\times 4000$.) (Courtesy of R. Wheelis, M.D.)

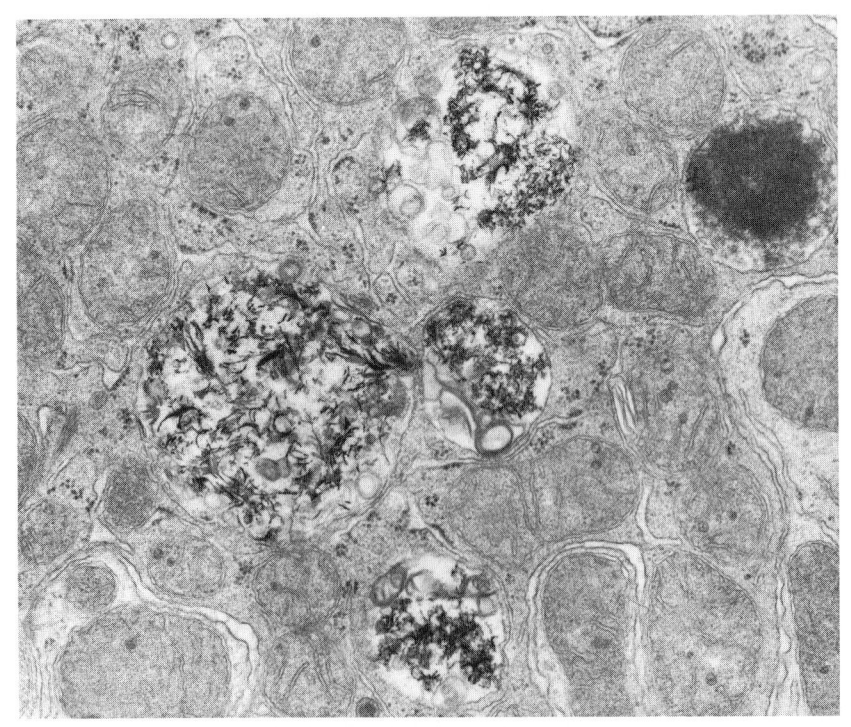

Figure 13-5 Same patient as in Figure 13-4. Lysosomes of the glomerular epithelial cells and those of the proximal tubule contain irregular "crystalloid" aggregates. The cells are otherwise unremarkable. ($\times 15,000$.) (Courtesy of R. Wheelis, M.D.)

Radiation

CLINICAL DATA

It has been appreciated only recently that the kidneys are probably the most radiosensitive abdominal organ. The exact pathogenesis of radiation damage to the kidney is unknown. Current evidence suggests that the degree of tissue damage can be correlated to the dose and the time interval which has elapsed after exposure to radiation. However, individual variations and preexisting renal lesions may affect the type of response.

Radiation damage usually can be traced to therapy for malignancy of the upper abdomen, the pelvis, or the testes, or total body irradiation. Heavy metal radioisotopes also have been implicated.

Renal functional changes appear when more than 400 rads are delivered to the kidney. Alterations include a decrease in renal plasma flow, glomerular filtration rate, and tubular function.

HISTOLOGY

GENERAL. The general process can be described as an initial cell swelling and a subsequent sclerosis involving all renal elements. The cell type which appears to be most frequently affected is the endothelial cell.

GLOMERULI. The changes vary from no alteration to severe mesangial sclerosis. Endothelial cell changes described consist of swelling, detachment from the basal lamina, and formation of new basal lamina, resulting in a "duplication" of the peripheral glomerular basal lamina.

TUBULES AND INTERSTITIUM. The earliest change is thought to be a thickening of the tubular basal lamina, although this has been shown only in experimental animals. In advanced renal disease, tubular atrophy, accompanied by dense interstitial fibrosis, is also a very conspicuous feature. Inflammatory cell infiltration, on the other hand, usually is sparse.

VESSELS. The vessel changes range from mild sclerosis to florid intimal injury with deposits of fibrin and other serum proteins in the wall, which result in vascular occlusion. A conspicuous feature of the vascular change is the absence of an inflammatory cell infiltrate.

CLINICAL COURSE AND PROGNOSIS

The reversibility of these changes depends on the total amount of irradiation and other, as yet unknown factors. Clinical manifestations usually occur after a latent period of 4 months to one year. Proteinuria, hypertension, and renal insufficiency of varying degree are the most common findings. Some patients, however, have a rapid progression of renal injury and present initially with oliguric renal failure.

TUBULO-INTERSTITIAL NEPHROPATHY IN METABOLIC DISORDERS

Hyperuricemia

CLINICAL DATA

Two renal syndromes may occur with hyperuricemia: (1) the formation of uric acid stones, and (2) the development of tubulo-interstitial disease. Approximately 10 to 20 per cent of patients with gout develop urolithiasis. In addition, as is common with stones of other types, complications include obstruction and infection with secondary tubulo-interstitial disease.

A form of intrarenal urolithiasis with acute renal failure has been described following the administration of potent cancer chemotherapeutic agents. Their use causes a rapid rise in plasma urate concentration due to the liberation of large amounts of nucleoprotein, which is metabolized to uric acid. Consequently, sodium biurate precipitates in the tubular lumen, causing obstruction. Pretreatment of the patient with allopurinol and proper attention to an alkaline diuresis, however, usually will prevent this complication.

Finally, tophaceous deposits in the kidney and in cartilaginous structures may occur in patients with chronic hyperuricemia, especially those prone to develop gout. These deposits may result in extensive renal scarring, but rarely lead to renal insufficiency.

HISTOLOGY

The sodium biurate usually is deposited in the interstitial tissues of the medullary papilla and produces a histologic picture of interstitial fibrosis and lymphocyte infiltration similar to that of chronic bacterial tubulo-interstitial nephritis. In addition, an associated finding in most biopsies is a moderate to marked degree of nephrosclerosis. Needle-shaped crystals may be demonstrated in tissue fixed in alcohol and never exposed to water. Large crystalline deposits may incite a foreign body reaction.

CLINICAL COURSE AND PROGNOSIS

There does appear to be a good correlation between the development of urate nephropathy and the severity of hyperuricemia. In a postmortem study of urate nephropathy, Talbott (1960) found histologic evidence of renal urate deposits in two-thirds of the examined group.

Reduction of plasma urate concentrations with allopurinol, uricosuric agents, or both, decreases the incidence of urate nephropathy. It is unknown whether such treatment alters the vascular lesion.

Cystinosis

CLINICAL DATA

Cystinosis is a rare metabolic inborn error transmitted by an autosomal recessive mode and manifested by the deposition of crystals of cystine throughout the body. Renal disease present within the first year of life is characterized by proximal tubular dysfunction.

The earliest manifestation of the disease is the appearance of aminoaciduria, and other tubular defects become evident soon thereafter, including glycosuria, hyperphosphaturia, renal tubular acidosis, and a concentration defect. In addition, rickets and growth failure are common. Eventual development of tubulo-interstitial disease is associated with a reduction in glomerular filtration rate and azotemia.

HISTOLOGY

The principal lesion in cystinosis is atrophy of the proximal tubule (swan-neck lesion) (Fig. 13–6). There is also an associated infiltration

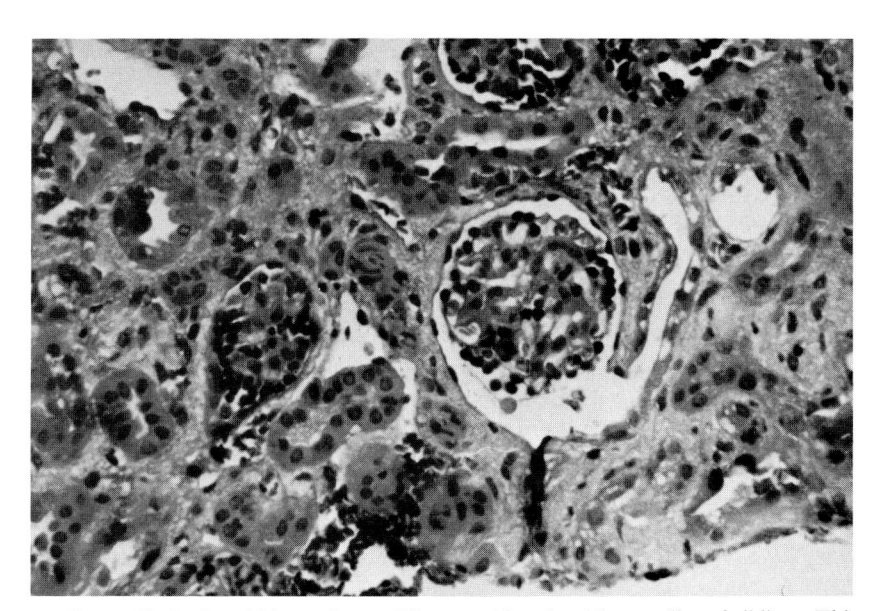

Figure 13–6 Renal biopsy from a 5½ year old male with two affected siblings. This glomerulus demonstrates an elongated segment of the first portion of the proximal tubule, which is lined by epithelial cells. Vacuoles also may be seen in these cells. The glomerulus has very prominent epithelial cells consistent with giant cells seen in this location. (H&E, ×300.)

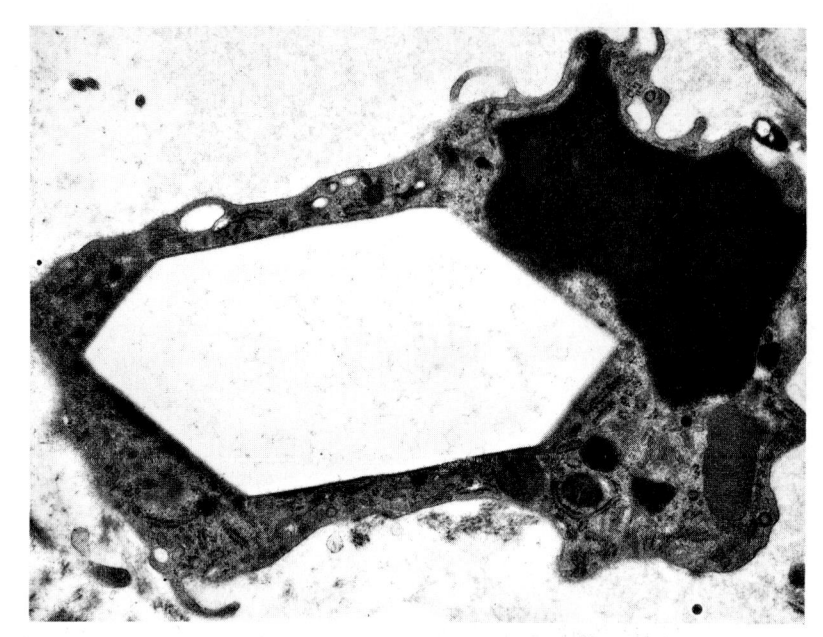

Figure 13-7 An interstitial cell from the same patient as in Figure 13-6. Rhomboid shaped crystals are noted within lysosomes of many interstitial cells. Similar crystals may be seen in glomerular epithelial and proximal tubular (neck) cells. (× 5000.)

of the interstitium with cystine-containing inflammatory cells (Fig. 13-7). Interstitial fibrosis, tubular atrophy, and interstitial inflammation advance rapidly, resulting in diffuse renal scarring early in life. Crystals have been described in epithelial cells of the glomerulus and proximal tubule as well.

CLINICAL COURSE AND PROGNOSIS

Renal failure usually appears in the first or second decade of life. The involvement of other visceral organs is noted by the presence of hepatomegaly, lymphadenopathy, and splenomegaly. Unfortunately, there is no specific treatment available. In some centers patients have been treated with chronic dialysis or renal transplantation.

HEREDITARY AND DEVELOPMENTAL TUBULO-INTERSTITIAL NEPHROPATHY

Cystic Disorders

The cystic disorders of the kidney represent types of dysplastic malformations, which may be single cysts varying in size from less than

1 cm to 10 cm or more in diameter, or multiple cysts. They may be either congenital or acquired, but in some instances a distinction cannot be made.

Polycystic Renal Disease

Polycystic renal disease is characterized by the presence of many bilateral cysts, which cause increase in the total renal size but at the same time reduce the functioning renal tissue by compression. The lesion occurs either in infancy or in middle life, with few cases being found between these peaks. This pattern, plus different modes of inheritance, suggests that the two conditions probably are unrelated etiologically. The adult form has an autosomal dominant inheritance, whereas the neonatal form appears to be an autosomal recessive variety. The two types of polycystic disease do not occur in the same family. Furthermore, the incidence of the adult type is less than 1 per 1000 population up to the age of 80 years, although it is estimated that a person with the dominant gene who lives to the age of 80 has a 100 per cent chance of being afflicted.

CLINICAL DATA

The two diseases are quite distinct clinically. The infantile form of polycystic disease is much rarer than the adult form, and usually causes very early death. Since adult polycystic disease often is slowly progressive over many years, it frequently is asymptomatic initially. In addition, even though the dominant gene has a high degree of penetrance, the variation in overt onset of the adult disease makes it difficult to predict the prognosis before symptoms are present.

The onset of symptoms in the adult form generally occurs when the patient is in his early forties, although the range is extremely variable, with onset sometimes occurring as late as the seventies. Males and females are affected equally, and a positive family history also is common. Symptoms usually are related to abnormalities due to the cysts, such as lumbar discomfort, pain, hematuria, infection, and colic, or those associated with a loss of renal function, including uremic symptoms. The presence of hypertension is common, with approximately half the patients having this finding at the time of diagnosis.

On examination, the patient may be found to have large, bilateral, and irregular abdominal masses, which are sometimes mistaken for hepatosplenomegaly. The urine shows mild proteinuria and varying degrees of hematuria, but red cell casts are infrequent. Pyuria is common as well, even in the absence of bacterial infection. In addition, the excretory urogram characteristically indicates large kidneys with irregular outlines owing to the many cysts. The calyces, infundibula, and pelves also are compressed and elongated by cysts, giving what is sometimes referred to as a "spidery" apppearance. Renal and hepatic radionuclide scans also show the typical "moth-eaten" appearance due to the cysts, which displace functional tissue.

HISTOLOGY

Kidney biopsies have been performed in cases of polycystic renal disease in an attempt to evaluate asymptomatic patients for the presence of early lesions. Thus far, however, no specific changes have been found. In clinically apparent cases, renal biopsy is contraindicated.

CLINICAL COURSE AND PROGNOSIS

There is great variation in the course of polycystic disease; some patients live for decades without adverse effects, while others have complications, with progressive uremia and rapid demise, unless specific therapy such as transplantation or dialysis is undertaken. In the absence of therapy, the average age at death is approximately 50 years, after a clinical course of about 10 years from the onset of symptoms.

Medullary Cystic Disease

Medullary cystic disease, first clearly described in 1945, also is known as familial juvenile nephronophthisis. Symptoms usually begin in the first two decades of life, although the disease has been observed as late as the sixth decade. Data concerning genetic transmission are scant, but extensive studies in several families suggest that autosomal dominant transmission is probable.

Clinical Data

Polyuria, which is caused by a vasopressin-resistant renal concentrating defect, is often the earliest symptom. Urinary sodium wastage also frequently is present, and commonly it is severe enough to require a sodium intake of several hundred milliequivalents daily in order to prevent extracellular volume depletion. In many patients, these symptoms develop slowly over a period of years and are so well compensated for that they are not considered abnormal. Uremic symptoms, however, are what bring these patients to the attention of a physician.

Laboratory findings for medullary cystic disease are similar to those expected in patients with chronic renal failure. For example, proteinuria is minimal or absent, and the urinary sediment is not remark-

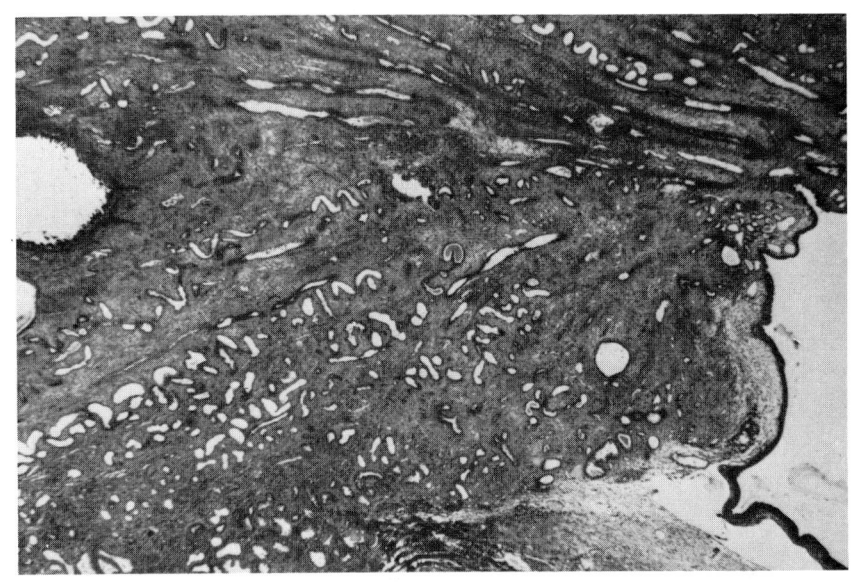

Figure 13–8 Low power photomicrograph of a kidney from a 9 year old girl who has an affected sister. The primary change is marked dilatation of kidney tubules, primarily collecting ducts in the medulla. The cortex remained relatively spared from this change but showed marked atrophy of the parenchyma. (H&E, ×20.)

able. The serum alkaline phosphatase level also generally is elevated owing to renal osteodystrophy. In addition, radiographic examination of the urinary system demonstrates only small kidneys.

HISTOLOGY

Since the principal lesion is in the collecting ducts (Fig. 13–8) renal biopsy of the cortex is unrevealing unless obstruction and infection occur.

CLINICAL COURSE AND PROGNOSIS

Progression of medullary cystic disease varies depending on the degree of renal dysfunction when the patient is first examined. As a rule, however, the disease progresses slowly but inexorably.

TUBULO-INTERSTITIAL DISEASE IN MALIGNANCY

The interstitial spaces of the kidney may be invaded by proliferative malignant cells in leukemia and lymphosarcoma. The interstitial infiltration involves the cortex more than the medulla. This infiltration is found in approximately half of autopsies in generalized lymphocytic lymphomas and in one-third of all malignant lymphomas. It produces an increase in size of the kidneys, often asymmetrical. Excretory urography reveals elongation and narrowing of the calyces due to this diffuse swelling. On balance, however, an increase in the size of the kidneys in a patient with diffuse malignant disease does not necessarily signify neoplastic infiltration, since such a finding is present at autopsy in only 50 per cent of patients with enlarged kidneys. Furthermore, despite the extensive interstitial involvement, there are few functional changes. Finally, proteinuria is absent or insignificant, and blood urea or creatinine concentrations rarely are elevated unless some other complication, such as uric acid nephropathy, hypercalcemia, or bacterial infiltration occurs.

ENDEMIC TUBULO-INTERSTITIAL NEPHROPATHY OF THE BALKANS

In certain well-defined regions in the Balkans, a chronic "Balkan nephropathy" has been described which has the characteristics of tubulo-interstitial nephritis. The onset is never acute, and the disease is discovered on routine examination by the presence of proteinuria or along with the findings of chronic renal insufficiency. Special clinical features include the absence of edema, the rarity of finding hypertension, and anemia of severe proportions. After initial presentation, renal function deteriorates rapidly, with chronic end stage disease appearing within two years after the first symptoms. The exact cause of the condition is unknown, although many observers suspect a virus or some environmental toxin. In addition, the disease is endemic, but it is not familial and there are no associated auditory or ocular defects, such as those which accompany other forms of familial nephritis.

HISTOLOGY

GENERAL. Most published data come from autopsy studies, and consequently end stage disease had been present. There are only a few reports on renal biopsies.

GLOMERULI. The glomeruli are not primarily affected, although they may show changes that can be attributed to ischemia secondary to marked loss of overall renal parenchyma, which results in small, scarred kidneys. The glomeruli therefore may show changes ranging from wrinkling of the basal lamina to ischemic obsolescence. These alterations are most marked near the capsule.

TUBULES AND INTERSTITIUM. The primary change in endemic tubulo-interstitial nephropathy of the Balkans is diffuse interstitial fibrosis and tubular atrophy. All areas of the kidney are affected, as are all tubular segments. There is also an accompanying scattered infiltrate of chronic inflammatory cells.

VESSELS. The vascular changes in this disease are not prominent and tend to reflect the degree of general parenchymal atrophy.

CLINICAL COURSE AND PROGNOSIS

This disease of unknown etiology has an unrelenting course to renal failure in about two years. No information is available about its recurrence in transplant recipients.

References

1. Bengtsson, U.: A comparative study of chronic nonobstructive pyelonephritis and renal papillary necrosis. Acta Med. Scand. *172* (Suppl. 388): 1, 1962.
2. Dalgaard, O. Z.: Bilateral polycystic disease of the kidneys. A follow-up of two hundred eighty-four patients with their families. Acta Med. Scand. *158* (Suppl. 328): 1, 1957.
3. Epstein, F. H.: Calcium and the kidney. Amer. J. Med. *45*:700, 1968.
4. Freedman, L. R.: Urinary tract infection, pyelonephritis, and other forms of chronic interstitial nephritis. *In* Strauss, M., and Welt, G. (eds.), Diseases of the Kidney. 2nd Ed. Little, Brown and Co., 1971, pp. 667–733.
5. Frei, E., III, Bentzel, C. J., Rieselbach, R., and Block, J. B.: Renal complications of neoplastic disease. J. Chron. Dis. *16*:757, 1963.
6. Hamburger, J., Richet, G., Crosnier, J., Funck-Bretano, J. L., Antoine, B., Ducrot, H., Mery, J. P., and Montera, H.: Nephrology (translated by Anthony Walsh). Philadelphia, W. B. Saunders Co., 1968.
7. Henderson, D. A.: The aetiology of chronic nephritis in Queensland. Med. J. Aust. *1*:377, 1958.
8. Leaf, A.: The syndrome of osteomalacia, renal glycosuria, amino-aciduria, and hyperphosphaturia (the Fanconi syndrome). *In* Stanbury, J. B., Wyngaarden, J. B., and Fredrickson, D. S. (eds.), The Metabolic Basis of Inherited Disease. New York, McGraw-Hill Book Co., 1960.
9. Mahoney, C. P., Striker, G. E., Hickman, R. O., Manning, G. B., and Marchioro, T. L.: Renal transplantation for childhood cystinosis. New Eng. J. Med., *283*:397, 1970.
10. Mostofi, F. K., and Berdjis, C. C.: The kidney. *In* Berdjis, C. C. (ed.), Pathology of Irradiation. Baltimore, Williams & Wilkins Co., 1971.
11. Murray, T., and Goldberg, M.: Chronic interstitial nephritis: etiologic factors. Ann. Intern. Med. *82*:453–459, 1975.
12. Potter, E. L., and Osathanondh, V.: Normal and abnormal development of the kidney. *In* Mostofi, F. K., and Smith, D. F. (eds.), The Kidney. Baltimore, Williams & Wilkins Co., 1966.
13. Relman, A. S., and Schwartz, W. B.: The kidney in potassium depletion. Amer. J. Med. *24*:764, 1958.
14. Schreiner, G. E.: Toxic nephropathy. *In* Beeson, P. B., and McDermott, W. (eds.), Textbook of Medicine. 14th Ed. W. B. Saunders Co., Philadelphia, 1975.
15. Spühler, O., and Zollinger, H. U.: Die chronischinterstitielle Nephritis. Z. Klin. Med. *151*:1, 1953.
16. Strauss, M. B.: Microcystic kidney disease. *In* Strauss, M. B., and Welt, L. G. (eds.), Diseases of the Kidney. 2nd Ed. Boston, Little, Brown and Co., 1971.
17. Talbott, J. H., and Terplan, K. L.: The kidney in gout. Medicine (Baltimore) *39*:405, 1960.
18. Tyler, F. H.: Urate nephropathy. *In* Strauss, M. B., and Welt, L. G. (eds.), Diseases of the Kidney. 2nd Ed. Boston, Little, Brown and Co., 1971.
19. Williams, H. E., and Smith, L. H., Jr.: Disorders of oxalate metabolism. Amer. J. Med. *45*:715, 1968.
20. Wolstenholme, G. E. W., and Knight, J. (eds.): The Balkan Nephropathy. Ciba Foundation Study Group No. 30. Boston, Little, Brown & Co., 1967.

Chapter Fourteen

Slowly Progressive Renal Vascular Disease

Introduction

Hypertension exists in from 15 to 20 per cent of the general population of the United States. Approximately 90 per cent of this group have no discernible cause for hypertension; the clinical syndrome in these patients is called "essential" or "idiopathic" hypertension. The remainder have secondary causes such as renal vascular disease (3 per cent), endocrinopathies (1 per cent), or chronic renal disease (1 per cent). Progression to marked blood pressure elevation (so-called malignant hypertension) most commonly is associated with pre-existing essential hypertension, but it may be seen in the other categories as well.

The relationship between renal vascular disease and hypertension has been studied and discussed frequently. Although narrowing of the larger branches of the renal artery, usually by atherosclerosis, can cause hypertension, the discussion in this chapter will be directed toward the relationship between hypertension and small artery and arteriolar changes.

As a result of an autopsy study of changes in small arteries and arterioles, Bell came to the following conclusions: (1) these arteries (interlobular size) show elastic reduplication which increases with age and which is independent of hypertension, although likely to be accelerated by it, (2) arteriolosclerosis increases with age, and (3) arteriolosclerosis accelerates as the blood pressure rises, even with pressure differences in the normal range.

Castleman and Smithwick performed a large number of renal biopsies during sympathectomy for the treatment of hypertension. They discovered that in 40 per cent of their patients only minor histologic indications of vascular injury were present, a finding that gave little support to the idea that small-vessel change is the cause of hypertension. In a review of previous studies and of his personal observations, Heptinstall (1954) concluded that arteriolosclerosis is a phenomenon of aging that is accentuated by hypertension, but hypertension probably plays no role in its initiation. It has been proven, however, that arteriolar necrosis is clearly related to elevated blood pressure.

Clinical Data

Slowly progressive renal vascular disease produces no symptoms in the majority of patients in its early stages. Proteinuria usually is absent, although it rarely may present in intermittent or moderate amounts (up to 2 g daily). In the absence of renal failure, the sediment contains only hyaline and fine granular casts, although occasionally intermittent microscopic hematuria might occur. Additionally, the earliest detectable abnormality in renal function is decreased tubular excretory function, which is manifested as reduction in renal plasma flow. Later, the glomerular filtration rate is affected as well. Hypertensive patients also have other renal functional abnormalities, such as an exaggerated natriuretic response to saline solutions, which is apparently a result and not a cause of increased blood pressure.

Histology

GLOMERULI. The glomeruli generally are unremarkable, except for evidence of ischemia manifested by collapse or "wrinkling" of some peripheral capillary loops (Figs. 14–1 and 14–2). This change may give the false impression that there is mesangial sclerosis, but the mesangial widening appears to be a result of the decreased size of the outer capillary loops in general, with complete collapse in selected areas (Fig. 14–3).

TUBULES AND INTERSTITIUM. The major alteration in the tubules and interstitium is scarring, which appears as irregular, zonal areas of increased interstitial connective tissue containing atrophied tubules and obsolescent glomeruli (Fig. 14–4). Small collections of lymphocytes also may be embedded in the connective tissue.

Elsewhere the tubules for the most part are not unusual, although there may be a mild, generalized thickening of their basal lamina. In the latter case there is a minor, diffuse increase in interstitial tissue (Fig. 14–5).

VESSELS. The interlobular arteries and afferent arterioles are the structures most conspicuously affected by slowly progressive renal vascular disease. The changes include an increase of extracellular material, as well as deposits of serum proteins. Additionally, the vascular alterations are accentuated in areas of interstitial scarring.

Text continued on page 187

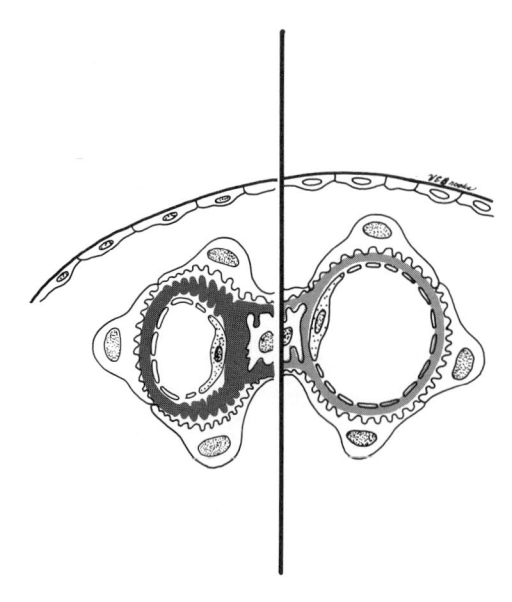

Figure 14-1 Diagram of an ischemic glomerulus. The major change is "wrinkling" of peripheral capillary loops, which is most pronounced near the mesangial regions.

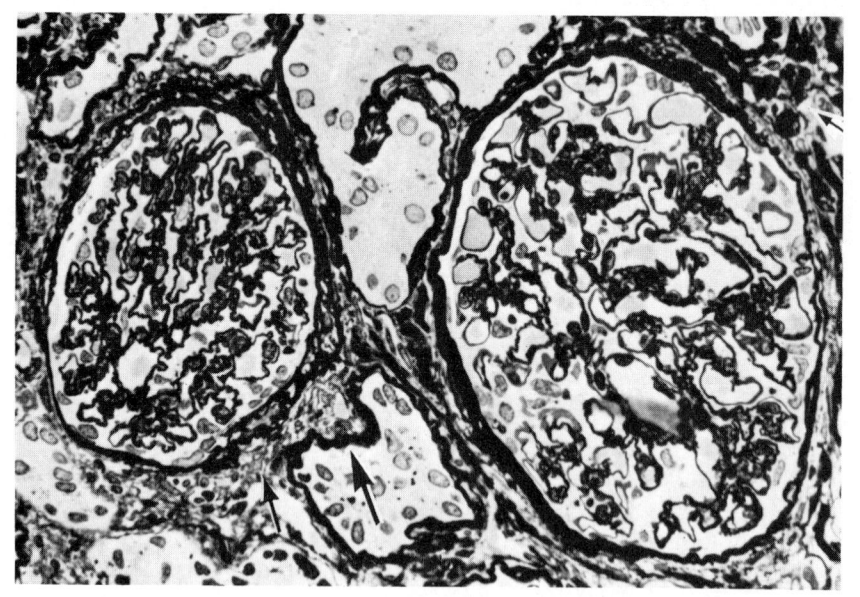

Figure 14-2 Specimen from a 72 year old man who was admitted to hospital because of the apparent acute onset of hypertension. The interstitial fibrosis (light arrows) and thickening of the tubular basal lamina (heavy arrow) suggest that this is a long-standing process. The glomeruli demonstrate varying degrees of wrinkling of the basal lamina. In the glomerulus on the right, wrinkling is most marked near the mesangial region, while the peripheral basal lamina for the most part appears normal. In the glomerulus on the left, the wrinkling extends throughout the basal lamina, even into the periphery. Note that in this glomerulus there is thickening and duplication of Bowman's basal lamina, which merges with the surrounding interstitial fibrosis. (Silver methenamine, ×300.)

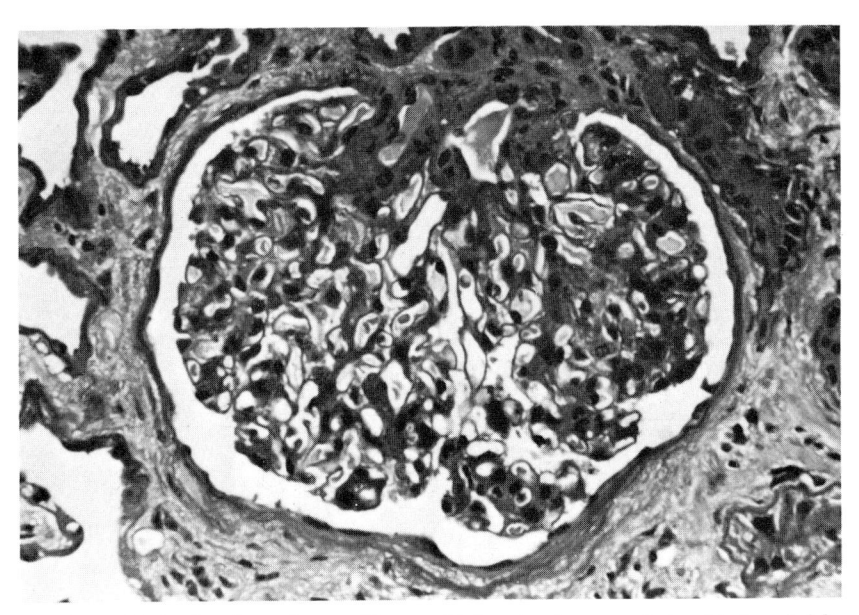

Figure 14–3 Specimen from a 57 year old female who was admitted to hospital for evaluation of hypertension and poor renal function. Note that in this section it is difficult to detect the wrinkling of the peripheral basal lamina. In fact, the mesangial areas appear to be increased. Only by silver methenamine staining can the wrinkling be fully appreciated and the mesangial sclerosis seen to be due to the accumulation of collapsed peripheral basal lamina. (H&E, ×300.)

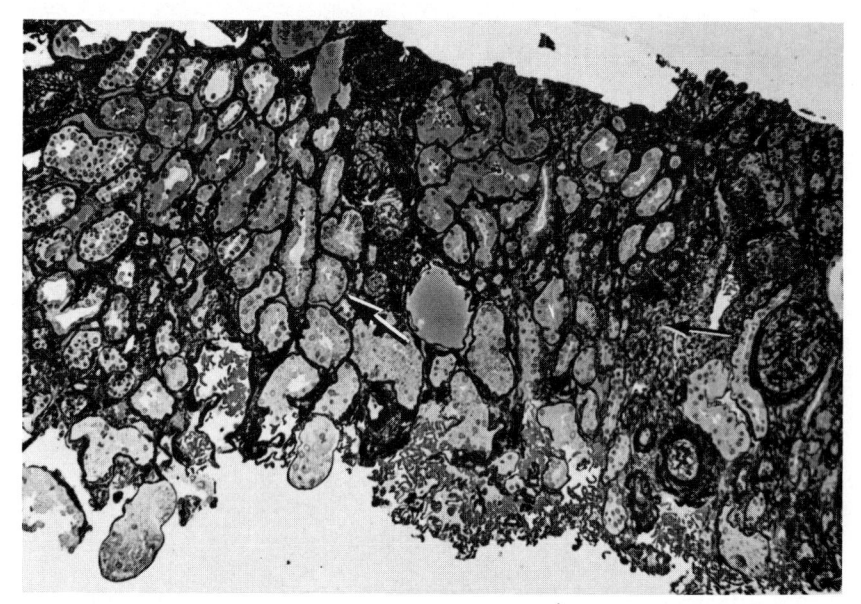

Figure 14-4 Low power photomicrograph of the same patient as in Figure 14-2. There are alternate areas of interstitial fibrosis with tubular atrophy (light arrow) and zones where the tubular and interstitium appear to be relatively preserved (heavy arrow). In the interstitial areas of fibrosis and tubular atrophy, Bowman's basal lamina is also thickened. (Silver methenamine, ×75.)

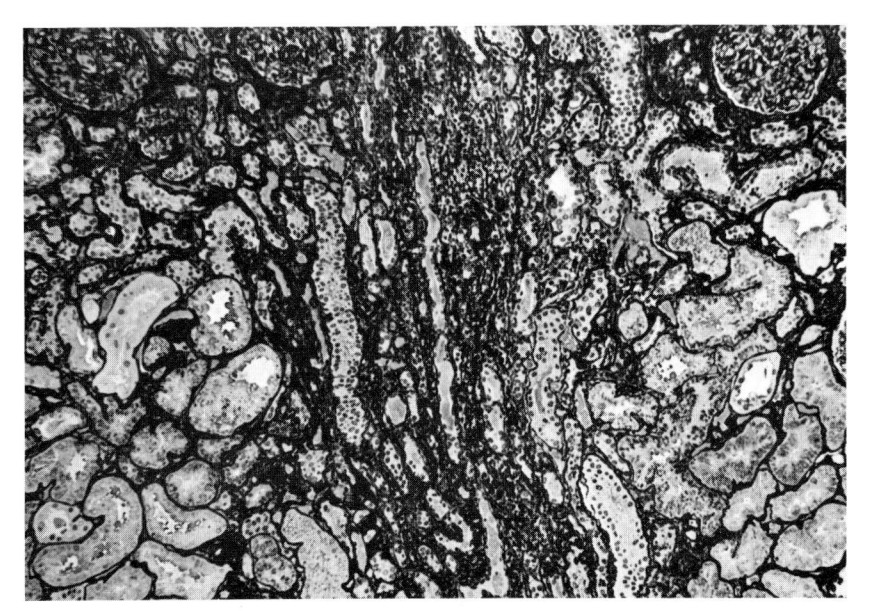

Figure 14-5 Another area from the same biopsy specimen as in Figures 14-2 and 14-4, demonstrating that in areas removed from the larger zones of fibrosis, the tubular basal laminae are slightly but generally thickened. (Silver methenamine, ×300.)

The extracellular material accumulation appears to be mostly in the form of multilayering of lamellae internal to the smooth muscle cell layers (Figs. 14-6, 14-7, and 14-8). This has been called duplication of the internal elastic lamella; in fact, the lamellae consist primarily of basal lamina and collagen (Fig. 14-9). There also is an increase in the basal lamina around the smooth muscle cells of the media, but this is a feature which is difficult to detect in the usual preparation.

In addition, a variable characteristic is the deposition of hyalin in the wall, usually between the endothelial and smooth muscle layer, occasionally forming an eccentrically placed mass or uniform "collar" (Figs. 14-10 and 14-11). This material may either interrupt or displace the continuity of the elastic lamella. At higher magnification the hyalin has a homogeneous, finely granular appearance (Fig. 14-12).

Clinical Course and Prognosis

For an understanding of the natural history of untreated hypertension, Perera's report (1955) is of value. He demonstrated that most patients: (1) are less than 50 years old when their blood pressure becomes elevated, (2) live approximately 15 years thereafter free of significant symptoms, and (3) during the next five years develop variable degrees of heart, brain, or kidney involvement. This disease is typified

Text continued on page 191

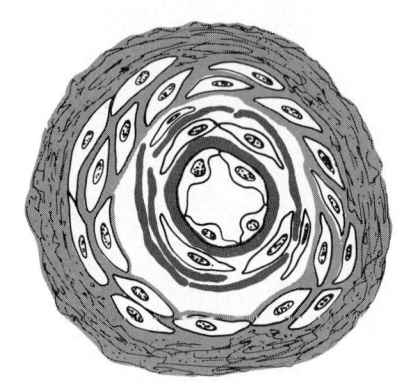

Figure 14-6 Diagram of a small artery, demonstrating multilayering of lamella internal to the smooth muscle cells of the media.

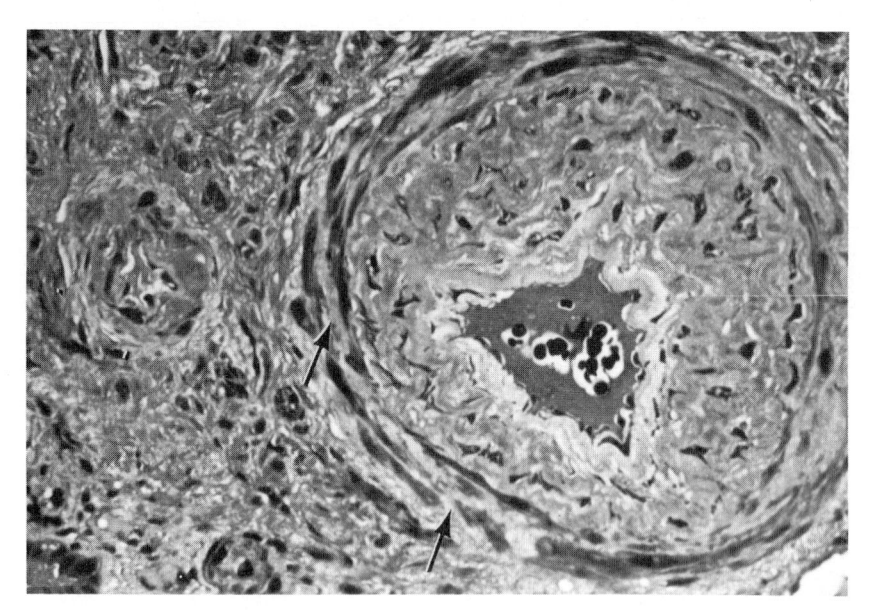

Figure 14-7 Artery from the same patient as in Figure 14-3. The smooth muscle cells of the media are surrounded by an increased amount of extracellular material (arrows). Internal to the media are multiple concentric layers of extracellular material, between which are interspersed elongated cells. The lumen is severely compromised. (H&E, ×300.)

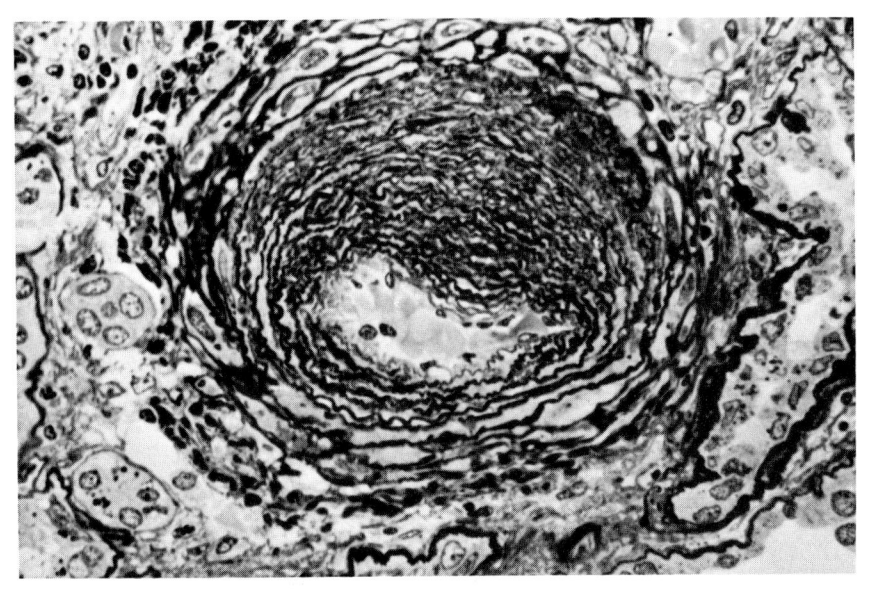

Figure 14-8 Silver stained preparation of an artery from the same patient as in Figure 14-3. Note that the laminated material internal to the media stains positively with silver methenamine. (× 300.)

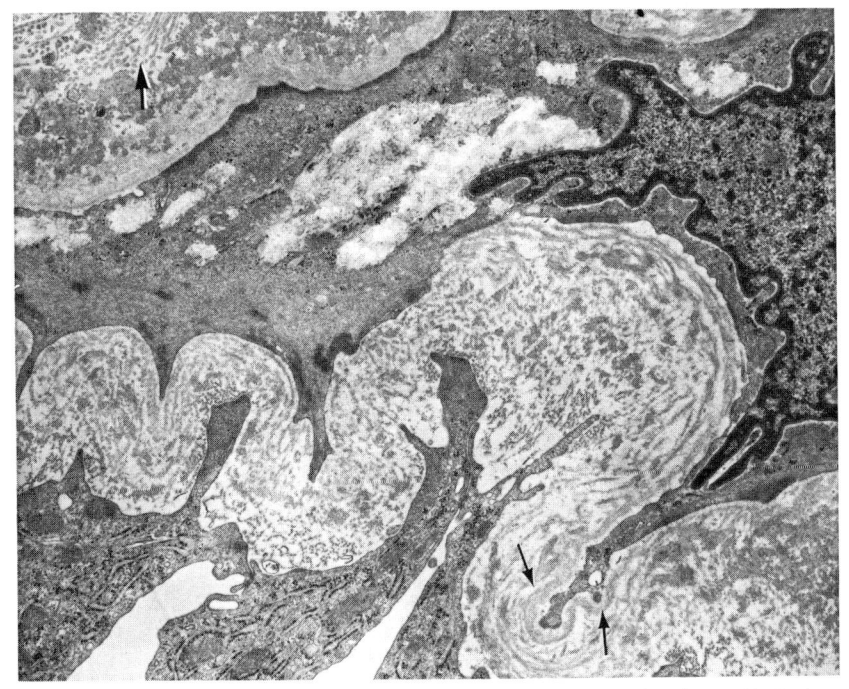

Figure 14-9 Electron micrograph from the same patient as in Figure 14-3, demonstrating that the extracellular material in the lamella consists of a considerable amount of identifiable collagen (light arrows) as well as fragments of basal lamina and cell debris (heavy arrow). (× 7500.)

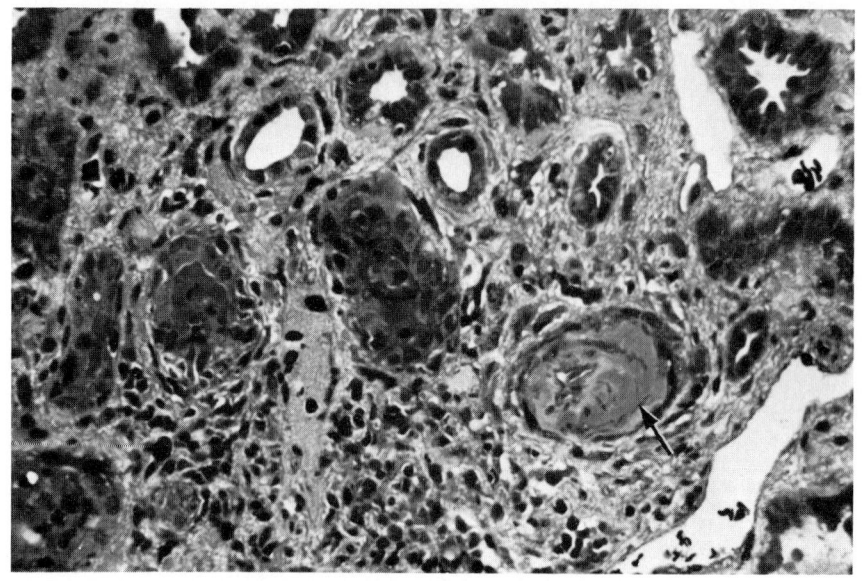

Figure 14-10 This biopsy specimen from a 63 year old man demonstrates rather marked deposition of a homogeneous, eosinophilic material in a subintimal location (arrow). The material appears to be deposited around the entire circumference of the vessel and at one point extends into the media. (H&E, ×300.)

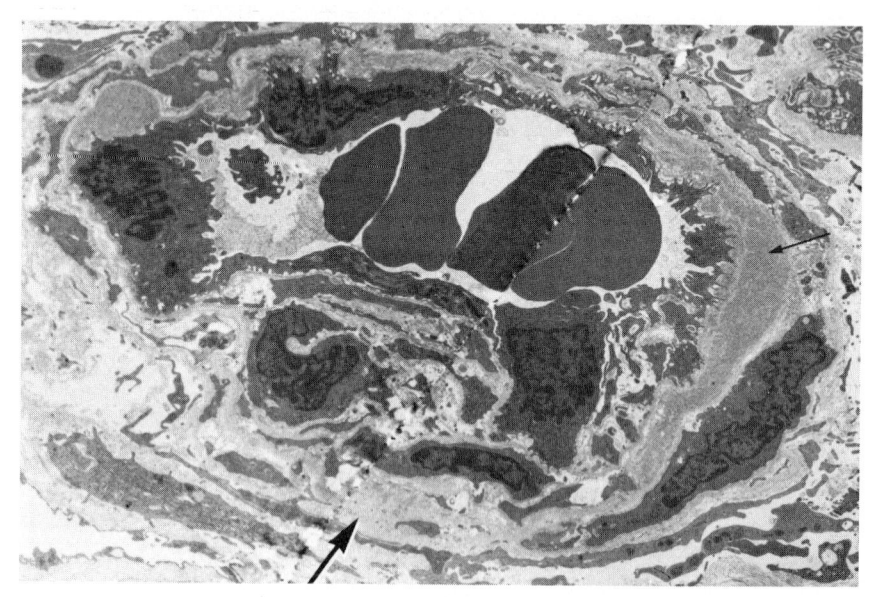

Figure 14-11 A low power electron micrograph of a small artery of a 51 year old man who had long-standing proteinuria and mild hypertension. The area between the intima and surrounding smooth muscle cells contains irregular quantities of a homogeneous, electron-dense material (light arrow) and a variable increase in the amount of extracellular material between smooth muscle cells (heavy arrow). (×1000.)

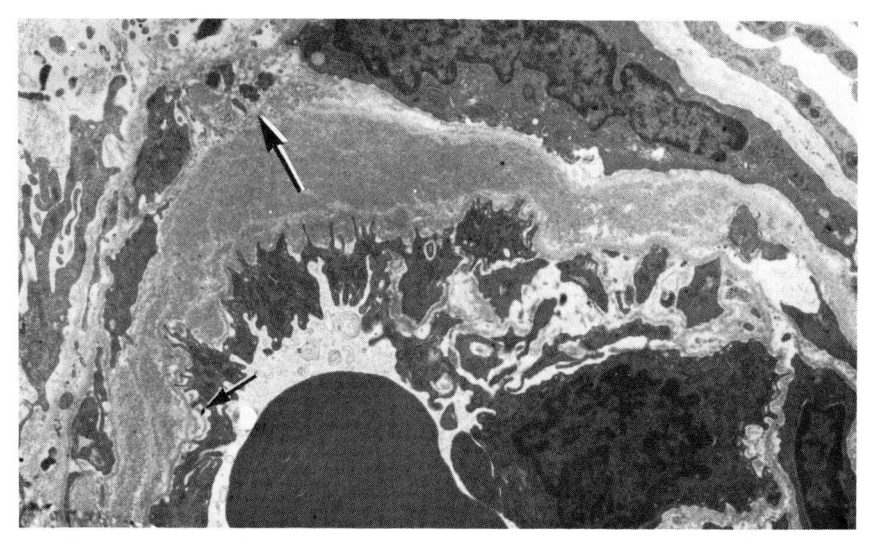

Figure 14–12 Higher magnification of Figure 14–11, demonstrating multilayering of the basal lamina beneath the endothelium (light arrow) and the homogeneous nature of the hyalin. Also demonstrable are collections of cell debris (heavy arrow). (× 2500.)

by marked individual variation. Some patients have rapid and extensive organ deterioration, whereas others have hypertension for more than 20 years without clinically significant complications.

The results of the Framingham study (Dawber and Kannel, 1961) indicated that stroke, coronary arteriosclerosis, and congestive heart failure are more common in the hypertensive population than in people with normal blood pressure. There also is evidence that hypertension increases the mortality from vascular diseases.

Although the majority of patients with hypertension have nephrosclerosis, only a few have serious impairment of renal function. Most patients with essential hypertension who develop uremia do so as the result of an acute acceleration of their disease to malignant nephrosclerosis (see Chapter 11).

The Veterans Administration Cooperative Study Group on Antihypertensive Agents (1970) has shown that treatment of hypertension significantly improves prognosis. Therapy has been most effective in preventing congestive heart failure and stroke. Unfortunately, reduction in the incidence and severity of coronary artery disease has not been as impressive.

References

1. Bell, E. T.: Renal Diseases. 2nd Ed. Philadelphia, Lea and Febiger, 1950.
2. Castleman, B., and Smithwick, R. H.: The relationship of vascular disease to the

hypertensive state: II. The adequacy of the renal biopsy as determined from a study of 500 patients. New Eng. J. Med. *239*:729, 1948.
3. Dawber, T. R., and Kannel, W. B.: Susceptibility to coronary heart disease. Mod. Concepts Cardiovasc. Dis. *30*:671, 1961.
4. Dustin, P., Jr.: Arteriolar hyalinosis. *In* Richter, G. W., and Epstein, M. A., eds.: International Review of Experimental Pathology. Vol. 1. New York, Academic Press, 1962.
5. Hamburger, J., Richet, G., Crosnier, J., Funck-Bretano, J. L., Antoine, B., Ducrot, H., Mery, J. P., and Montera, H.: Nephrology (translated by Anthony Walsh). Philadelphia, W. B. Saunders Co., 1968.
6. Heptinstall, R. H.: Renal biopsies in hypertension. Brit. Heart J. *16*:133, 1954.
7. Perera, G. A.: Hypertensive vascular disease: Description and natural history. J. Chron. Dis. *1*:33, 1955.
8. Veterans Administration, Cooperative Study Group on Antihypertensive Agents. J.A.M.A. *202*:1028, 1967; *213*:1143, 1970.

Section IV

NEPHROTIC SYNDROME

Chapter Fifteen

Infantile Nephrotic Syndrome

Introduction

The infantile nephrotic syndrome is defined as that type which occurs during the first year of life. The histologic lesion associated with the disease varies according to the geographic location of the children. In Finland, for example, where there is a high incidence of the syndrome, virtually all patients have microcystic disease, whereas in France and Canada primary glomerular disorders are more common.

Clinical Data

In North American children, the nephrotic syndrome is likely to be associated with either microcystic disease or primary mesangial disease. It is significant that the distinction between these conditions often is uncertain clinically. Although family history, premature birth, placentomegaly, presence of other minor congenital abnormalities of the face and limbs, early age of presentation, and lower plasma albumin level all tend to suggest microcystic disease, none of these features is pathognomonic.

Differentiation ultimately depends on histologic examination. Although patients with microcystic disease all die within a few months of developing the nephrotic syndrome, those with primary mesangial disease tend to survive. Since the characteristic tubular changes of microcystic disease become progressively more apparent with the passage of time, a delay of one or two months from the onset of nephrotic syndrome before performing a biopsy might be expected to facilitate their recognition. In the planning of long-term management, however, an earlier search may be needed in order to allow for estimates of prognosis and genetic counseling.

Although in microcystic disease the light microscopic picture is dominated by proximal tubular dilatation, glomerular abnormalities also are evident on electron microscopy. Microdissection of nephrons previously has demonstrated that microcystic tubules often are abnormally narrow distal to the dilated segments. The ultrastructural changes observed in the proximal tubular cells could be either the cause of the tubular dilatation and narrowing or the result of tubular atrophy, but no evidence suggesting an immunologic pathogenetic mechanism has been found (Lange et al., 1963; Kouvalainen, 1963; Hoyer et al., 1967; Griswold and McIntosh, 1972).

The children with primary glomerular disease are not a homogeneous group. The reported abnormalities vary from podocyte fusion to diffuse sclerosis. Additionally, since the presence of prominent glomerular epithelial cells in infants may confuse the assessment of glomerular cellularity, thin histologic sections and confirmatory electron microscopy are essential to differentiate this condition from minimal change nephrotic syndrome (Churg et al., 1970). The presence of obsolescent glomeruli in increased numbers also could facilitate that distinction.

We recently have had the opportunity to review the patients with infantile nephrotic syndrome who had been entered into an ongoing study at the University of Washington over a period of 13 years. The cases all showed marked local or diffuse mesangial cell proliferation, with varying degrees of glomerular sclerosis. Only one patient had immunoglobulin deposition. Two-thirds of these patients are still alive.

The majority of patients were boys, and there was no predilection for race. Consanguinity is not a feature of either the microcystic or the primary glomerular varieties of the syndrome, but placentomegaly, prematurity, and low birth weight are common features in patients with the microcystic lesion. Although there is no consistent pattern of associated anomalies in the infantile syndrome, we discovered a large number of apparently unrelated findings in our patients. In the microcystic group, one patient had low-set ears, Meckel's diverticulum, and patent ductus arteriosus; one displayed talipes calcaneovalgus; another had pyloric stenosis; one had proximally displaced thumbs, misshapen ears, a small snub nose, and Meckel's diverticulum. In the primary mesangial disease group, one child displayed protruding, low-set ears, frontal bossing, a depressed nasal bridge, and short limbs, as well as a systolic murmur at the left sternal edge. Chest x-ray, Venereal Disease Research Laboratory test (VDRL), chromosome analysis, and tests for urinary amino acids and mucopolysaccharides were normal.

The most striking laboratory findings are proteinuria, hypoalbuminemia, and normal blood urea nitrogen or creatinine.

Histology

MICROCYSTIC DISEASE. Microcystic disease is characterized by variable proximal tubular dilatation with the appearance of low-lying proximal tubular epithelial cells (Figs. 15–1 and 15–2). The number and prominence of the dilated tubules increase with time. In addition, the electron microscopic features are striking in that the basal infoldings, microvilli, and mitochondria are small and sparse in all proximal tubules. The tubular basement membranes often are thick and duplicated, while the dilated lumina are empty or contained hyaline casts or red blood cells. The distal tubules generally are normal on light and electron microscopy, and the interstitial regions are widened by edema and mononuclear cell infiltration.

Bowman's spaces often are dilated, especially in early biopsies, where the podocytes were seen to be fused, the lamina densa of the glomerular capillary basement membranes was focally duplicated, and the lamina rara interna irregularly was widened by fine, flocculent, electron-dense material (Fig. 15–3). The mesangial matrix also is expanded mildly to moderately, the epithelial cells were increased in number, and the endothelial cells were prominent, with many mitochondria and multiple processes projecting into the capillary lumina.

PRIMARY MESANGIAL DISEASE. The patients with primary mesangial disease are not entirely a homogeneous group. Their major changes are glomerular. The mesangial matrix always is expanded, often markedly, in association with either a local (generally axial) or diffuse increase in the number of mesangial cells (Fig. 15–4). The podocytes are partially or completely fused, the lamina densa of the glomerular capillary basal laminal focally duplicated, the lamina rara interna irregularly widened by fine, flocculent, electron-dense material, and the epithelial cells increased in number; occasionally the endothelial cells are prominent and have surface projections. The tubular alterations are restricted to atrophy, which is proportional and presumably secondary to glomerular obsolescence. Red blood cell casts, hyaline casts, and free red cells also are present in the lamina. The interstitial regions contain mononuclear cells and connective tissue approximately proportional to the degree of glomerular obsolescence. The interstitial vessels generally are normal.

Clinical Course and Prognosis

It has been our experience that nearly all children with the microcystic disease succumb to infection within the first year, whereas those with other lesions often do quite well. The microcystic patients, for example, all died of complications from infection at a mean age of

Text continued on page 200

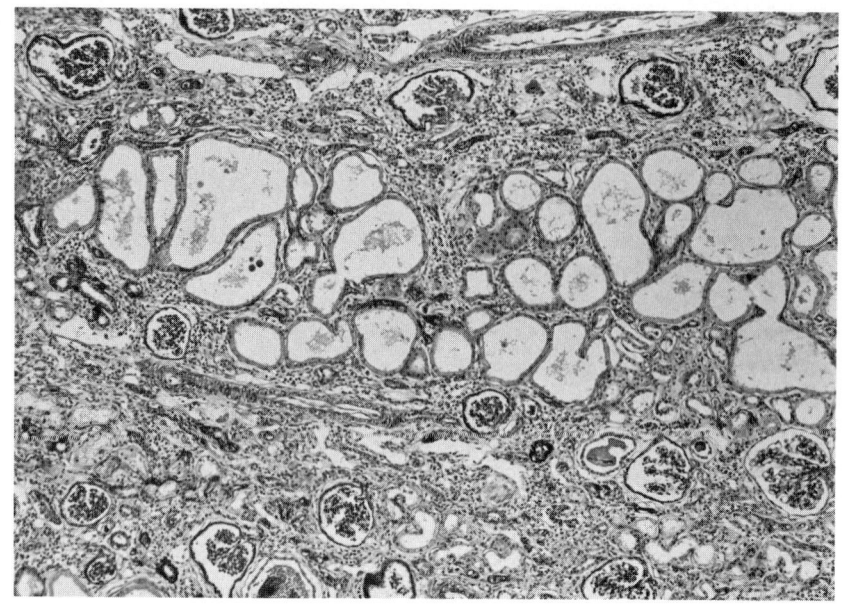

Figure 15–1 Low power photomicrograph of an autopsy specimen from a 2½ month old child who was noted to have proteinuria at birth. Within 1 month the child was grossly edematous and had multiple episodes of skin and pulmonary infection. At this magnification the principal abnormality appears to be marked dilatation of many of the tubules. The glomeruli do not appear to be abnormal. (H&E, × 75.)

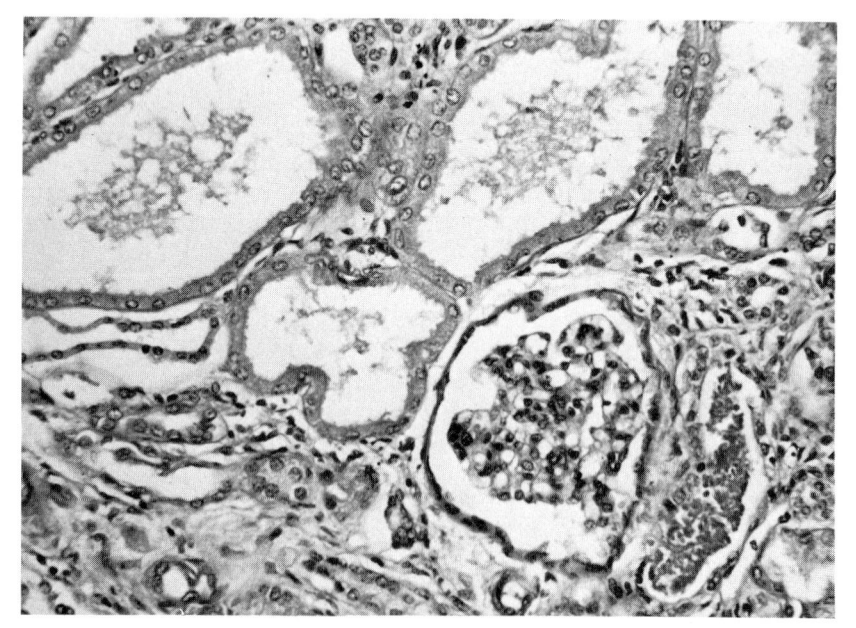

Figure 15–2 Higher power micrograph of the same patient as in Figure 15–1. The glomerulus appears normal. The tubules are dilated and have low-lying epithelium. The tubule at the lower right contains granular material. (H&E, ×300.)

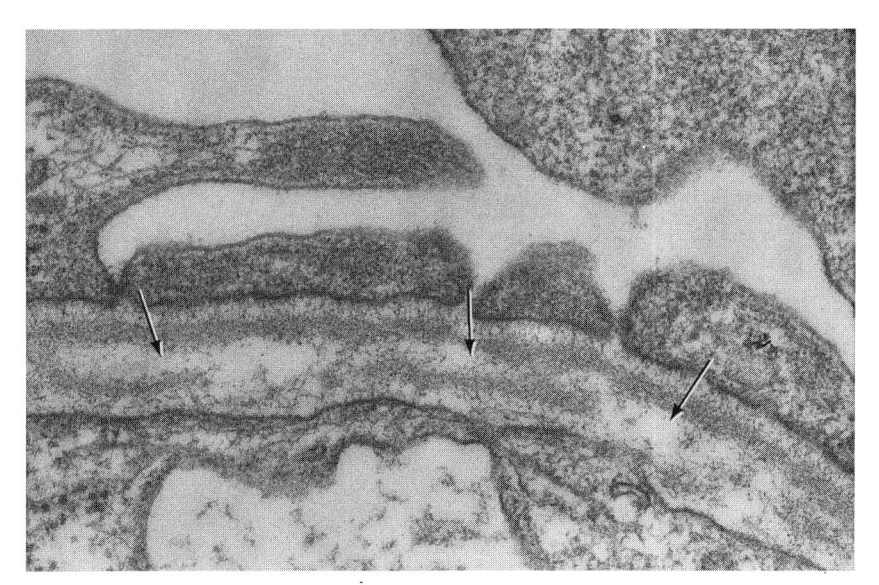

Figure 15-3 Electron micrograph from the same patient as in Figures 15-1 and 15-2. The basal lamina is duplicated in an irregular fashion. There also is a quantity of flocculent, electron-dense material resembling basal lamina (arrows) lying beneath the endothelium cells. The endothelial cell cytoplasm is swollen and quite prominent throughout. The epithelial cells have a normal appearance in this area. The basal lamina changes are quite irregular, having the multilaminated appearance in only a small fraction of the total peripheral capillary loop. ($\times 30,000$.)

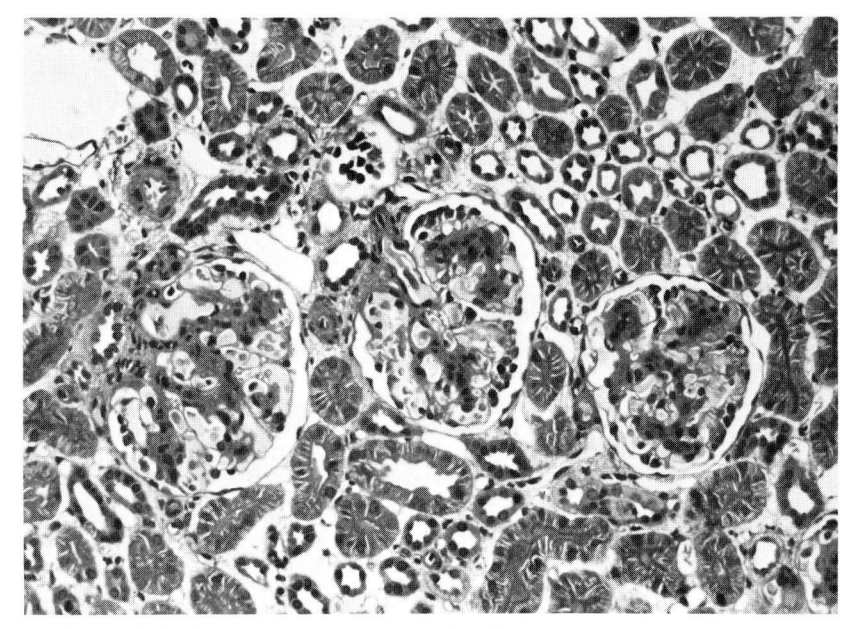

Figure 15-4 Specimen from a 4 month old child who was noted to have proteinuria at his 6 week checkup. Red cells and red blood cell casts were seen in the urine. The glomeruli in this biopsy are seen to be the primary site of involvement. There is an increased amount of mesangial matrix, as well as an increased number of mesangial cells. The surrounding tubules and interstitium appear relatively normal. This child is now 4 years old and has normal renal function. (H&E, $\times 300$.)

15 weeks (range: 6 weeks to 11 months), and none had developed chronic renal failure before death.

At the same time, four of the patients with primary mesangial disease remained alive, with normal renal function, at a mean age of 58 months (range: 17 months to 9 years). Currently, none is nephrotic, although one has mild hypertension. Two patients died, one suddenly of undetermined causes at the age of 20 months, having received no corticosteroid or immunosuppressive therapy, and the other from coliform meningitis at the age of 22 weeks while being treated with prednisolone and cyclophosphamide.

Because neither corticosteroid nor immunosuppressive treatment has been shown to cause consistent reduction in proteinuria, and since deaths in several series commonly have been demonstrated to be due to infectious complications, this therapeutic regimen should be employed sparingly. Furthermore, since infantile nephrotic syndrome associated with primary mesangial disease often has a favorable immediate prognosis, any treatment which predisposes to its most ominous complication appears risky. Similarly, it is difficult to support a policy of early renal transplantation for all neonatal patients with nephrotic syndrome in anticipation of inevitable mortality during early childhood without careful histologic study of renal tissue and function. Meticulous supportive and antibiotic therapy, however, might be predicted to be of greater ultimate benefit. Finally, precise morphologic differentiation of the two disease groups commonly involved will also improve genetic counseling, thereby decreasing the likelihood of additional children with microcystic disease being born.

References

1. Churg, J., Habib, R., and White, R. H. R.: Pathology of the nephrotic syndrome in children. Lancet *1*:1299, 1970.
2. George, C. R. P., Hickman, R. O., and Striker, G. E.: Infantile nephrotic syndrome. Clin. Nephrol. 5:20, 1976.
3. Grupe, W. E., Cuppage, F. E., and Haymann, W.: Congenital nephrotic syndrome with interstitial nephritis. Amer. J. Dis. Child. *111*:482, 1966.
4. Habib, R., and Bois, E.: Hétérogénéité des syndromes néphrotiques à début précose du nourrisson (syndrome néphrotique "infantile"). Etude anatomo-clinique et génétique de 37 observations. Helv. Paediat. Acta *28*:91, 1973.
5. Hallman, N., Norio, R., and Rapola, J.: Congenital nephrotic syndrome. Nephron *11*:101, 1973.
6. Hoyer, J. R., Michael, A. F. Good, R. A., and Vernier, R. L.: The nephrotic syndrome of infancy: clinical, morphologic, and immunologic studies of four infants. Pediatrics *40*:233, 1967.
7. Kaplan, B. S., Bureau, M. A., and Drummond, K. N.: The nephrotic syndrome in the first year of life: Is a pathologic classification possible? Pediatrics *85*:615, 1974.
8. Norio, R.: Heredity in the congenital nephrotic syndrome. Ann. Paediat. Fenn. *12*:1, (Suppl. 27) 1966.
9. Oliver, J.: Microcystic renal disease and its relation to "infantile nephrosis." Am. J. Dis. Child. *100*:312, 1960.
10. Paatela, M.: Renal microdissection in infants with special reference to the congenital nephrotic syndrome. Ann. Paediat. Fenn. *9*:1, (Suppl. 21) 1963.

Chapter Sixteen

Primary Nephrotic Syndrome

Introduction

Nothing is more confusing in nephrology than the clinical syndrome of nephrosis and its relationship to other renal and systemic diseases. The classical definition of nephrotic syndrome includes proteinuria (in excess of 2 g/day/m^2), hypoalbuminemia, hypercholesterolemia, and edema. Since the last three characteristics probably are due to the heavy proteinuria, a more simplified approach would be to limit the definition to heavy protein excretion. However, some patients might excrete large amounts of protein without manifesting the other abnormalities, whereas others may excrete less protein and have all the classic findings. Therefore, strict definitions may be misleading.

A myriad of etiologies, histologic features, and clinical presentations have been linked to the nephrotic syndrome. In fact, virtually every form of glomerular disease, and even some nonglomerular forms, has been implicated. In an attempt to overcome this confusing situation, we have subdivided this *syndrome* into three categories (Table 16-1): (1) nephrotic syndrome associated with systemic diseases, (2) primary nephrotic syndrome, often referred to as the idiopathic nephrotic syndrome, and (3) nephrotic syndrome associated with other renal syndromes, such as glomerulonephritis. Since the term "idiopathic" has become associated with one particular histologic lesion by pediatricians (minimal lesion) and with another by internists (membranous lesion), and thus is a source of confusion, we will use the designation "primary nephrotic syndrome." More thorough reviews of nephrosis associated with other renal and nonrenal syndromes are discussed in the appropriate chapters.

TABLE 16-1

Nephrotic syndromes associated with systemic diseases:
   Diabetes mellitus (Chapter 21)
   Systemic lupus erythematosus (Chapter 17)
   Amyloid (Chapter 23)
Primary nephrotic syndrome:
   Infantile nephrotic syndrome (Chapter 14)
   Minimal lesion nephrosis
   Proliferative lesion nephrosis
     Pure proliferative
     Membranoproliferative
       With subendothelial deposits
       With dense intramembranous deposits
   Sclerosing lesion nephrosis
     Focal and global sclerosis
     Membranous lesion
Nephrotic syndrome associated with other renal syndromes (the *nephritic* nephrotic):
   Glomerular disease of acute onset with/without rapid progression (Chapters 7 and 8)
   Slowly progressive glomerular disease (Chapter 11)

NEPHROTIC SYNDROME ASSOCIATED WITH SYSTEMIC DISEASE

Diabetes is probably the most common systemic disease associated with the nephrotic syndrome. When a diabetic patient becomes nephrotic, the renal lesion is advanced and functional impairment is evident (Chapter 21). In addition, a patient with systemic lupus erythematosus who also is nephrotic often has a more severe and progressive form of nephritis (Chapter 17). Furthermore, the deposition of amyloid material in the glomeruli usually is advanced when the patients present with nephrosis. *Accordingly, when the nephrotic syndrome is associated with systemic disease, it has a poor prognosis simply because it signifies advanced or severe renal damage.*

NEPHROTIC SYNDROME ASSOCIATED WITH OTHER RENAL SYNDROMES

The term "nephrosis" can be used to differentiate the patient who has heavy proteinuria with normal urine sediment and renal function from the patient who has an abnormal urine sediment and renal insufficiency and who presumably had a significant glomerular lesion. Patients who have the nephrotic syndrome in association with other renal syndromes nearly always have renal insufficiency at the time of onset of heavy proteinuria or develop significant renal functional abnormalities shortly thereafter. The patient with nephritis can have significant proteinuria and therefore can be *nephrotic* as well, the occurrence of these two findings together signifying severe or advanced renal disease. Furthermore, patients with glomerular disease of acute onset who have an associated heavy proteinuria, and consequently are nephrotic as well, tend to have advanced renal lesions and a poor prognosis (Chapters 7 and 8). Similarly, when a patient with slowly progressive glomerular disease enters a nephrotic stage, this often signals the terminal phase of his disease.

PRIMARY NEPHROTIC SYNDROME

INTRODUCTION

In nephritic patients, heavy proteinuria occurs when the disease is far advanced, and is therefore an ominous sign. This stands in sharp contrast to patients with the primary nephrotic syndrome, in whom heavy proteinuria and its consequences are the main clinical features, and in whom renal failure rarely is a presenting problem. Renal insufficiency may occur in the primary nephrotic syndrome, but only after a fairly long course of nephrosis.

The following discussion of the *primary nephrotic syndrome* will center on three histologic characteristics: (1) minimal lesion (lipoid nephrosis), (2) proliferative lesion, and (3) sclerosing lesion (Table 16-2). It is difficult to use clinical grounds alone to determine the nature of the injury; therefore, renal biopsy is indicated strongly in the evaluation of the primary nephrotic syndrome.

The clinical presentation of primary nephrotic syndrome often is not helpful in determining the underlying pathologic process. The most common complaint is edema, which in children frequently is periorbital. Constitutional complaints such as anorexia, weakness, and malaise also are common.

Edema is the most frequent physical finding, whereas hypertension is less common, even in the more progressive forms of this syndrome, until renal function is significantly reduced. Renal function usually is normal, and the degree of hypoalbuminemia tends to correlate with the severity of proteinuria. Hyperlipidemia frequently occurs to remarkable levels, and usually mimics the pattern of a Frederickson Type II hyperlipidemia. (The most helpful clinical data for distinguishing the type of lesion present prior to biopsy are summarized in Tables 16-2 and 16-3).

MINIMAL LESION

CLINICAL DATA

The minimal lesion is the most common cause of nephrotic syndrome in children and accounts for over 90 per cent of cases in the first decade of life. In fact, age is the most important factor in the diagnosis of minimal lesion. Males are affected more commonly than females.

TABLE 16-2. Distinguishing Features of Primary Nephrotic Syndrome

	Minimal Lesion	Proliferative Lesions — Pure proliferative	Proliferative Lesions — Membranoproliferative	Sclerosing Lesions — Focal Sclerosis	Sclerosing Lesions — Membranous Sclerosis
Incidence*					
Children	70%	5%	10%	10%	5%
Adults	20%	40%	5%	5%	30%
Sex preponderance	Male (70%)	Equal	Slight female	Male (65%)	Male (70%)
Urinalysis					
Hematuria (0–4+)	0	2+, casts common	3+, many casts	1+, rare casts	1+, rare casts
RBC casts					
Proteinuria, selectivity	Moderate, massive, selective	Moderate, nonselective	Moderate, nonselective	Moderate, massive, nonselective	Moderate, massive, nonselective
Complement levels					
C3	Normal	Normal	Low	Normal	Normal
C4	Normal	Normal	Normal	Normal	Normal
Response to treatment	Good	Rare	Rare	Rare	Rare
Spontaneous remission	Common	Rare	Rare	Rare	Common
Relapse	Frequent	Frequent	Frequent	Frequent	Frequent
Prognosis	Good	Poor; progressive to renal failure	Poor; progressive to renal failure	Poor; progressive to renal failure	Poor; slow progression to renal failure
Histology					
Light microscopy	Normal	Proliferation of intraglomerular cells with varying degrees of sclerosis	Mesangial proliferation and increased mesangial matrix; focal thickening of GBL; often lobular pattern	Focal, segmental sclerosis progressing to complete sclerosis	Diffuse, regular thickening of GBL
Electron microscopy	Fusion of pedicels	Confirms light microscopic finding	Mesangial and intramembranous deposits; splitting of GBL	Confirms light microscopic findings	Regular subepithelial or intramembranous deposits
Immunofluorescence	Negative	Various patterns	C3 in mesangium and peripheral GBL	IgM, IgG, C3 in sclerotic areas	IgG, C3 in regular deposits

*Per cent of cases of PNS in each histologic group based on review of multiple surveys.

Protein excretion can be massive but usually there is a predominance of albumin (selective proteinuria). Oval fat bodies are easily found in the urine, but red cells or red cell casts are very rare.

HISTOLOGY

LIGHT MICROSCOPY. On routine light microscopy, no abnormality is detected except for what appears to be a continuous layer of cytoplasm over the external side of the glomerular basal lamina (Figs. 16-1, 16-2, 16-3). The proximal tubules also may contain an increased number of vacuoles, but this is an irregular feature.

ELECTRON MICROSCOPY. On electron microscopy, however, the usual pedicellar architecture with interdigitation of adjacent cell processes is found to be effaced over large areas of the capillary loops (Fig. 16-4). The cell junctions also appear to be abnormal in that the usual filtration membrane is difficult to demonstrate. The remainder of the glomerulus is unaffected.

CLINICAL COURSE AND PROGNOSIS

The course of minimal lesion nephrosis is characterized by a good response to corticosteroids (90 per cent in children and 66 per cent in adults), but also by frequent relapses (60 to 90 per cent in children, 30 per cent in adults). Occasionally, patients become steroid resistant (no longer respond to previously effective doses) or steroid dependent (steroid dosages cannot be tapered to an acceptable level without relapse). In these situations, however, other cytotoxic agents, such as cyclophosphamide and chlorambucil, have proved effective in inducing prolonged remissions. Progression of this lesion to end-stage renal failure is rare and probably represents misinterpretation of the original histologic lesion.

PROLIFERATIVE LESIONS

CLINICAL DATA

The proliferative lesions are a heterogeneous group of mixed types and varying etiologies that are grouped together simply because they share the histologic features of proliferation of intraglomerular cells.

One distinct group has been identified, however, and information about its pathogenesis clarified: membranoproliferative glomerulonephritis (MPGN). Two histologically distinct subtypes have been described, those with subendothelial deposits (SED) and those with dense intramembranous deposits (DIMD). Although each may have different etiologies, their clinical presentations are very similar and biopsy is

Text continued on page 208

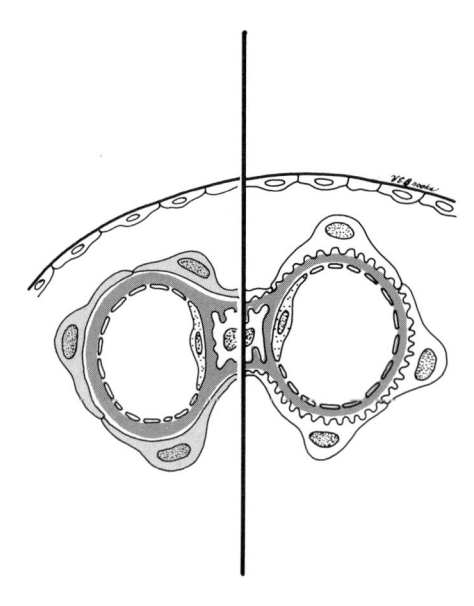

Figure 16–1 Diagram showing effacement of the normal architecture of the podocytes and the formation of a continuous layer over the external surface of the basal lamina.

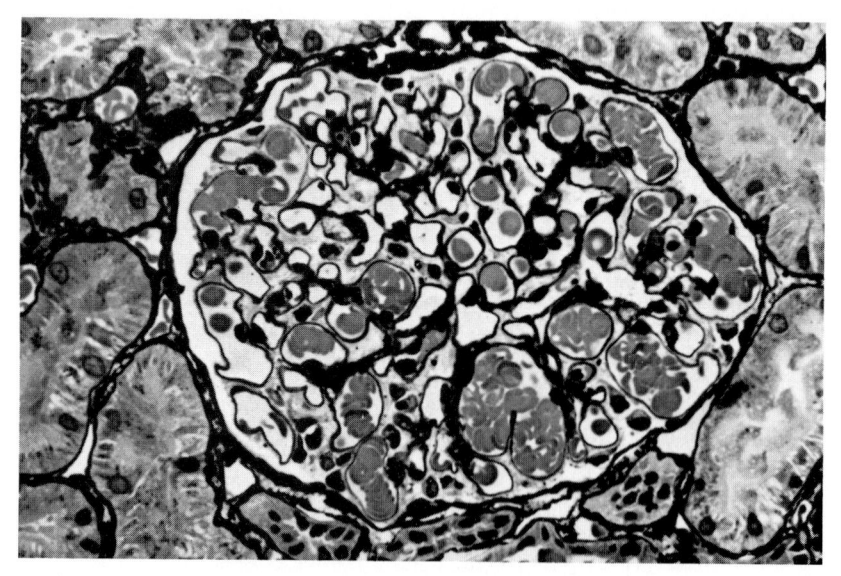

Figure 16–2 Specimen from a 4 year old child who was admitted to hospital because of marked, generalized edema. The urine sediment contained only oval fat bodies, and renal function was normal. The basal lamina and mesangial regions are unremarkable. The capillary spaces are widely patent throughout. (Silver methenamine, × 300.)

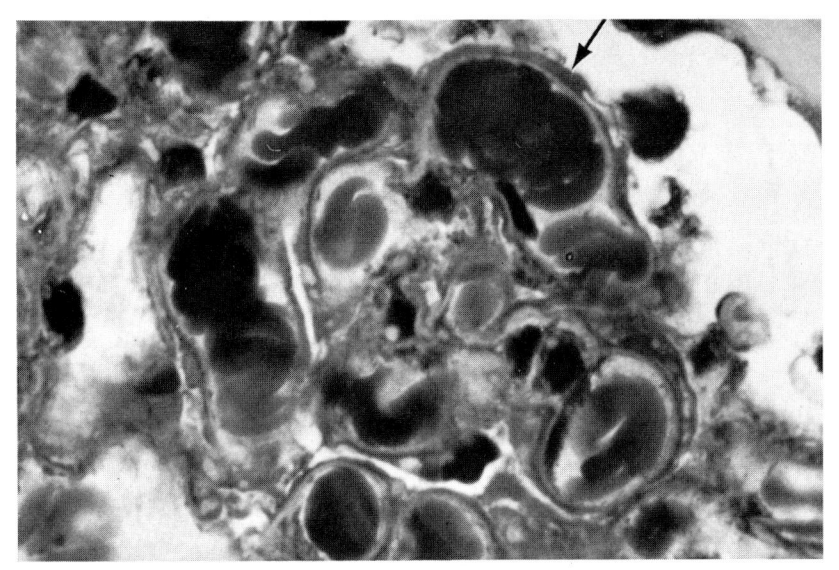

Figure 16–3 Same patient as in Figure 16–2. At high power the epithelial cell foot processes can be seen to be completely effaced over the majority of the peripheral capillary loops. The lucent basal lamina adjacent to the red cells in the capillary lumen is clearly outlined by a continuous sheet of epithelial cell cytoplasm (arrow). (H&E, ×1200.)

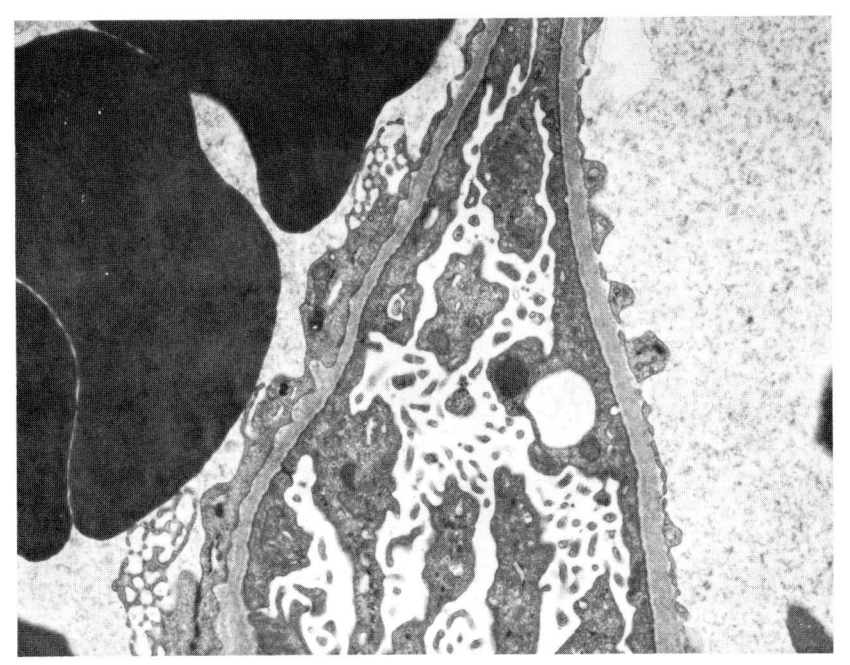

Figure 16–4 Electron micrograph from same patient as in Figures 16–2 and 16–3. The epithelial cells form a continuous sheet rather than occurring in pedicels. Note that cell junctions are widely spaced. The basal lamina and underlying endothelium are not affected. (×5000.)

necessary to determine the type of lesion. Previous infection is reported in about 50 per cent of each type of lesion, although streptococcal infection is relatively rare. Nephrotic syndrome is the mode of presentation in over 80 per cent of cases, although an occasional patient may present with renal insufficiency, hypertension, and an abnormal urine sediment (i.e., a nephritic picture). Hematuria, often macroscopic, is the rule and red cell casts are easily identified. Although hypocomplementemia was thought to be common in this histologic category of the disease, it is most often associated with MPGN with DIMD. MPGN is thought to represent a disease in which the "alternate pathway" of complement activation is involved. The "classic pathway," whereby complement is activated by antigen-antibody complexes, requires the interaction of the initial components of complements (C1, C4, and C2). Activation of these components leads to C3 activation, which in turn initiates the attack sequence of complement (C5 to C9) leading to chemotaxis, cell adherence, and lysis.

The attack sequence also can be initiated independently of the classic pathway by other plasma components through an alternate pathway. One such component, called C3-nephritic factor, has been found in the serum of patients with MPGN with DIMD. This disease is mediated by the immune system, but instead of involving the antibody system, it appears to reflect an abnormality of the effector complement system. Table 16–3 summarizes the clinical and histologic differences between these two morphologically different entities.

HISTOLOGY

PURE PROLIFERATIVE LESION

Light Microscopy. When all other renal and nonrenal syndromes associated with proliferation of glomerular cells are excluded, only a small group of patients who are nephrotic and have this morphologic lesion remain. The proliferation also commonly affects only the mesangial cells (Figs. 16–5, 16–6).

The lesion may be difficult to detect unless a careful cell count is performed, since the glomeruli may appear to be normocellular. More often, however, there is a clear increase in cell numbers (Figs. 16–5, 16–6). The type most often involved are mesangial cells. There frequently also is an increase in the amount of mesangial matrix. The sclerosis is most prominent near the vascular pole. Late in the process the mesangial matrix is diffusely increased.

Electron Microscopy. Electron microscopy, however, shows an increased number of cells, which are mainly of mesangial origin. There often is an increase in mesangial matrix as well (Fig. 16–7).

Fluorescence Microscopy. Few studies report findings on fluorescence microscopy in this condition, and there appears to be no consistent or characteristic pattern.

PRIMARY NEPHROTIC SYNDROME 209

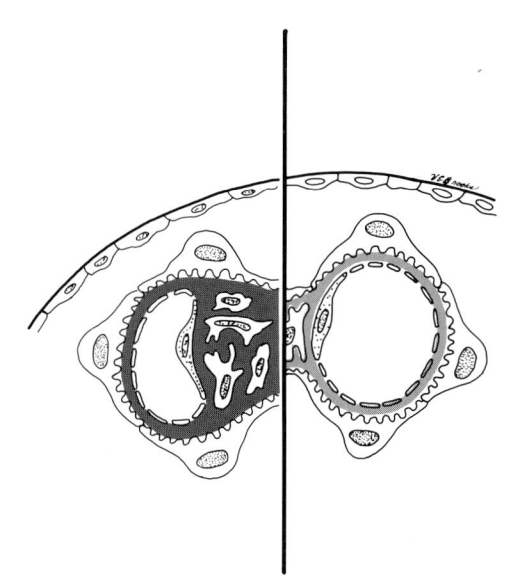

Figure 16–5 Diagram of a glomerulus showing proliferation of mesangial cells and increase in mesangial matrix.

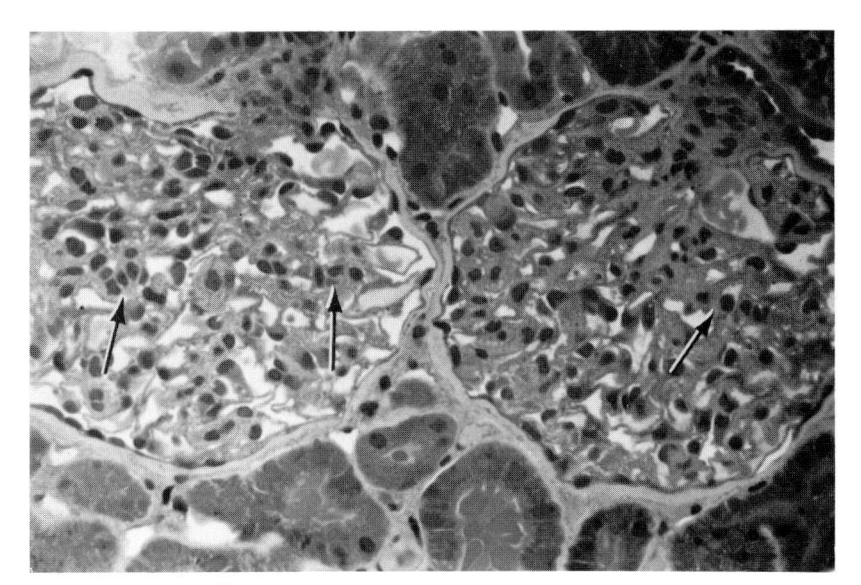

Figure 16–6 Specimen from an 8 year old boy who has had the nephrotic syndrome for 3 years. Steroid therapy decreased but did not eradicate the proteinuria. Renal function is normal, and the urine sediment contains only oval fat bodies. The glomeruli contain 130 to 150 cells. These increased numbers of cells are in the mesangial regions (arrows). (H&E, ×300.)

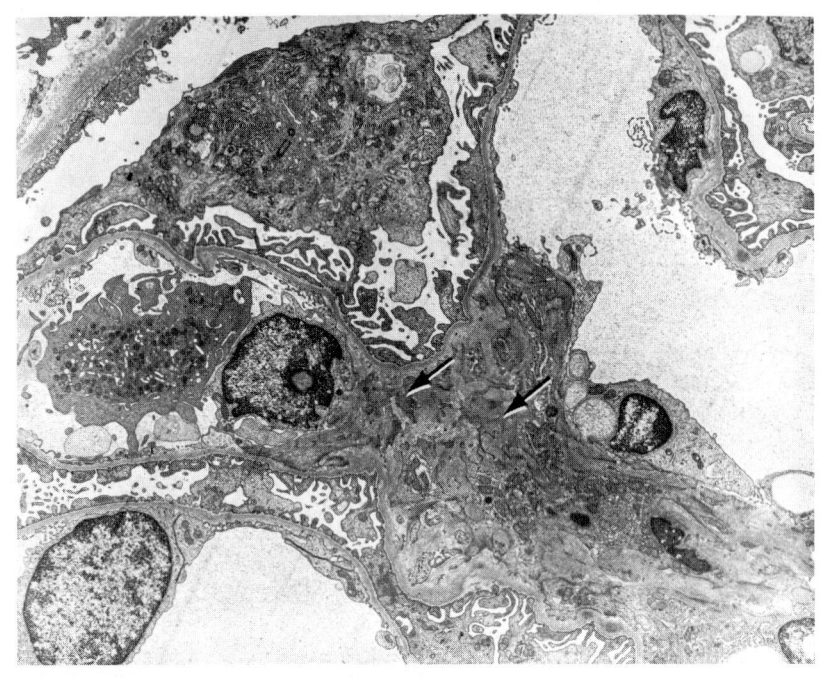

Figure 16-7 Electron micrograph from the same biopsy specimen as in Figure 16-5. The mesangial regions contain an increased amount of cell cytoplasm and a slight increase in mesangial matrix. The endothelial and epithelial cells are unremarkable. By immunofluorescence small amounts of IgG and IgM were found to be present in the mesangial region. There are small electron-dense deposits in a similar distribution (arrows). (×1500.)

TABLE 16-3. Clinical and Morphologic Characteristics of Membranoproliferative Glomerulonephritis (MPGN)

	MPGN with SED*	MPGN with DIMD†
Mesangial proliferation	++	+
Mesangial sclerosis	+	+
Mesangial deposition		
C1q	+	Rare ⎫ Also basal lamina of
C3	+	+ ⎬ tubules and Bowman's
Properdin	+	Rare ⎭ capsule
IgG	+	Rare
Mesangial interposition	+	Rare
Basal lamina deposits		
Subendothelial	+	Rare
Intramembranous	Rare	+
Subepithelial	Rare	+
Epithelium proliferation	Rare	Common
Serum C3	Variably decreased	Commonly decreased
Serum C1q and C4	Variably decreased	Normal
C3 nephritic factor	Rarely present	Common
	Classic pathway activation	Alternate pathway activation

*SED, subendothelial deposits.
†DIMD, dense intramembranous deposits.

MEMBRANOPROLIFERATIVE LESION

Light Microscopy. Two forms of membranoproliferative glomerulonephritis have been described; these are quite similar by light microscopy but are clearly differentiated by fluorescence and electron microscopy (Table 16-3). The most common type is characterized by desposits in the subendothelial space and in the mesangium (Figs. 16-8, 16-9). This was the first recognized form. The second is differentiated by dense, more or less uniform, linear "sausage-shaped" deposits within the substance of the glomerular basal lamina and in the basal lamina of Bowman's capsule and tubules (Figs. 16-12 and 16-13).

The common features of these types of glomerular injury are enlarged glomeruli with hyperplasia of mesangial cells and mesangial sclerosis. In both forms of this syndrome but especially in association with subendothelial deposits, the capillary loops are markedly compressed. Proliferation of epithelial cells, at times forming crescents, is much more frequent when dense intramembranous deposits are present. In the type with subendothelial and mesangial deposits, the mesangial cells may often be seen to extend out around the peripheral capillary loops, giving an appearance of a double basal lamina. This "double contour" or "tram tracking" appearance was the most characteristic and differentiating feature presented in early papers on membranoproliferative glomerulonephritis. It is typified by the irregularity with

Text continued on page 216

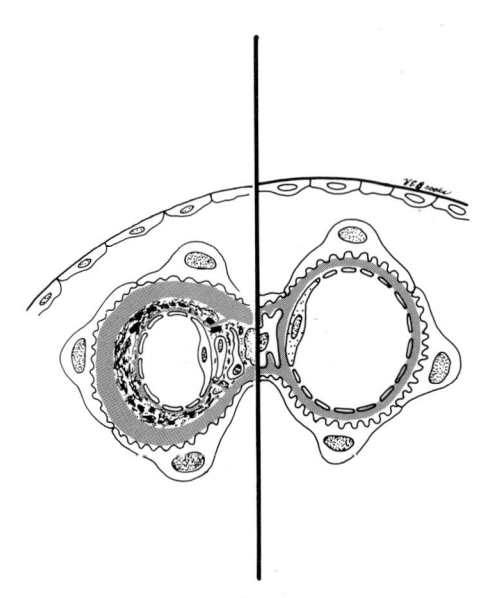

Figure 16–8 MPGN with SED. Diagram demonstrating a double-layered peripheral lamina between which are found both deposits and cytoplasmic extensions of mesangial cells. There also are deposits in the mesangial regions and an increased number of mesangial cells.

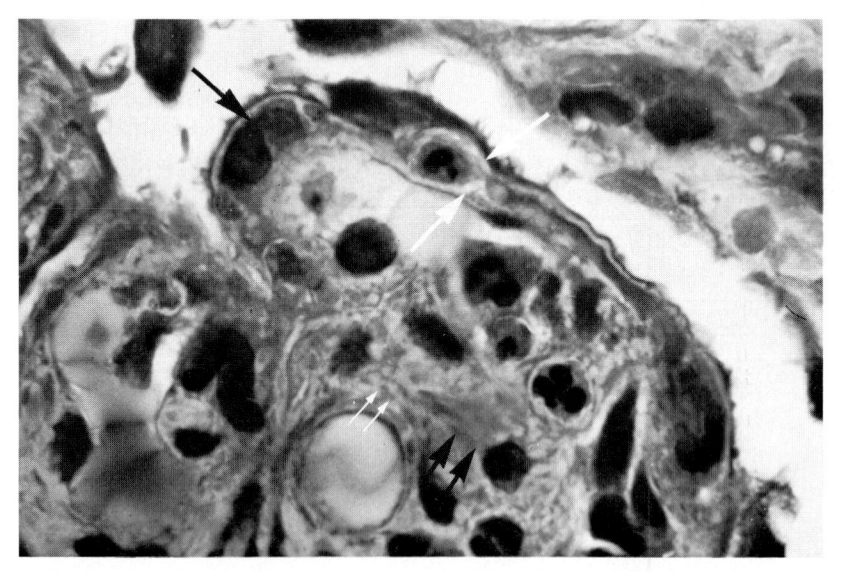

Figure 16–9 Specimen from a 14 year old boy who was found to have edema, proteinuria, hematuria, red cell casts in the urine, hypocomplementemia and decreased platelet survival. A high power light micrograph demonstrates continuous epithelial cell cytoplasm on the urinary aspect of the basal lamina, duplication of the basal lamina (opposing light arrows), cell nuclei, and cytoplasm between the layers of the basal lamina in the periphery of the capillary loop (single heavy arrow), an increase in the amount of mesangial matrix (double light arrows), and the presence of deposits in the mesangial region (double heavy arrows). There are two readily identifiable neutrophils in the center of the field. (H&E, ×1200.)

PRIMARY NEPHROTIC SYNDROME 213

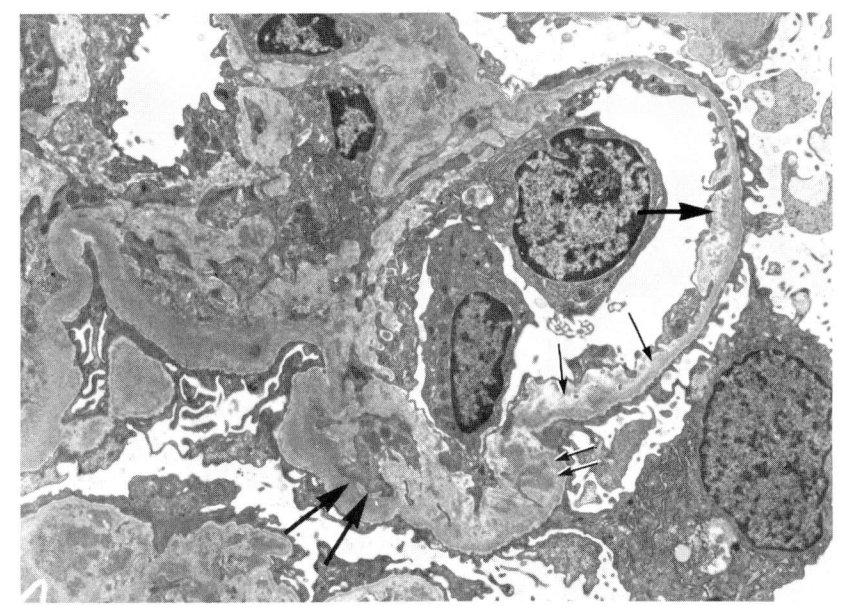

Figure 16-10 Same patient as in Figure 16-9. The lamina densa is identifiable around the entire periphery of the capillary loop. On the subendothelial aspect there are irregular deposits of flocculent material (single light arrows) and a second layer of basal lamina (heavy arrow). In other zones there are deposits (double light arrows) and extensions of mesangial cell cytoplasm toward the periphery (double heavy arrows). In the mesangial region there are increased numbers of cells as well as deposits. The endothelial cytoplasm is prominent and quite irregular in thickness. The epithelial cells are unremarkable. (× 2500.)

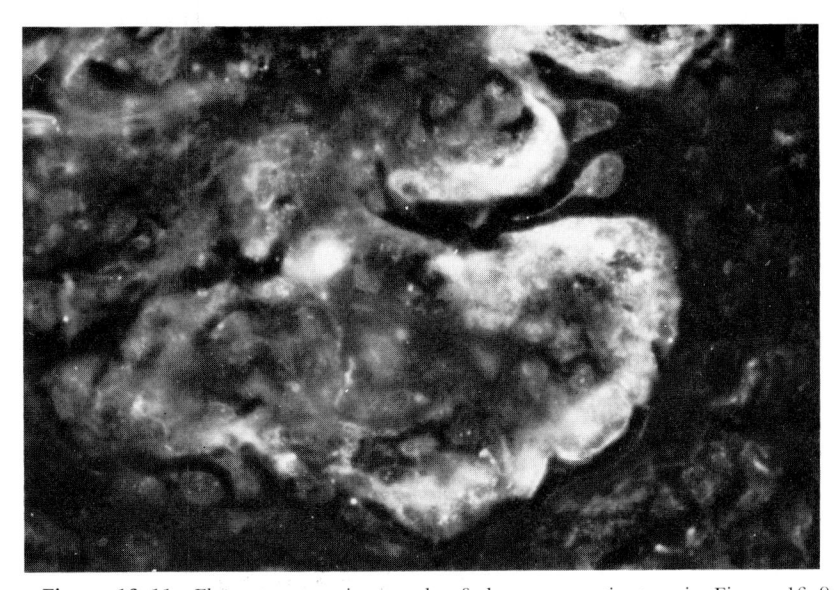

Figure 16-11 Fluorescence micrograph of the same patient as in Figure 16-9. There is extensive deposition of C3 and IgG in the peripheral basal lamina, as well as in the mesangial matrix. (× 1200.)

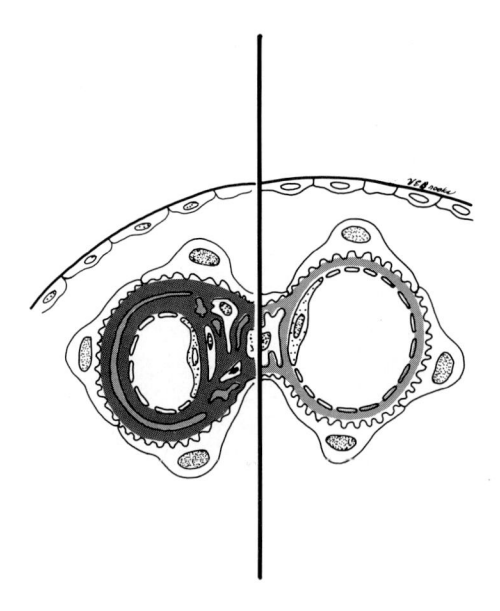

Figure 16-12 A diagram demonstrating effacement of the normal epithelial architecture with the formation of a nearly continuous sheet of cytoplasm over the urinary aspect of the basal lamina. Within the basal lamina is a dense continuous deposit, which is also seen in the mesangial region. There is an increase in mesangial cells and in the amount of mesangial matrix.

Figure 16-13 Biopsy from an 18 year old man rejected by the armed services because of proteinuria. Creatinine clearance is normal and 24 hour protein excretion is 7.8 g. Total hemolytic complement is markedly decreased. The glomerular basal lamina are outlined by a continuous dense deposit. Capillary spaces are markedly reduced and the mesangial regions are expanded by an increase in both mesangial substance and the number of mesangial cells. Bowman's capsule is unremarkable. (H&E, ×300.)

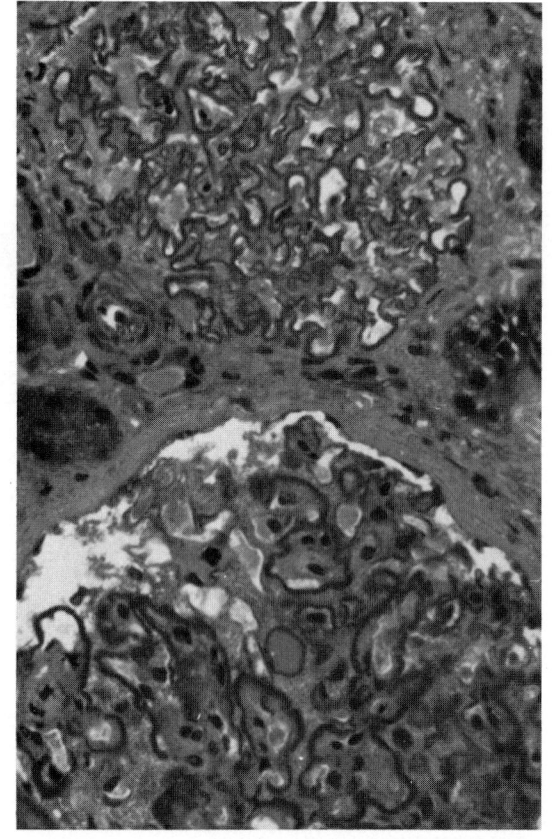

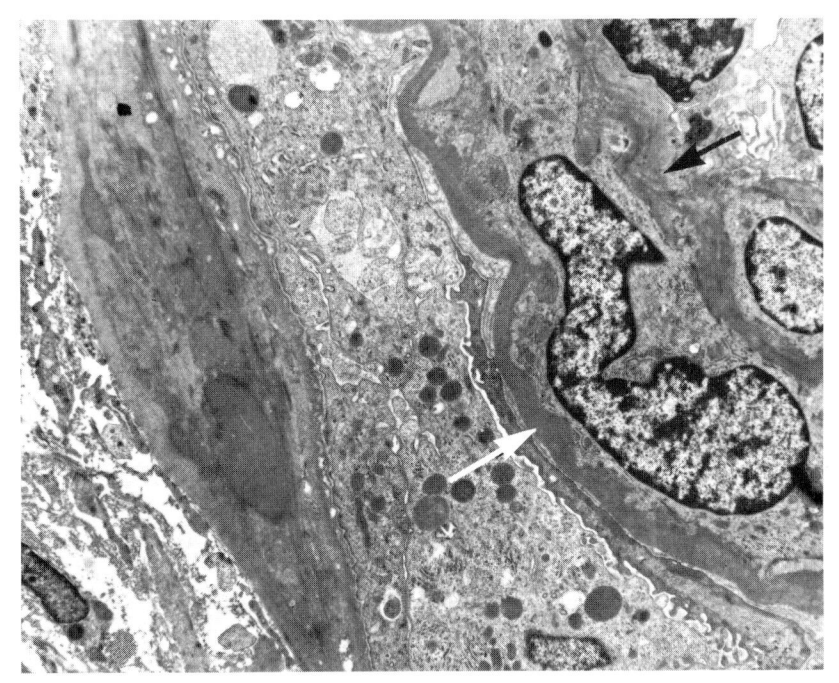

Figure 16–14 Electron micrograph from same patient as in Figure 16–13. The peripheral basal lamina is replaced by a very electron-dense deposit (light arrow). The capillary lumen is separated from this layer by interposed mesangial cells and a second layer of basal lamina (heavy arrow). Bowman's basal lamina contains deposits as well. The visceral epithelial cell layer is present as a continuous sheet over the urinary surface of the basal lamina. (×1500.)

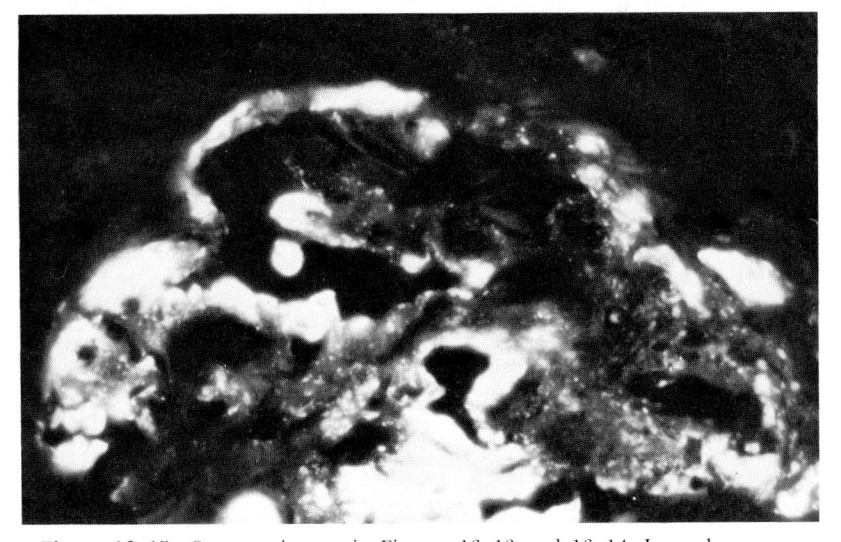

Figure 16–15 Same patient as in Figures 16–13 and 16–14. Large homogeneous deposits of complement components are seen in the peripheral basal lamina and in the mesangial regions. The mesangial deposits tend to be more granular and irregular in contour. Deposits of IgG and IgM are present in small amounts and in irregular configuration in the mesangial regions. (×500.)

which it involves the peripheral capillary loops. Most often the true lamina densa is unaltered.

These two types have considerable overlap and may not be distinguishable in the individual case. The entity "lobular glomerulonephritis" should be placed in this group, since it shares many clinical or histologic features. This condition, however, is characterized by fewer basal lamina deposits and more pronounced mesangial sclerosis (Figs. 16-15, 16-16, 16-17). Whether it remains as a separate entity or as a stage of the other two remains a topic for future investigation.

Fluorescence Microscopy. The deposits in the subendothelial and mesangial forms of the disease consist primarily of IgG and complement components (Fig. 16-11). The dense accumulations consist of ribbon-like strands of C3 (Fig. 16-14). These deposits may also be found irregularly distributed in the basal lamina of Bowman's capsule and of the tubules.

Electron Microscopy. In both types there is a marked increase in the size of the mesangial regions due to an increase in the number of cells and in amount of mesangial matrix and deposits. The basal lamina is duplicated in both types. In MPGN with SED the layers encase cell

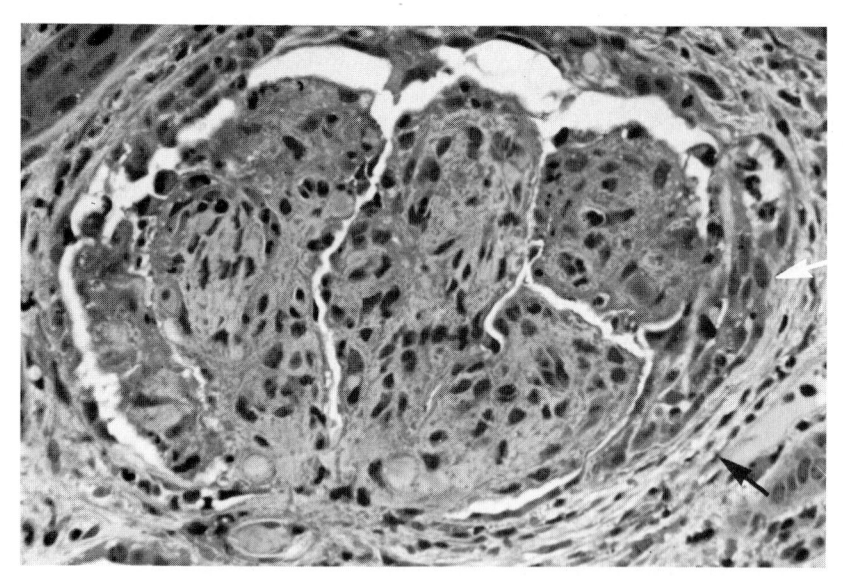

Figure 16-16 Specimen from a 14 year old boy who presented with nephrotic syndrome and azotemia, which had developed and rapidly progressed over a 6 month period. On admission, blood pressure was 150/100, and the patient had moderate peripheral edema. The 24 hour protein level was 6.8 g and the urine sediment was telescopic. Creatinine clearance was 21 ml/min and total hemolytic and C3 complement were low. The illustrated glomerulus is very distorted. The capillary spaces are nearly completely obliterated. The overall architecture is simplified and the central or mesangial regions consist of concentrically arranged masses of extracellular material and elongated cells. There also is moderate epithelial cell proliferation (light arrow). The surrounding Bowman's basal lamina appears to be duplicated (heavy arrow). (H&E, ×300.)

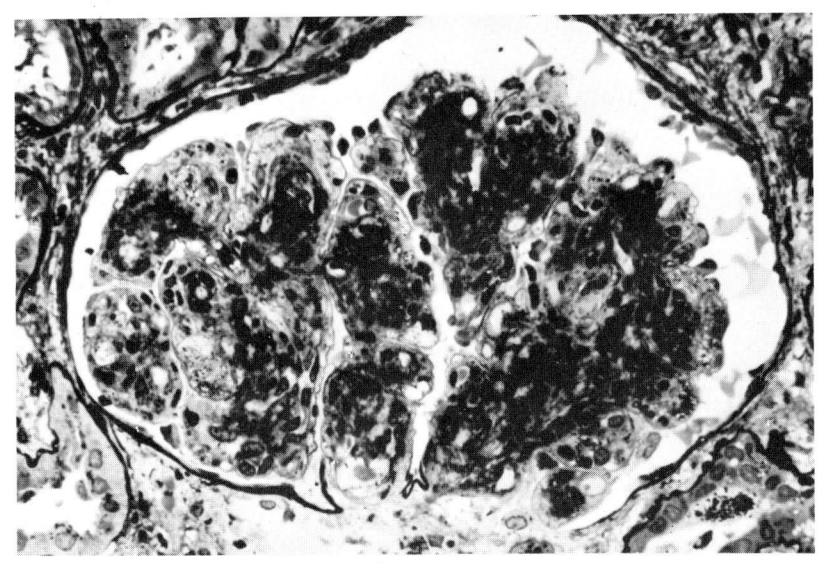

Figure 16-17 Same patient as in Figure 16-16. In this silver stain the dense sclerosis in the mesangial regions can be appreciated. (Silver methenamine, ×300.)

cytoplasm (? mesangial) and deposits. In MPGN with DIMD there are large, homogeneous deposits, which may completely encircle a capillary loop. More commonly, they occur in multiple segments. Additional basal lamina deposits are seen in both types, especially in MPGN with DIMD, where they are found in Bowman's capsule and in tubular basal lamina.

Additional features of both types are endothelial cell hypertrophy and surface villation, loss of epithelial cell foot processes, and infiltration of the mesangium and peripheral capillaries by monocytes and neutrophils.

CLINICAL COURSE AND PROGNOSIS

PURE PROLIFERATIVE LESION. While the minimal lesion and sclerosing lesion groups of nephrosis are quite distinct clinicopathologic syndromes, that occurring with the proliferative lesion is a conglomeration of pathologic lesions and varied clinical syndromes.

For the most part, patients with the proliferative lesion have a poor prognosis. Although occasionally reports of good response to corticosteroid therapy have been reported, a controlled study in Great Britain failed to show that therapy influences the course of this lesion.

MEMBRANOPROLIFERATIVE GLOMERULONEPHRITIS. There is a relatively poor prognosis associated with either histologic type, but the progression to renal failure is more rapid when associated with dense intramembranous deposits. Unfortunately, this lesion recurs almost universally in the transplanted kidney, whereas a recurrence of MPGN with subendothelial and mesangial deposits is relatively rare.

Kincaid-Smith (1973) has reported success in treatment of the membranoproliferative lesion, with a combination of cyclophosphamide, dipyridamole, and anticoagulants. We recently have studied a group of patients with this lesion, measuring several parameters of hemostasis: platelet survival time, fibrinogen turnover, and plasminogen turnover. Platelet survival time is uniformly shortened in this disease. In addition, cross transfusion studies, in which patients' platelets survived normally in healthy recipients but normal donor platelets were destroyed prematurely, demonstrated that this results from an extraplatelet cause. Fibrinogen and plasminogen utilization were only slightly increased; and therapy with dipyridamole and acetylsalicylic acid, heparin, and sodium warfarin, whether used alone or in combination, produced no consistent changes in platelet and fibrinogen survival. Further, none produced significant improvement in renal function during brief periods of administration. Consequently, controlled trials would be required to adequately assess the efficacy of drugs and the role of coagulation abnormalities in the disease.

SCLEROSING LESIONS

CLINICAL DATA

The membranous and focal sclerosing lesions also are thought to be mediated by the immune system. The membranous lesion, for instance, may represent a form of immune complex disease, for the lesion is reproducible in animals with repeated, graded doses of antigen. In addition, it is associated with some forms of chronic antigenemia in humans, such as chronic forms of hepatitis and malaria, and with gold administration. The presence of IgG and often C3 on the capillary loops further supports this hypothesis.

The focal sclerosing lesion was originally thought to represent instances of progression from the minimal lesion, but that theory has not been borne out. The deposition of immunoglobulins in the sclerotic areas suggested a primary disease of immune etiology, although this too is unproved. These lesions are relatively uncommon in children but other than an increased incidence of microscopic hematuria, rare red cell casts, and hypertension, the clinical presentation is very similar to the minimal lesion nephrotic syndrome.

HISTOLOGY

FOCAL AND GLOBAL SCLEROSIS

Light Microscopy. Sclerosis, defined by PAS positivity and staining by the methenamine silver technique, consists of an increase in the amount of extracellular material. This may occur in either the mesangial region or the peripheral basal lamina, or be manifested as obliteration of the capillary tuft (Fig. 16-19). The feature which differentiates this from other sclerosing diseases, however, is the tendency for the sclerosis to vary within and among glomeruli. In early lesions, considerably fewer than half the glomeruli are involved, and even in advanced cases the segmental nature of the lesions often is recognizable (Fig. 16-20). Synechiae also are a feature of the lesion, particularly apparent in its early stages (Fig. 16-21). Lipid and hyaline deposits are present in many of the larger sclerotic areas.

Electron Microscopy. In the sclerotic areas there is a homogeneous mass of extracellular material, which displaces and fills capillary loops and mesangial regions (Fig. 16-22). Cell debris and protein "deposits" may also be present in this general area.

Fluorescence Microscopy. In contrast to benign recurrent hematuria, in which the deposition of IgA is noted to be diffuse, deposits of IgM for all practical purposes are limited to the sclerosing lesions. In addition, C3 complement and IgG usually are present.

MEMBRANOUS LESIONS. The membranous lesion is defined morphologically by uniform thickening of the capillary wall owing to the subepithelial deposits on the glomerular basal lamina. These are separated from one another by subepithelial projections of the lamina densa. The resulting picture on cross section shows relatively regular "spikes" of the basal lamina projecting toward the urinary space, between which are deposits that can be identified readily.

Text continued on page 223

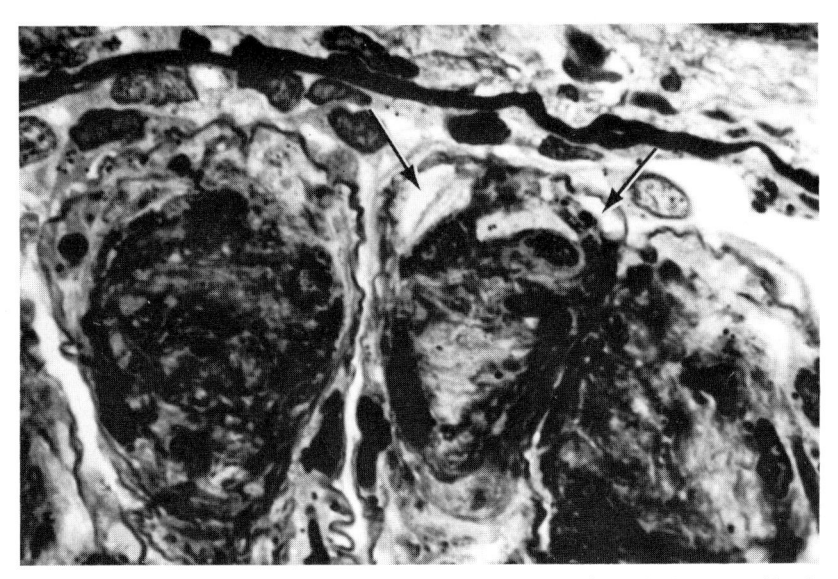

Figure 16-18 Same patient as in Figures 16-16 and 16-17. At higher magnification the marked mesangial sclerosis and small capillary loops (arrows) can be appreciated. The peripheral basal lamina is wrinkled but otherwise unremarkable. (Silver methenamine, ×1200.)

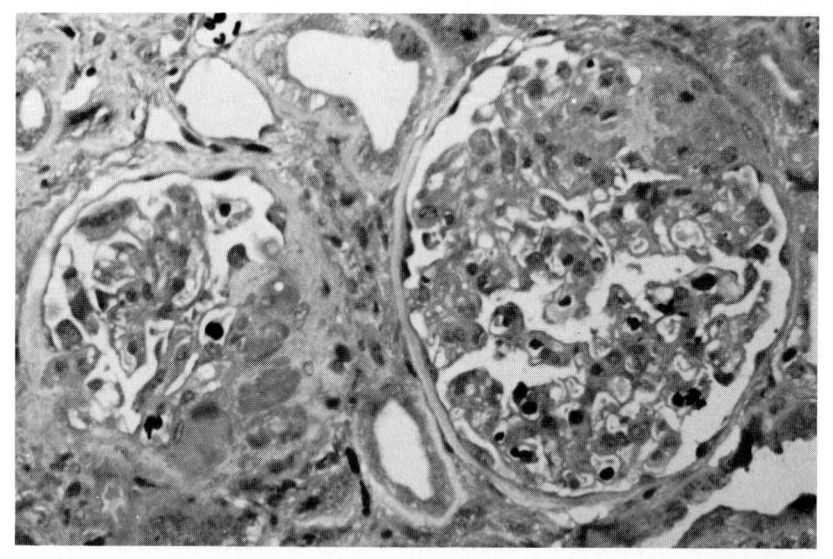

Figure 16-19 Biopsy from a 38 year old man with a 6 year history of intermittent proteinuria and edema initially responsive to steroids and azathioprine. At the time of biopsy he had 24 g of protein/24 hours in the urine. Creatinine clearance was 66 ml/min. Urine sediment revealed a small number of red cells and granular cells. The two glomeruli demonstrate varying degrees of sclerosis, with approximately 20 to 50 per cent of the total structure being involved. The glomerular architecture in the areas of sclerosis is completely effaced. Elsewhere there is mild mesangial sclerosis, but these areas appear otherwise unremarkable. (H&E, × 300.)

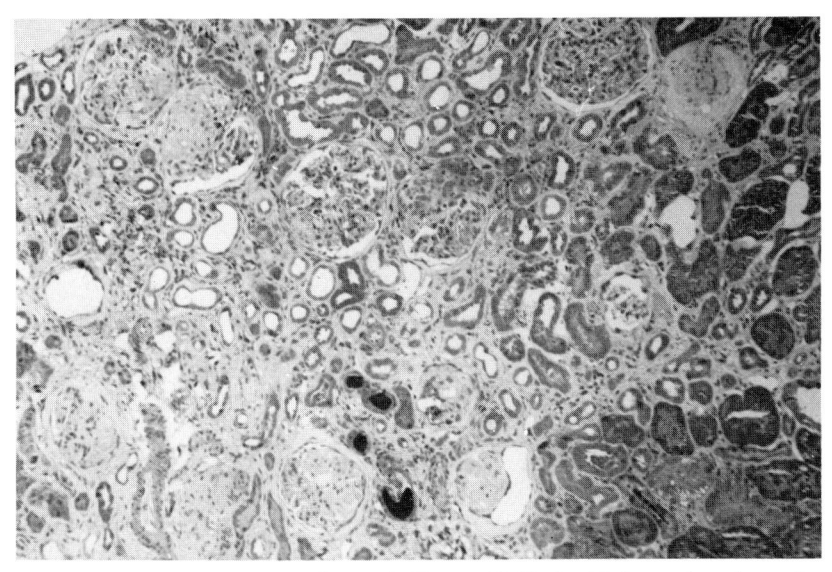

Figure 16-20 The same patient as in Figure 16-19. In this low power photomicrograph the irregularity of glomerular involvement can be seen. The glomeruli on the left are much more extensively involved than those on the right. Those on the left are in a juxtamedullary position (H&E, ×75.)

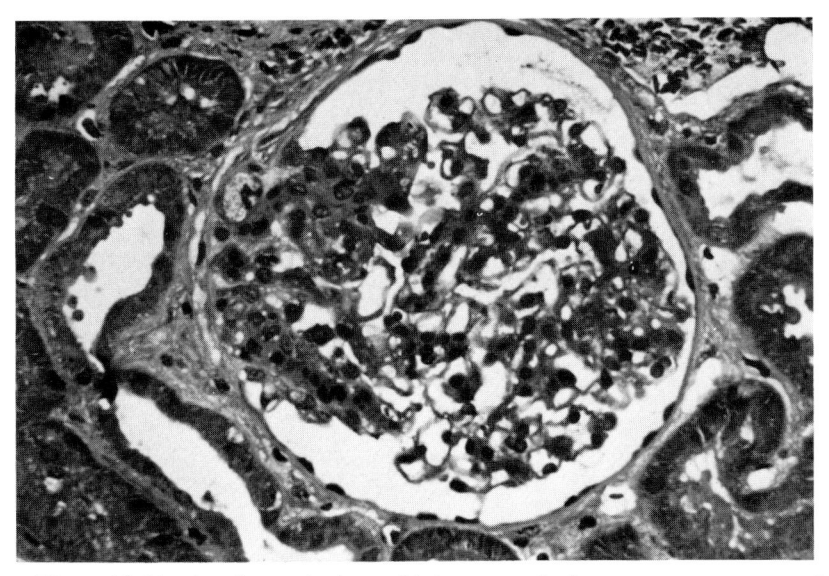

Figure 16-21 A well-organized synechia is present. Such structures most commonly occur opposite the vascular pole. In this case there is mesangial hypercellularity and sclerosis. (Paraffin, H&E, ×300.)

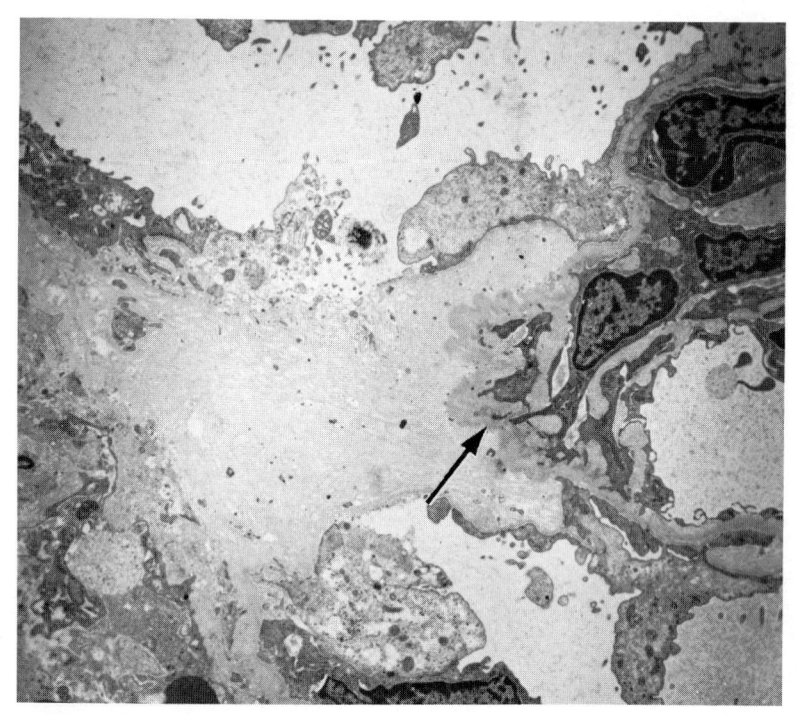

Figure 16–22 In the areas of sclerosis the basal lamina (arrow) can be seen to be either collapsed, as in this picture, or extended around masses of extracellular material, which are less dense. In this case the sclerosis connects the peripheral capillary loops with Bowman's capsule. (×1500.)

Light Microscopy. The light microscopic membranous lesions have been divided into four stages:

Stage 1. The capillary walls may appear to be normal in routinely stained sections; however, very fine stippling of the glomerular basal lamina might be evident when silver stains are used, particularly on oblique views, since the deposits do not take up the stain and thus appear as negative images (Figs. 16-23 and 16-24). It often is apparent, however, that this change is present in a relatively small number of the capillary loops.

Stage 2. The capillary wall thickening usually is detectable in routine sections. Silver stains also demonstrate "spike" formation over multiple capillary loops, but the mesangial regions are unremarkable (Figs. 16-27 and 16-28).

Stage 3. The capillary walls are thickened considerably, resulting in diminished size of the capillary lamina. "Spike" formations may still be present, but the predominant feature is an increase in the amount of extracellular material in the peripheral basal lamina resulting in a thickened contour (Figs. 16-31 and 16-32). The deposits may be surrounded by basal lamina and appear to be incorporated into a thickened basal lamina.

Stage 4. At this point, many glomeruli are obsolescent, and it might be difficult to determine the nature of the original lesion. Characteristically, however, the obsolescent glomeruli tend to be enlarged rather than shrunken and retracted.

Electron Microscopy

Stage 1. The deposits on the epithelial side of the basal lamina appear to be relatively small and irregularly spaced (Fig. 16-25). The projections of the lamina densa toward the epithelial cells also are rudimentary and in many areas are difficult to detect. The glomerular basal lamina itself is not thickened.

Stage 2. The subepithelial deposits are regular and readily apparent (Fig. 16-29). The spike-like projections of the lamina densa are well formed, and the overlying epithelial cells contain many organelles in the cytoplasm, but the pedicels are absent.

Stage 3. The basal lamina is thickened greatly. In addition, the deposits seem to lie within the substance of the basal lamina, and in many areas they are completely enclosed by lamina densa (Fig. 16-33). The epithelial cells also are evident, as noted in Stage 2. Multiple profiles of hyaline substance can be seen and the peripheral basal lamina is thickened.

Stage 4. The deposits within the basal lamina are less apparent (Figs. 16-35 and 16-36). The basal lamina also is thickened diffusely and markedly, and it could be difficult to distinguish this lesion from others in the broad category of chronic glomerulonephritis.

Fluorescence Microscopy. Subepithelial deposits of IgG and, less frequently, complement components (from 20 to 40 per cent in most

Text continued on page 231

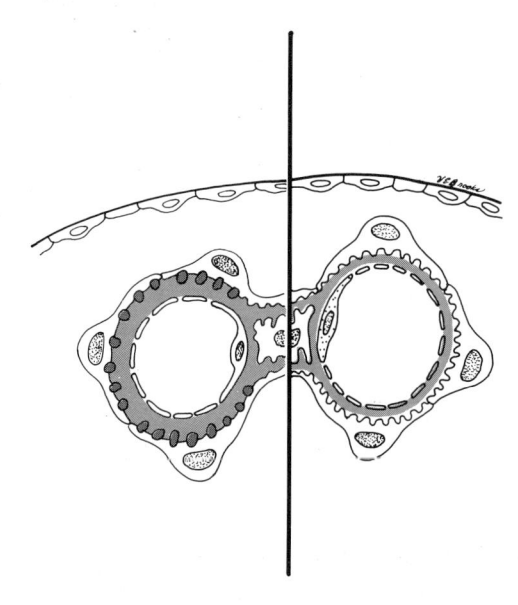

Figure 16-23 Diagram demonstrating multiple small subepithelial deposits. The epithelial cell layer is a continuous sheet over the basal lamina and deposits. The lamina densa contains small extensions, which protrude between the deposits. The endothelial cells and capillary lumen are unremarkable, as is the mesangial matrix.

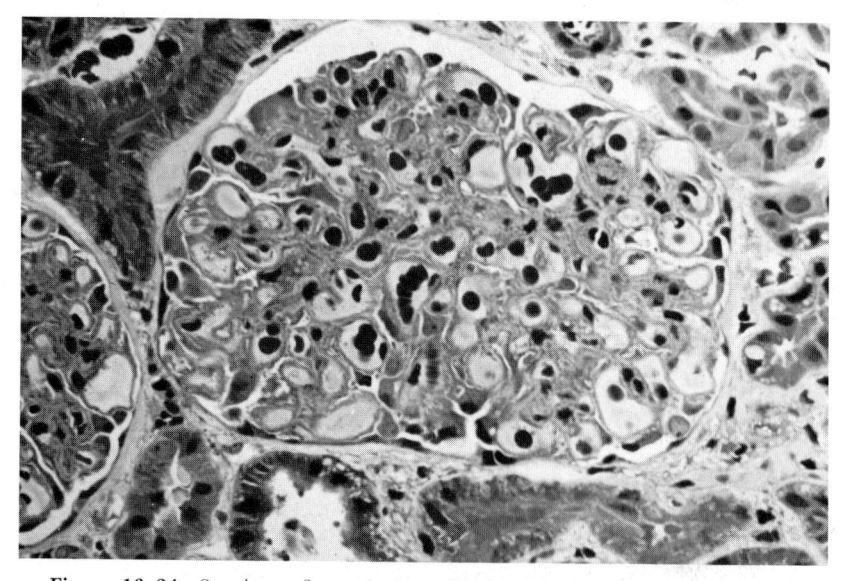

Figure 16-24 Specimen from an 11 year old girl who was admitted because of proteinuria, hypoalbuminemia (1.5 g/dl), and hematuria. Creatinine clearance was normal. The major histologic finding is a diffuse thickening of the capillary membranes which on silver staining was found to be made up of spikes of lamina densa between which are homogeneous protein deposits. (H&E, ×300.)

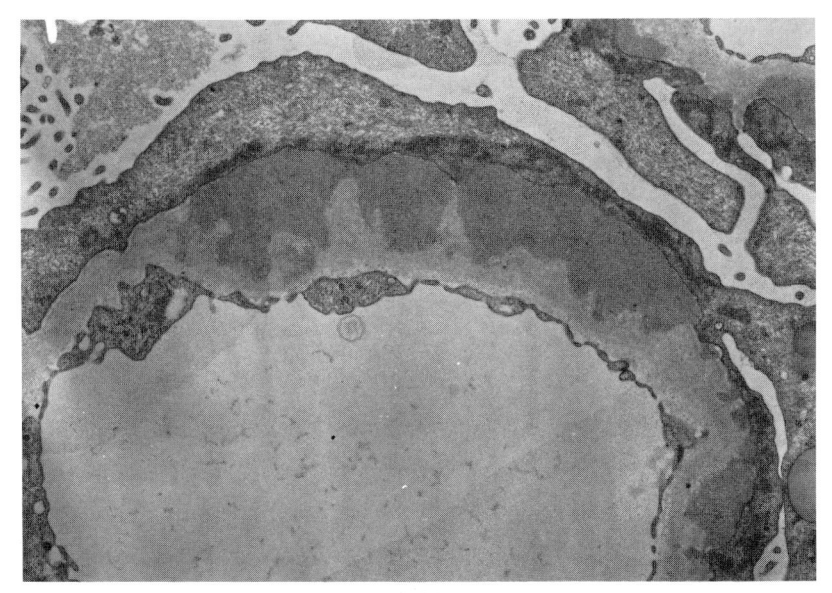

Figure 16-25 Electron micrograph from same patient as in Figure 16-24. On the subepithelial aspect of the lamina densa are large irregularly shaped deposits. Between the deposits are extensions of the lamina densa toward the overlying epithelial cells. The epithelial cell layer over the peripheral basal lamina is continuous. The endothelial cell cytoplasm and capillary space are unremarkable. ($\times 6000$.)

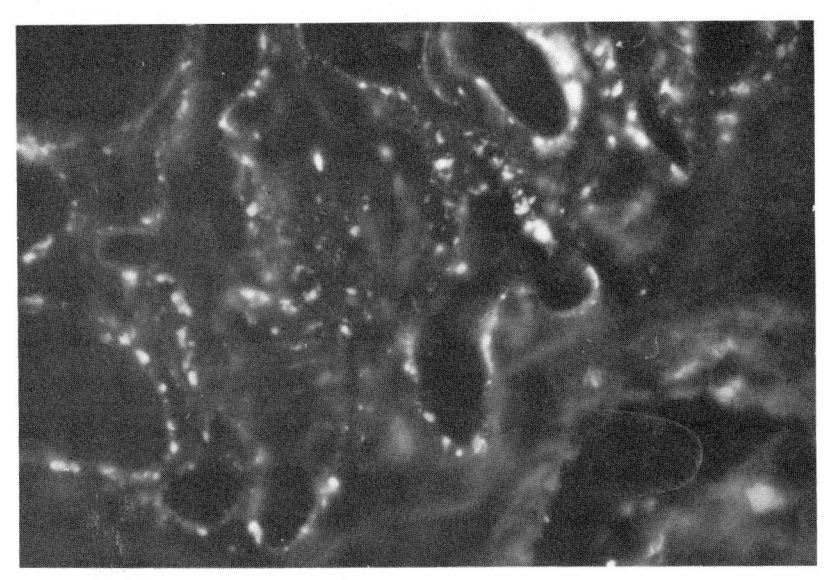

Figure 16-26 Fluorescence micrograph from same patient as in Figure 16-24. There are multiple irregularly shaped deposits of protein containing IgG and small amounts of C3 over the peripheral aspects of the glomerular basal lamina. The mesangial matrix is free of this material. ($\times 1200$.)

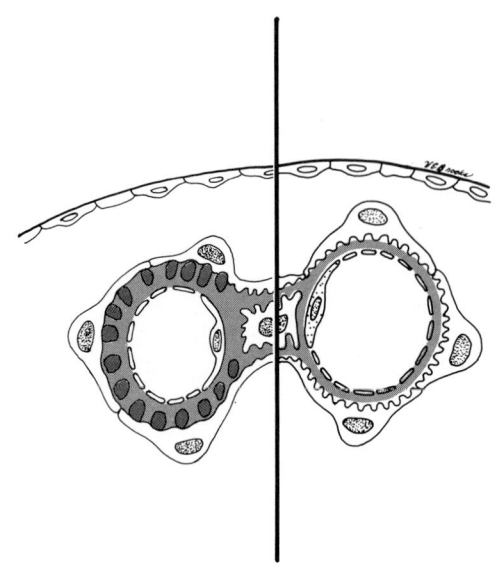

Figure 16–27 Diagram demonstrating larger subepithelial deposits, further incorporated into the basal lamina (stage 2).

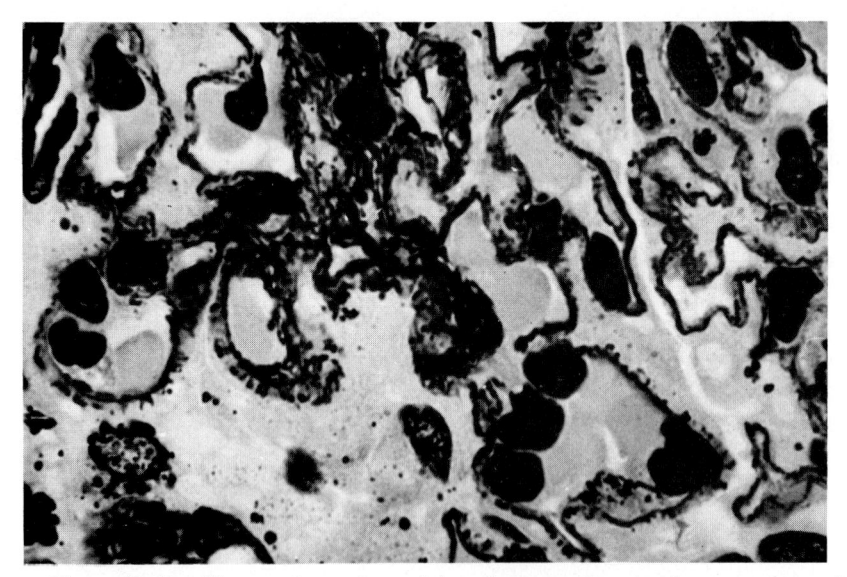

Figure 16–28 Silver methenamine staining, demonstrating that in more advanced lesions the subepithelial "spikes" are very regular in distribution on the basal lamina and quite obvious. (Silver methenamine, ×1200.)

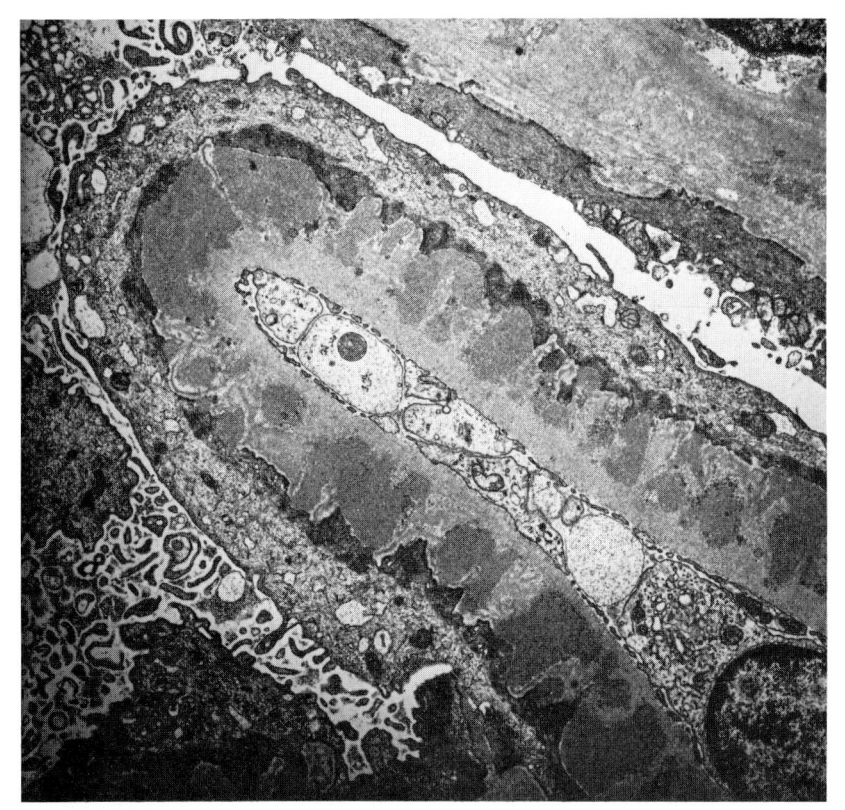

Figure 16–29 An electron micrograph of the same biopsy specimen as in Figure 16–28. Compared with Figure 16–27, the deposits are larger and much more uniform, and the lamina densa covers the distance from the base to the apex of the deposit nearly completely. The overlying epithelial cell layer is continuous. (× 7500.)

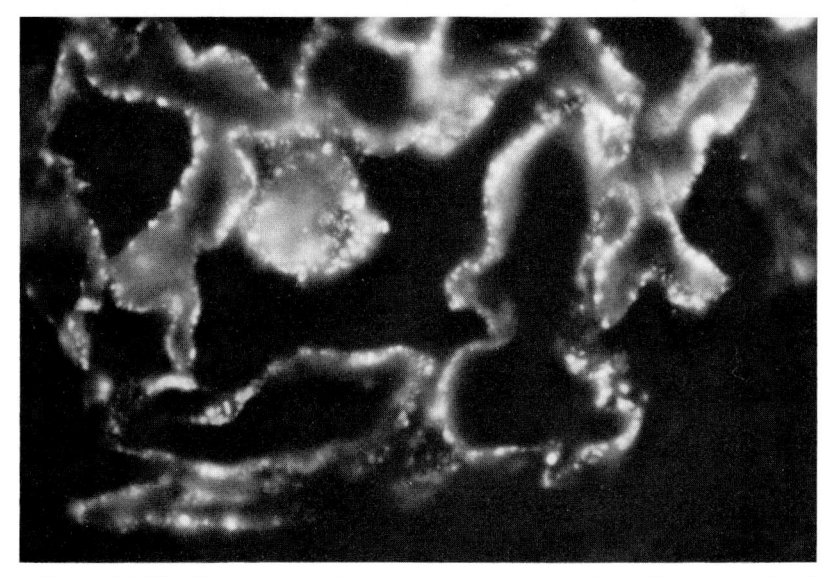

Figure 16–30 Fluorescence micrograph demonstrating the uniform granular distribution of immunoglobulin (IgG) on the peripheral basal lamina. There are no deposits in the mesangium. (×1200.)

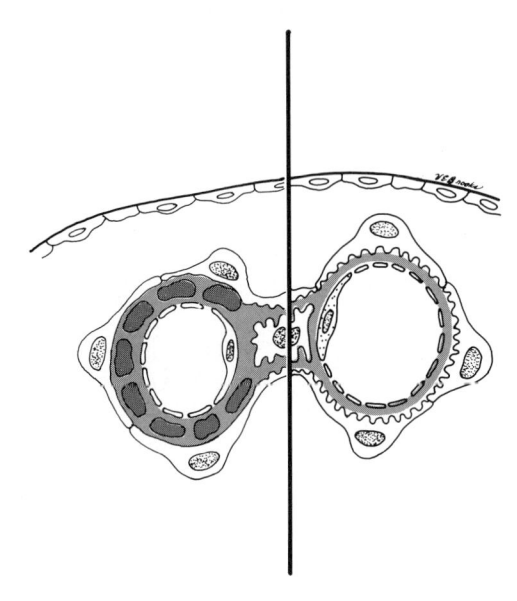

Figure 16-31 Diagram of a stage 3 lesion. In this case, the deposits become surrounded by and incorporated within basal lamina. The mesangial regions are not affected.

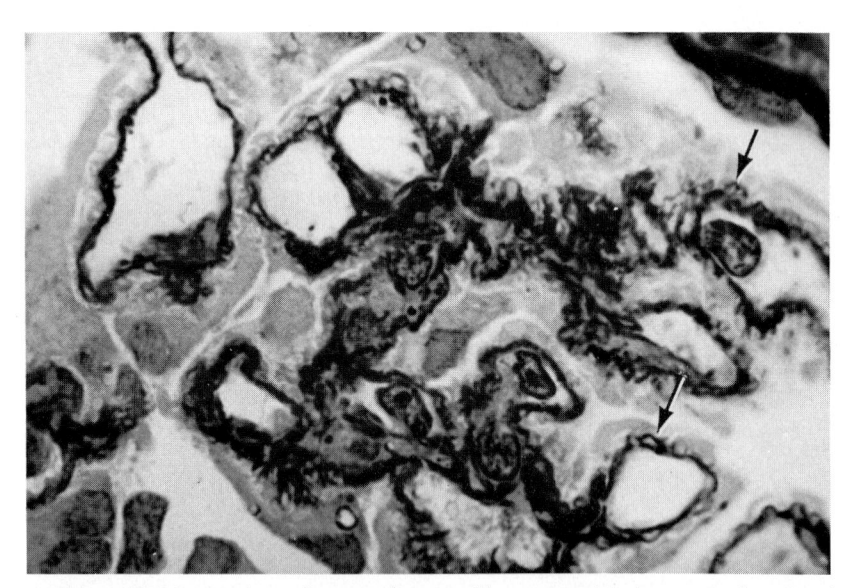

Figure 16-32 Specimen from a 27 year old woman with documented nephrotic syndrome for 1 year who had a 24-hour urinary protein excretion varying from 4 to 14 g. Creatinine clearance was 45 ml/min. The basal lamina in this biopsy seems to be severely distorted by multiple subepithelial projections, some of which appear to surround lucent areas of deposits (arrows). Note again that the mesangial regions are unaffected. (Methenamine silver, ×1200.)

PRIMARY NEPHROTIC SYNDROME 229

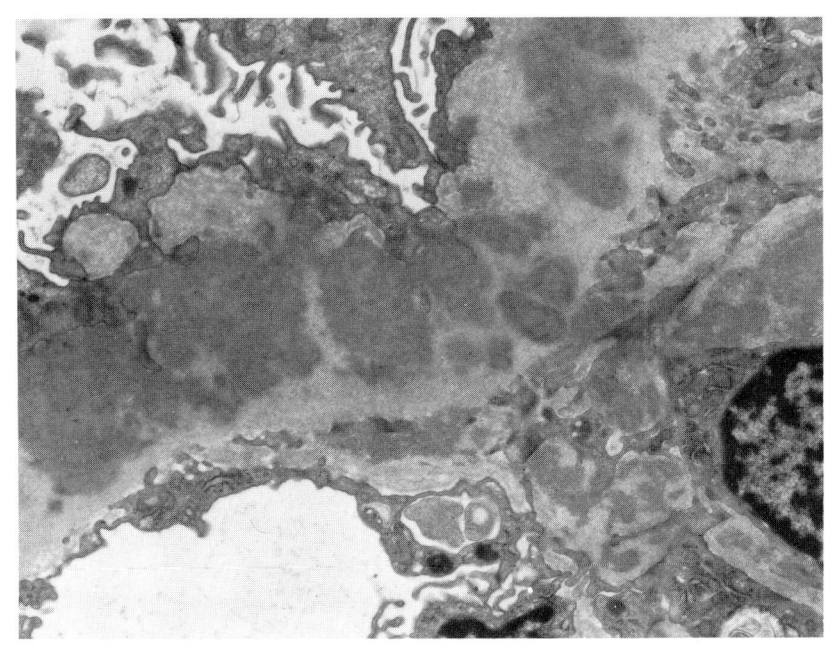

Figure 16–33 Electron micrograph of a biopsy specimen similar to Figure 16–32, showing large electron-dense deposits, many of which are completely incorporated into the basal lamina. (×10,000.)

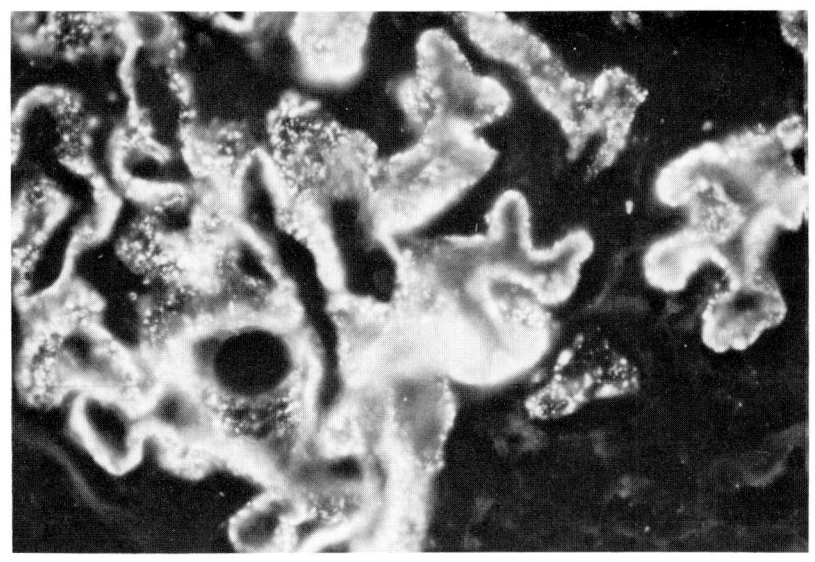

Figure 16–34 Fluorescence micrograph utilizing labeled anti-IgG, demonstrating a uniform diffuse and fairly heavy granular deposition of immunoglobulin on peripheral basal lamina, sparing the mesangial regions. (×1200.)

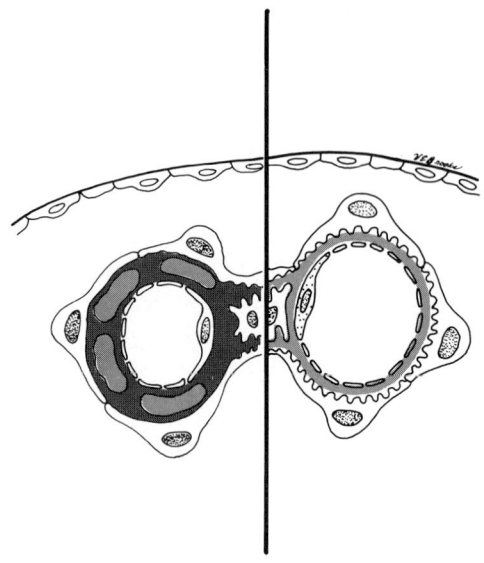

Figure 16-35 Diagram of a stage 4 lesion. The basal lamina is extensively thickened and contains large deposits, which are not as dense as in previous stages.

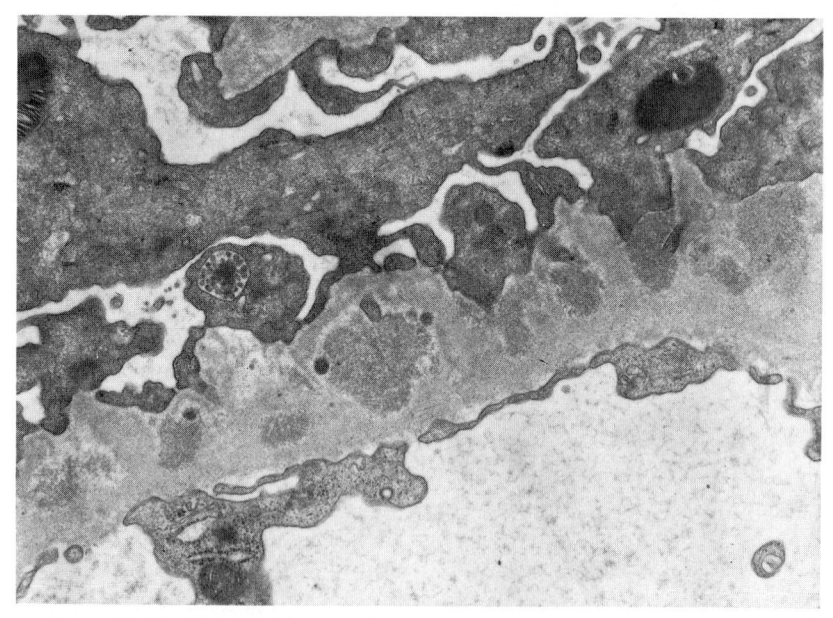

Figure 16-36 Electron micrograph of a biopsy from a 24 year old male who had had nephrotic syndrome for approximately 2 years. The basal lamina is markedly and irregularly thickened. Electron-dense deposits are evident. ($\times$ 7500.)

series) are present in a regular beaded fashion, but rarely deposits are evident in the mesangial regions unless associated with the clinical syndrome of systemic lupus erythematosus (Figs. 16-26, 16-30, and 16-34). These changes are diffuse and obvious even when light microscopic changes are minimal. As the disease progresses the deposits become less distinct, but even in obsolescent glomeruli, they may be seen.

CLINICAL COURSE AND PROGNOSIS

The histologic lesions in sclerosing lesion nephrosis are separable in their clinical course and prognosis.

FOCAL SCLEROSING AND GLOBAL SCLEROSING LESIONS. These processes occur with highest frequency in childhood. In recent studies by Habib and associates (1975), the response to chemotherapy also generally was poor. Of 46 patients treated with corticosteroids, for example, 20 per cent responded but were steroid dependent, 13 per cent had a partial remission, and 67 per cent were steroid resistant. Immunosuppressant therapy was somewhat more effective in the group responding to steroids. Progression to renal failure occurred in a period of from four to seven years, and unfortunately recurrence of this lesion in transplanted kidneys is quite common (Chapter 26).

The focal anatomic distribution, the only occasional response to therapy, and the higher incidence in childhood make the differential diagnosis of these abnormalities from minimal lesion difficult. The majority of those who are found to be non-responders or who have frequent relapses, however, and who initially were included in the minimal lesion group, ultimately are shown to have a focal or global sclerosing lesion.

MEMBRANOUS LESIONS. In most series the peak age of incidence is in the fifth decade, with a nearly equal male-to-female ratio. The usual mode of onset (seen in virtually all patients at some time during their illness) is as the nephrotic syndrome, characterized by a prolonged course with a reasonably high incidence of spontaneous remission. As discussed in the following paragraphs, this may be related to the pathologic lesion.

First, the survival rate at 5 years varies, but has been reported to be 80 to 90 per cent. There also seems to be reasonably good evidence that the pathologic changes described in specimens are in fact sequential, and that they relate to the clinical picture. Additionally, those patients who have minor lesions (nephrotic syndrome of less than 3 years and Stage I changes by biopsy) are most likely to have spontaneous remissions. The data of Habib and associates (1974), for example, suggest that spontaneous remission occurs very frequently in children. In their group of patients, the nephrotic syndrome was mild and transient, and never lasted more than 1 year. Gluck and associate (1973), however, also reported that some patients developed a mildly elevated blood urea nitrogen level even though the nephrotic syndrome had disappeared, which suggests that the disease was progressing despite remission of the proteinuria.

There is apparent disagreement over the effect of the adrenal corticosteroid therapy on the clinical outcome, but the high rate of spontaneous remission, and the fact that not all patients were biopsied in most of the reported series, makes the data difficult to interpret. Most authors agree, however, that steroid therapy does not seem to affect the frequency of remission.

The association of membranous glomerulonephritis with tumors, various drugs, hepatitis, and IgG (and occasionally C3) glomerular deposits also has suggested to many investigators that this is an *immune* type of disease, although antigens have never been identified with certainty.

References

1. Black, D. A. K., Rose, G., and Brewer, D. B.: Controlled trial of prednisone in adult patients with the nephrotic syndrome. Brit. Med. J. *3*:421, 1970.
2. Cameron, J. S.: Histology, protein clearances and response to treatment in nephrotic syndrome. Brit. Med. J. *4*:352, 1968.
3. Cameron, J. S., Turner, D. R., Ogg, C. S., Sharpstone, P., and Brown, C. B.: The nephrotic syndrome in adults with "minimal change" glomerular lesions. Quart. J. Med. *43*:461, 1974.
4. Forland, M., and Spargo, B. H.: Clinicopathological correlations in idiopathic nephrotic syndrome with membranous nephropathy. Nephron *6*:498, 1969.
5. Gluck, M. C., Gallo, G., Lowenstein, J., and Baldwin, D. S.: Membranous glomerulonephritis. Ann. Intern. Med. *78*:1012, 1973.
6. Habib, R.: Focal glomerular sclerosis (Editorial). Kidney Internat. *4*:367, 1973.
7. Habib, R., Gubler, M. C., Loirat, C., Ben Maiz, H., and Levy, M.: Dense deposit disease: A variant of membranoproliferative glomerulonephritis. Kidney Internat. *7*:204, 1975.
8. Habib, R., Kleinknecht, C., and Gubler, M. C.: The nephrotic syndrome. *In* Royer, P., Habib, R., Mathieu, H., Broyer, M., eds. Walsh, A.: Pediatric Nephrology, Philadelphia, W. B. Saunders Co., 1974.
9. Hayslett, J. P., Kashgarian, M., Bensch, K. G., Sprago, B. H., Freedman, L. R., and Epstein, F. H.: Clinicopathological correlations in the nephrotic syndrome due to primary renal disease. Medicine *52*:93, 1973.
10. Heptinstall, R. H.: Pathology of membranous glomerulonephritis. *In* Kincaid-Smith, P., Mathew, T. H. and Becker, E. L., eds.: Glomerulonephritis, Morphology, Natural History, and Treatment. Part I. New York, John Wiley & Sons, 1973.
11. Kincaid-Smith, P.: The natural history and treatment of mesangiocapillary glomerulonephritis. *In* Kincaid-Smith, P., Mathew, T. H., and Becker, E. L., eds.: Glomerulonephritis, Morphology, Natural History and Treatment. New York, John Wiley & Sons, 1973.
12. Matalon, R., Katzl, Gallo, G., Waldo, E., Cabaluna, C., and Eisinger, R. P.: Glomerular sclerosis in adults with nephrotic syndrome. Ann. Int. Med. *80*:488, 1974.
13. Ooi, Y. M., Vallota, E. H. and West, C. D.: Classical complement pathway activation in membranoproliferative glomerulonephritis. Kidney Internat. *9*:46, 1976.
14. Rosen, S.: Membranous glomerulonephritis: current status. Hum. Pathol. *2*:209, 1971.

15. Schreiner, G. E.: The nephrotic syndrome. *In* Strauss, M. B. and Welt, L. G., eds.: Diseases of the Kidney. 2nd Ed. Boston, Little, Brown & Co., 1971.
16. West, C. D.: Editorial review: Pathogenesis and approaches to therapy of membranoproliferative glomerulonephritis. Kidney Internat. 9:1, 1976.
17. White, R. H. R., and Glasgow, E. F.: Focal glomerulosclerosis—a progressive lesion associated with steroid-resistant nephrotic syndrome. Arch. Dis. Child. 46:877, 1971.

Section V

RENAL DISEASES ASSOCIATED WITH SYSTEMIC SYNDROMES

Chapter Seventeen

Systemic Lupus Erythematosus

Introduction

Renal involvement is present in the majority of patients with systemic lupus erythematosus. Since uremia is the leading cause of death in this syndrome, when there is evidence of nephritis, renal biopsy should be performed early as a guide to prognosis and therapy. Patients may have histologic evidence of renal involvement varying from no apparent injury to a florid inflammatory process affecting all of the renal parenchyma.

The reason for the variability in kidney involvement is unknown, but like other forms of immune complex disease, it probably depends on several factors. These include the size of the immune complex, characteristics of the antibody, the availability of antigen, and the immune response of the individual. Common to all patients with renal involvement is the presence of immune deposits of DNA and anti-DNA antibody in the glomerular capillary loops, which initiate the events of inflammation. The etiology of systemic lupus erythematosus is not known, although a viral agent has been suggested.

Some investigators believe that high-dose glucocorticoids generally are effective in treating lupus nephritis regardless of the type of involvement; others think that steroid administration should be guided by the initial renal histology and the response of the individual patient, including changes in urine sediment, kidney function, histology, or serum complement. We hold the latter view.

TABLE 17-1 Organ System Involvement in Systemic Lupus Erythematosus

Manifestation	Frequency (Per Cent)
Systemic: Fever, malaise, anorexia and weight loss	85
Skin and mucous membranes: "Butterfly" rash, ulcerative lesions, purpura, urticaria	75–85
Arthropathy: Arthritis, tenosynovitis	60
Cardiovascular: Pericarditis, myocarditis	50
Neurologic: Seizures, encephalitis	30
Renal: Proteinuria, hematuria, azotemia, hypertension	60

Clinical Data

Systemic lupus erythematosus affects predominantly women, with onset in the third decade. Multisystem involvement is the rule; however, this varies among patients (Table 17-1).

The diagnosis of systemic lupus erythematosus is confirmed serologically by the finding of antinuclear antibodies, or more specifically anti-native DNA antibodies in the serum. The absence of antinuclear antibodies virtually rules out the diagnosis, whereas increased levels of antinative DNA antibodies strongly suggests significant renal involvement.

Proteinuria, hematuria and cellular casts are the most consistent urinary findings in patients with lupus nephritis. In some cases, however, significant histologic renal pathology may be present without urinary abnormalities.

The renal biopsy is essential in order to determine the type and extent of the renal involvement. In addition, in this syndrome, renal biopsy is a necessary guide to therapy. It has only limited usefulness in the diagnosis of systemic lupus erythematosus, which is best made clinically and serologically.

Histology

Patients with lupus nephritis have renal lesions that encompass the entire spectrum of glomerular pathology. Even though the basic groups show considerable overlap, it is helpful to categorize and subdivide the *general* changes seen in a population of these patients. In order that this categorization have some validity, however, it is crucial to assess quantitatively and describe accurately each patient's renal biopsy, and to use these findings, together with all available data, to develop a management plan.

On the basis of quantitative examination of glomerular pathology, renal biopsies can be separated into three broad categories: (1) those with no lesion, (2) those with proliferative changes, and (3) those that primarily have an increased amount of extracellular material. When light, fluorescence, and electron microscopic findings are analyzed, the variations fall into two general categories: (1) those in whom only a small number of glomeruli are affected, and (2) those in whom nearly all glomeruli are affected. The final analysis of the histology is an assessment of the severity of the pathologic process.

GLOMERULI

NO LESION. Only 10 per cent of patients with systemic lupus erythematosus in most series have no demonstrable glomerular lesions by light microscopy. Although a number of these patients may have cytoplasmic aggregates of microtubules visible on electron microscopy, their significance and exact origin have not been defined clearly (Fig. 17–1).

FOCAL PROLIFERATIVE LESION

Those cases in which fewer than 10 per cent of glomeruli are involved have been termed *focal* glomerulonephritis. This abnormality is present in about 30 per cent of biopsies from patients with lupus nephritis. The cellular proliferation also may affect only a small number of the tufts (segmental) within individual glomeruli (Fig. 17–2). Although proliferation is usually restricted to intraglomerular cells, occasionally there might be proliferation of epithelial cells as well (Fig. 17–3). Deposits generally are limited to the mesangial regions and often will be present even in the glomeruli which appeared unaffected when examined by light microscopy. The presence of subendothelial deposits appears to be associated with progression of this focal lesion to the clinically more significant diffuse lesions. This occurs in about 10 per cent of cases. By electron microscopy localized areas of mesangial sclerosis and proliferation with rare deposits are visible (Fig. 17–4).

DIFFUSE PROLIFERATIVE LESION

The *diffuse* proliferative lesion is present in approximately 50 per cent of biopsy specimens from patients with lupus nephritis. It may vary from minor mesangial cell proliferation to diffuse proliferation of all glomerular cell elements, including epithelial cells, which form crescents. Even in widespread involvement, however, an underlying variability in hypercellularity between various parts of the individual glomeruli is visible (Fig. 17–5). The tufts often are widened and filled with proliferating endothelial and mesangial cells and neutrophils. Necrosis with karyorrhexis and apparent intravascular thrombosis ("hyaline thrombi") may be seen in patients with severe disease (Fig. 17–6). In a small number of specimens, hematoxylin bodies may also be evident as

Text continued on page 242

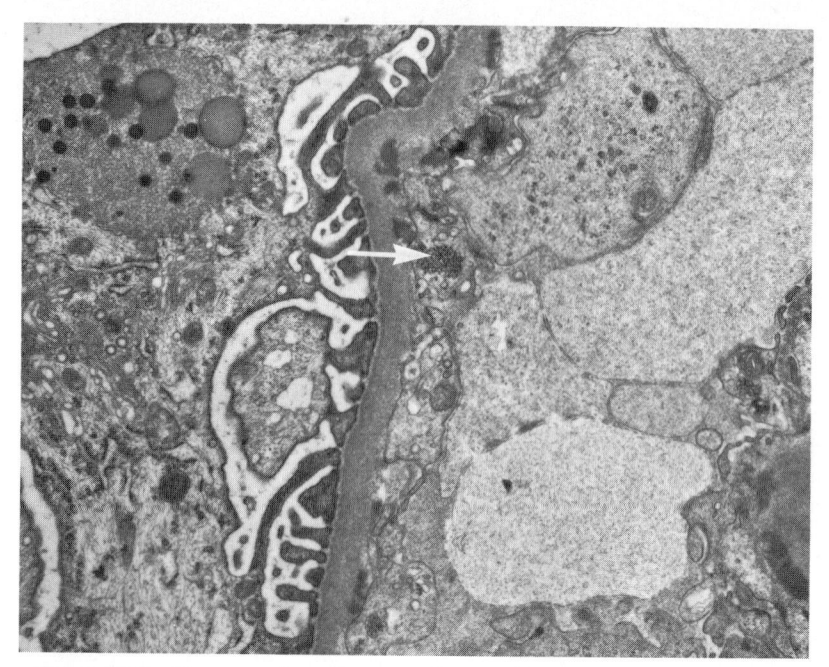

Figure 17-1 Biopsy specimen from an 18 year old female who was found to have discoid lupus and minimal proteinuria. Renal biopsy demonstrated diffuse, mild deposits of IgG and C3. In addition, endothelial cells of vessels of multiple sizes demonstrated profiles of tangled "myxovirus" (arrow). Two years later this patient was admitted to hospital in renal failure and had disseminated lupus erythematosus, from which she did not recover. (× 3200.)

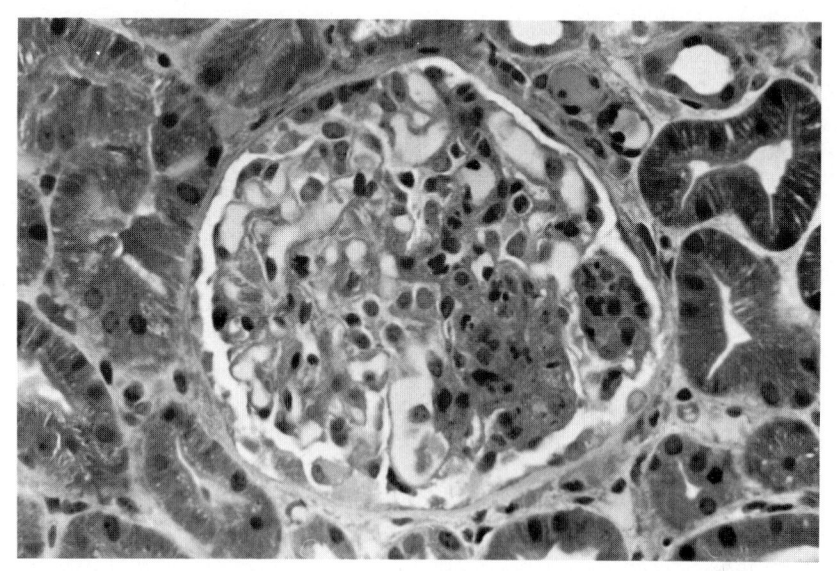

Figure 17-2 Specimen from an 11 year old male who complained of polyarthralgia, fever, and malaise. Serum studies documented the diagnosis of SLE. Serum creatinine level was 0.9 mg/dl, 24-hour urine protein, 1.2 g. Five of 23 glomeruli demonstrated the localized proliferation of intraglomerular cells noted in the right lower quadrant of this glomerulus. There are neutrophils as well as other circulating cells within the capillary lumen and in the mesangial regions. By immunofluorescence large deposits of IgG, C3, and IgA were noted in the mesangial regions of all glomeruli. (H&E, × 300.)

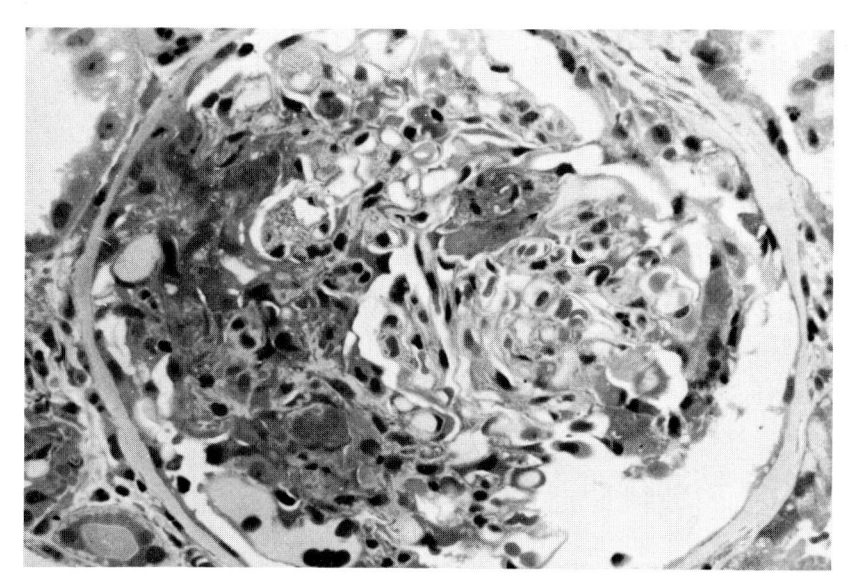

Figure 17-3 Specimen from a 42 year old female with SLE in which a number of the glomeruli demonstated proliferation of epithelial cells in multiple areas around the periphery of glomerular tuft. This is most easily demonstrable in this photomicrograph at approximately the two o'clock position. (H&E, ×300.)

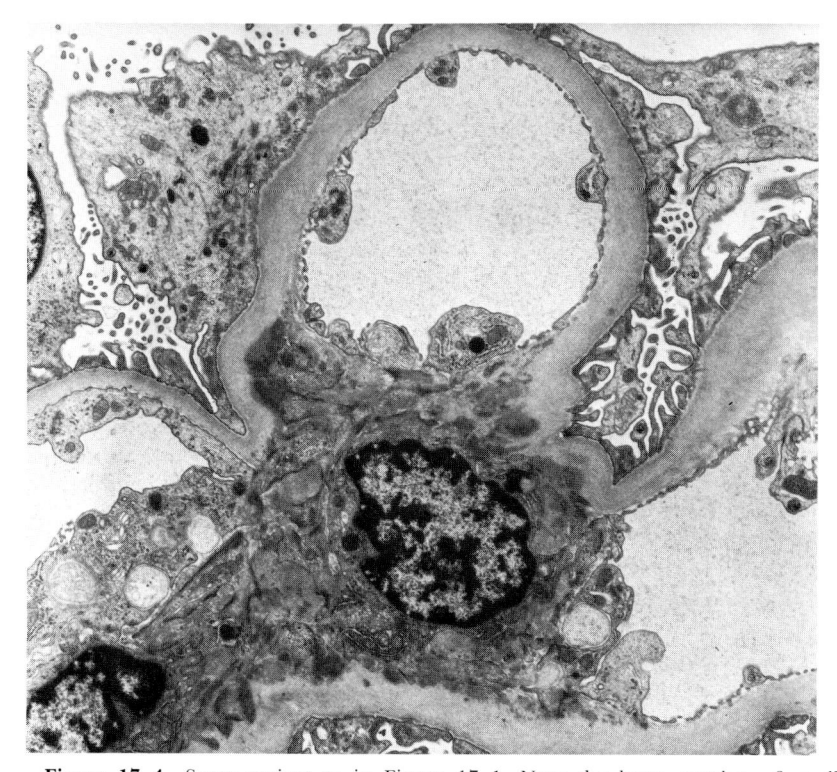

Figure 17-4 Same patient as in Figure 17-1. Note the large number of small electron-dense deposits lying within the mesangial matrix. Also note that the mesangial cells do not appear to contain this material. (×3000.)

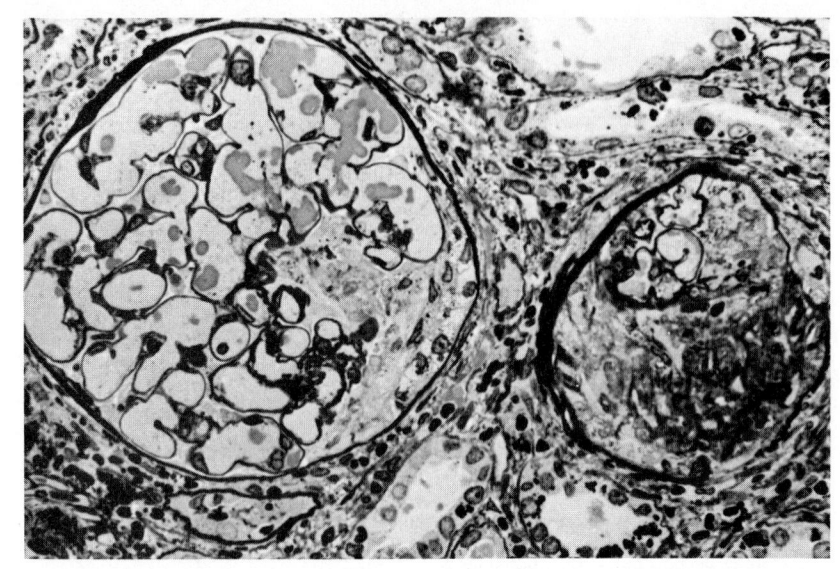

Figure 17-5 Biopsy specimen from a 21 year old woman who was admitted to hospital with a 9 month history of gradually increasing arthritis and a 4 day history of rapidly advancing central nervous system signs and the onset of acute renal failure. The glomerulus on the right contains a large cellular crescent which is undergoing earlier organization. That on the left contains epithelial proliferation in its right lower portion, whereas the rest of this particular glomerulus is relatively unaffected. Thus, even in the presence of severe renal failure and advanced histologic changes variability of the injury is still apparent. (Silver methenamine, ×300.)

amorphous masses of bluish-staining material surrounded by neutrophils. Although they are quite specific for lupus erythematosus, in the experience of most investigators these structures are rare.

In addition, deposits may be seen lying in the subendothelial space and mesangial regions, but they are irregular in distribution and on H & E staining of methacrylate-embedded material are easily distinguishable from the basal lamina (Fig. 17-7 and 17-8). In paraffin-embedded tissue, the basal lamina cannot be resolved separately from the cell cytoplasm, and therefore gives the impression of localized, prominent capillary wall thickening, a finding which led to the designation "wire loop lesion." This pattern is not specific for systemic lupus erythematosus, however, since it can be seen associated with other chronic immune complex diseases as well.

FLUORESCENCE MICROSCOPY. Deposits of IgM and C3 most commonly are found in the subendothelial and mesangial regions (Fig. 17-10), but they also may be seen in a subepithelial location in patients who have a stable or slowly progressive course. These deposits are irregular within and among glomeruli. IgA and fibrinogen seldom occur in significant quantities. Several investigators have postulated that subendothelial deposits are associated with florid proliferation and thus with an active, aggressive disease. In contrast, however, subepithelial

Text continued on page 246

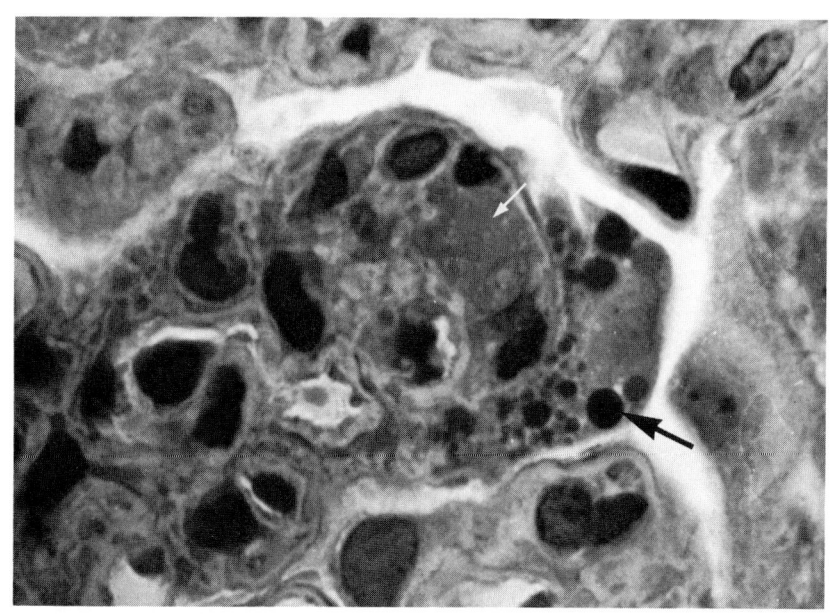

Figure 17-6 Same patient as in Figure 17-5. Note that the glomerular capillary lumen in this case is occluded by cells and a mass of amorphous protein (light arrow). The epithelial cells contains numerous protein droplets (heavy arrow). (H&E, ×1200.)

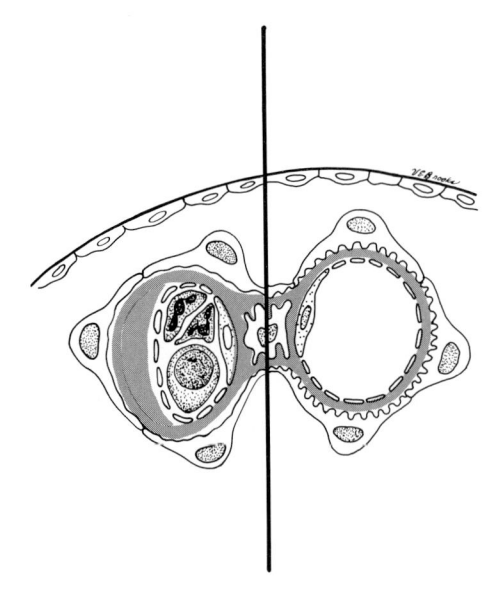

Figure 17-7 Drawing showing large subendothelial deposits and adherent leukocytes.

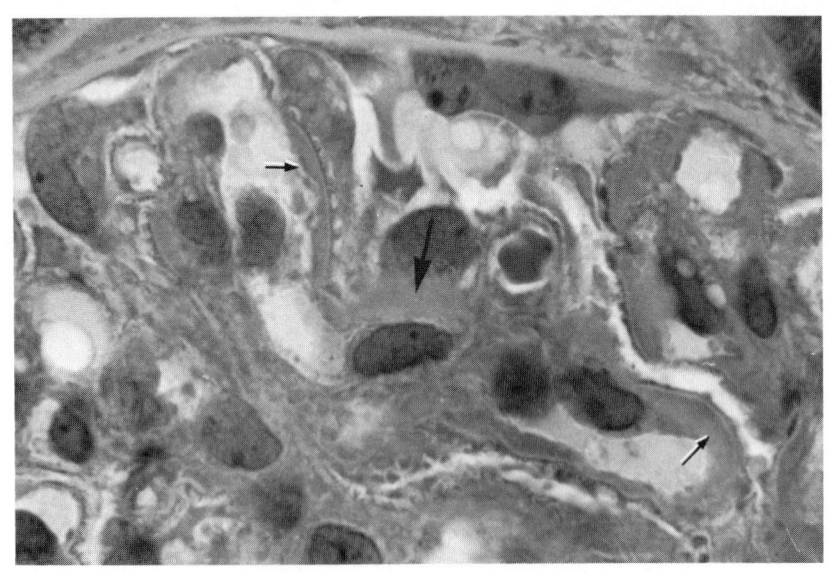

Figure 17-8 Specimen from a 26 year old woman who presented with mild renal failure, arthritis, and malaise. She had an active urine sediment and was excreting 3.4 g of protein every 24 hours in the urine. All 11 glomeruli were hypercellular and contained up to eight neutrophils per glomerulus and demonstrated large subendothelial deposits (light arrows). Deposits are also clearly apparent within the mesangial regions (heavy arrow). (H&E, ×1200.)

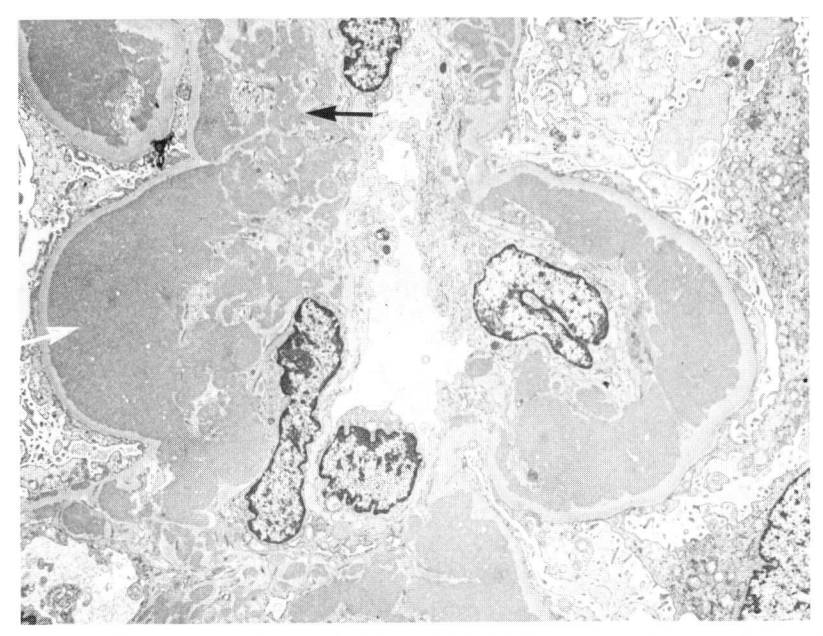

Figure 17-9 Same patient as in Figure 17-8. This low power electron micrograph substantiates the light microscopic impression of both subendothelial (light arrow) and mesangial (heavy arrow) deposits. (× 5000.)

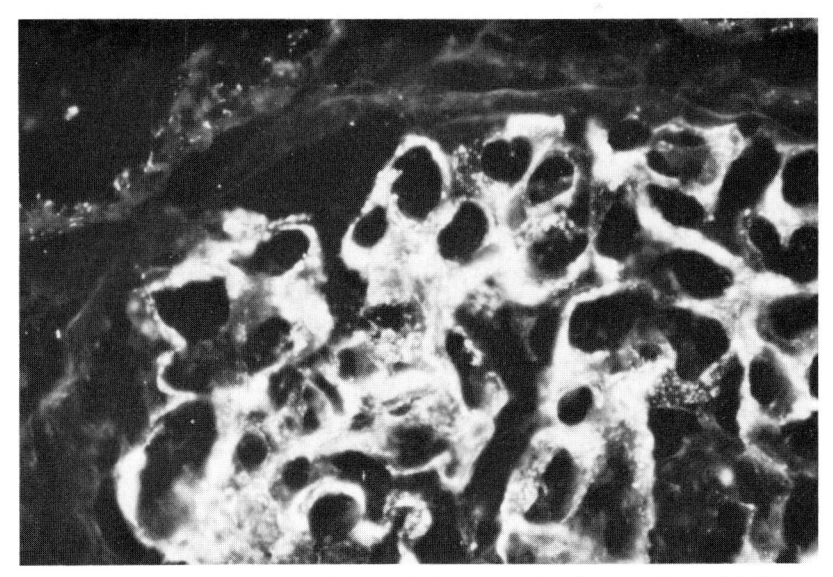

Figure 17-10 Fluorescence micrograph demonstrating the deposition of IgG in the mesangial regions and in the glomerular basal lamina. Same patient as in Figures 17-8 and 17-9. (× 300.)

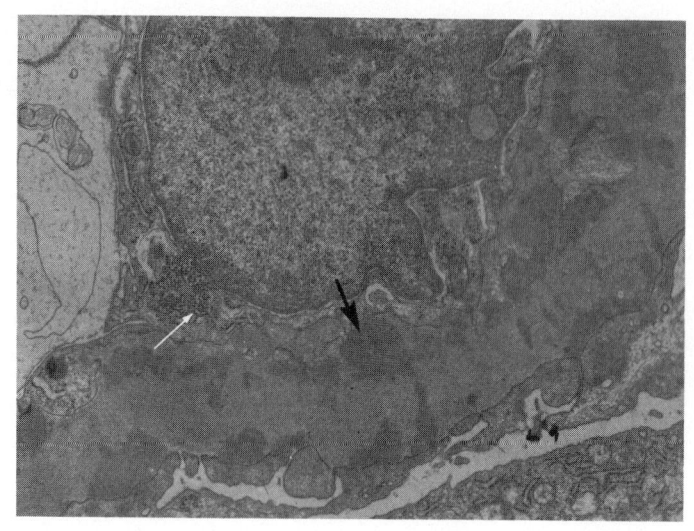

Figure 17-11 Specimen from a 42 year old male who presented with nephritis, depressed serum complement levels and elevated antinuclear antibody titers. Serum creatinine level was 1.3 mg/dl. The urine analysis results were essentially benign except for 0.9 g/24 hr protein excretion. By light microscopy numerous deposits were noted in the mesangial, subepithelial, and subendothelial regions. Note here that there are several profiles of "myxovirus" (light arrow). In addition, some of the deposits have the "fingerprint" pattern (heavy arrow). (×6300.)

deposits are thought to be present in patients with a more prolonged disease and less evidence of cellular proliferation.

ELECTRON MICROSCOPY. Localized areas of mesangial sclerosis and proliferation with rare deposits are visible in the *focal lesion,* and the pattern of deposits noted by light and fluorescent microscopy of the *diffuse lesions* can be confirmed. In patients with an acute onset of the disease, large and electron-dense, homogeneous masses of material lie in the subendothelial space adjacent to the lamina densa and in the mesangial matrix (Fig. 17-9). A number of electron microscopic peculiarities have been noted in biopsies of these patients: first, the microtubules previously described (Fig. 17-1), deposits in an organized pattern resembling a fingerprint (Fig. 17-11), and finally, crystalline structures within the deposited material. However, none of these has been shown to be specific for lupus erythematosus, and their significance is unclear.

SCLEROSING LESIONS

GENERAL FINDINGS. The sclerosing lesions of lupus erythematosus are similar to those seen in patients with so-called membranous and membranoproliferative glomerulonephritis and occur in about 15 per cent of patients with lupus nephritis.

LIGHT MICROSCOPY. The glomeruli are seen to have diffusely and more or less uniformly thickened peripheral capillary loops (Fig. 17–12). High power views reveal large deposits within the substance of the basal lamina (Fig. 17–13). Deposits may be seen in the mesangial region as well, and in these instances there is an increased number of mesangial cells. Hypercellularity and mesangial deposits are uncommon in patients with membranous glomerulonephritis who do not have systemic lupus erythematosus.

ELECTRON MICROSCOPY. Electron-dense deposits are visible between the subepithelial spikes of the lamina densa (Fig. 17–14). The amount of deposit often is so prominent that the architecture of the glomerulus is severely distorted. In addition, the epithelial cell foot processes are fused throughout. The subendothelial region and endothelial cells are normal in appearance, but the mesangial area may contain electron-dense deposits and an increased number of cells.

FLUORESCENCE MICROSCOPY. Deposits of immunoglobulin and complement are found diffusely in a regular subepithelial pattern in peripheral capillary loops and in the mesangium (Fig. 17–15).

INTERSTITIUM

Those patients who have no change or only a small number of glomeruli involved infrequently have alterations in the interstitium unless there is associated hypertension and ischemia. Patients with the diffuse proliferative response, however, often have an infiltrate consisting of lymphocytes, plasma cells, and a small number of acute inflammatory cells, which lie irregularly scattered among tubules and may be found in any location (Fig. 17–16). Their presence also has been correlated with activity of the disease.

VESSELS

Vascular lesions have seldom been described in patients with this syndrome. In those patients with the diffuse proliferative lesion and pronounced deposits, however, immunoglobulins similar to those seen in the peripheral glomerular basal lamina may be evident in afferent arterioles (Fig. 17–17).

Clinical Course and Prognosis

Although renal involvement in systemic lupus erythematosus is common, progression of the disease to uremia appears to be related to the type of reaction provoked in the kidney by the deposition of DNA–anti-DNA complexes. Each of the three common histologically defina-

Text continued on page 251

248 SYSTEMIC LUPUS ERYTHEMATOSUS

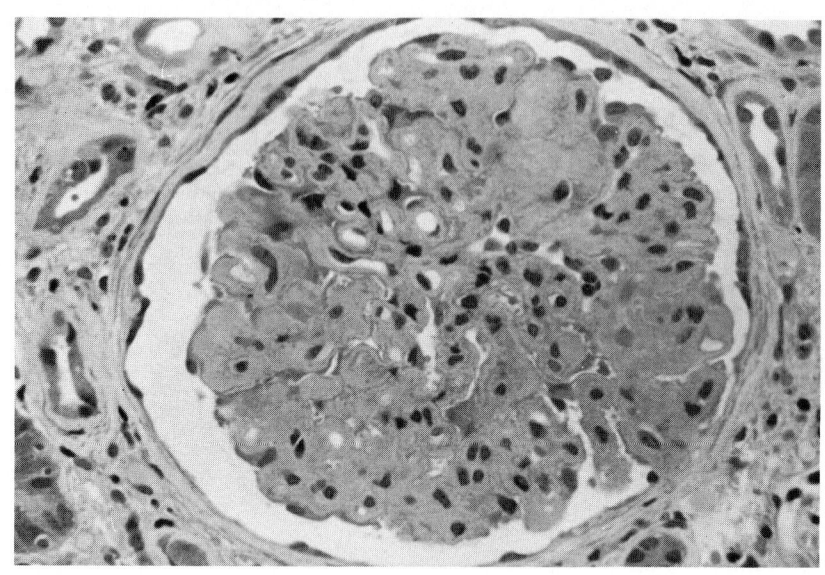

Figure 17-12 Specimen from a 49 year old female who was admitted to hospital for evaluation of nephrotic syndrome. She had had unexplained anemia for 10 years and a 4 year history of hypertension and proteinuria. She recently developed a skin rash, Raynaud's phenomenon, and abdominal pain. Serologic tests for lupus erythematosus were positive. Renal function was essentially normal. All 43 glomeruli revealed a diffuse thickening of the peripheral capillary loops, such as is present in this photomicrograph. There was also a mild increase in interstitial connective tissue and mild tubular atrophy. (H & E, ×300.)

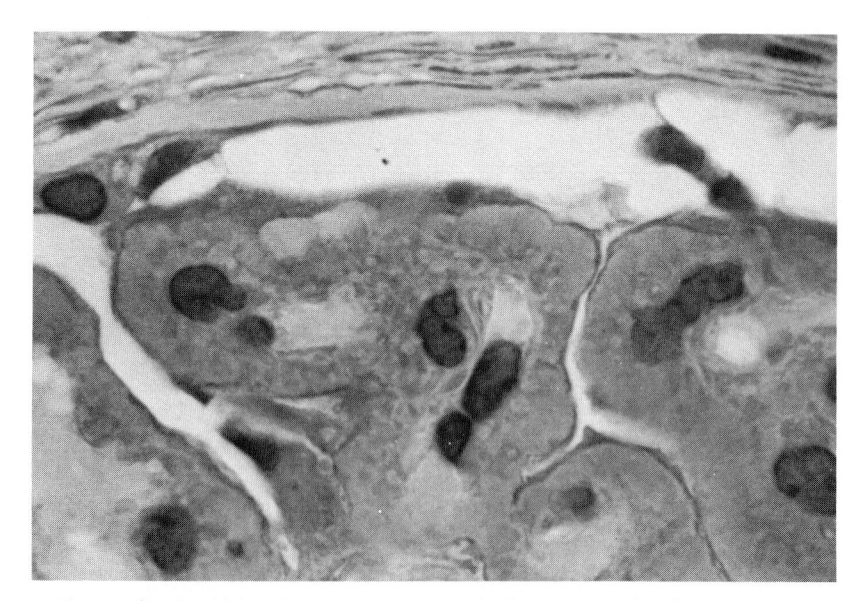

Figure 17-13 High power photomicrograph from the same patient as in Figure 17-12. Note that the glomerular basal lamina is difficult to resolve and it appears to be infiltrated with multiple large deposits. (H&E, ×63).

Systemic Lupus Erythematosus 249

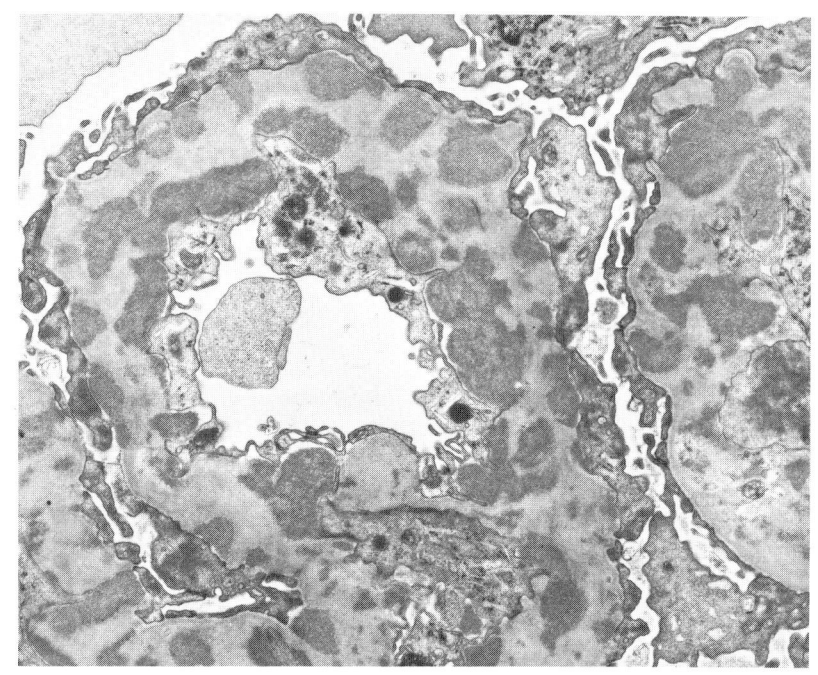

Figure 17-14 Electron micrograph of specimen from the same patient as in Figures 17-12 and 17-13. The glomerular basal lamina is severely distorted by a large number of electron-dense deposits on the endothelial side and on the epithelial side of the basal lamina. They also occur within the mesangial matrix. ($\times 4800$.)

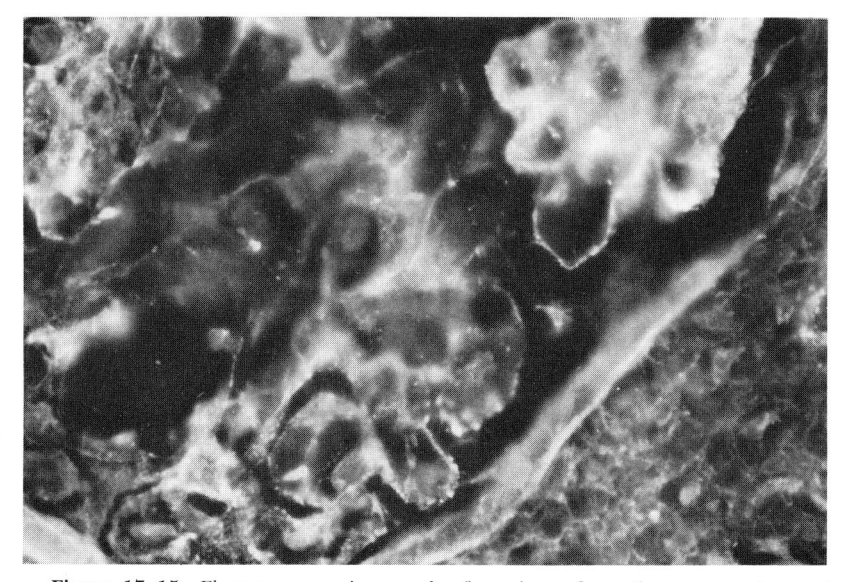

Figure 17-15 Fluorescence micrograph of specimen from the same patient as in Figures 17-12, 17-13, and 17-14. Peripheral granular deposits of IgG are present throughout. Note also that the mesangial regions contain large amounts of immunoglobulin. Deposits of C3, IgA, and IgM are also present in similar distribution. ($\times 300$.)

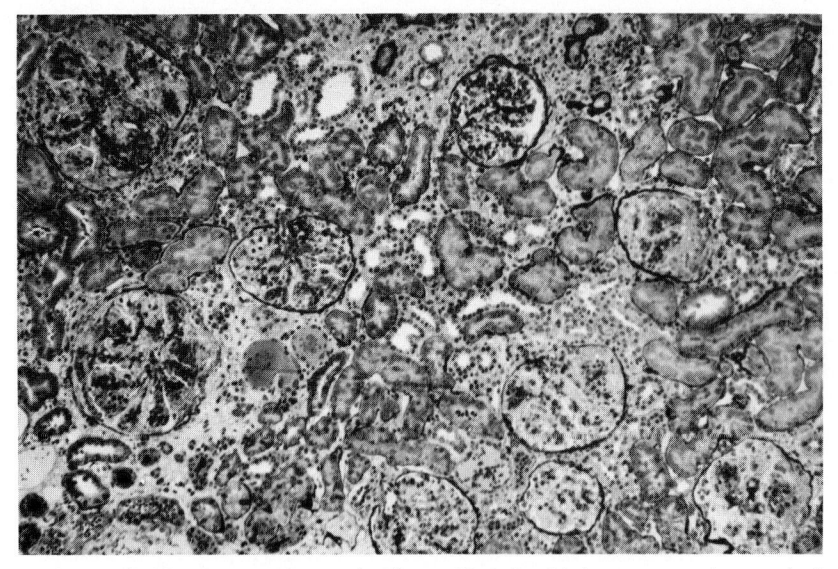

Figure 17–16. Same patient as in Figure 17–8. In this low power micrograph the variability of involvement of glomeruli, as well as the presence of interstitial infiltration with mononuclear inflammatory cells, is apparent. (Silver methenamine, ×20.)

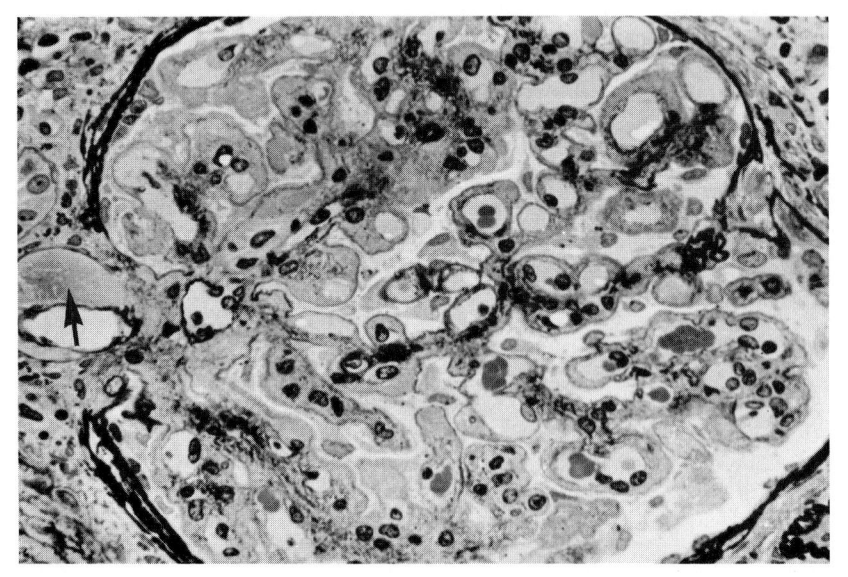

Figure 17–17 Same patient as in Figures 17–12, 17–13, 17–14, and 17–15. In this patient the afferent arteriole contains large deposits (arrow). Note the synechia at the two o'clock position. (Silver methenamine, ×300.)

ble abnormalities described in the histology section of this chapter has its own prognosis and response to treatment.

FOCAL PROLIFERATIVE LESION

Patients with the focal lesion usually have clinical evidence of mild renal involvement (Table 17-2), including microscopic hematuria and proteinuria, whereas renal insufficiency, hypertension, and nephrotic syndrome are unusual. Furthermore, in our experience no patients progressed to renal insufficiency, although other investigators have reported progression in about 10 per cent of cases, especially if subendothelial deposits were present initially.

These data would indicate that therapy directed at this renal lesion is not indicated, since it is, for the most part, benign and nonprogressive.

DIFFUSE PROLIFERATIVE LESION

The diffuse proliferation lesion is the most common type of renal involvement. Unlike the focal or sclerosing lesion, it is associated clinically with signs of active immune complex deposition. This is most reliably measured in the serum by the presence of antibody to native DNA and suppression of hemolytic complement (CH_{50}) or individual complement components (C3, C4). In addition, these serologic findings correlate well with the activity of the disease and response to treat-

TABLE 17-2   Clinical Pathologic Correlation in Lupus Nephritis

Clinical Feature	Histologic Lesion		
	Proliferative		Sclerosing
	Focal	*Diffuse*	
Incidence	30%	50%	20%
Urinary sediment:			
Hematuria	Microscopic	4+, often microscopic	Microscopic
RBC casts	Rare	Many	Rare
Nephrotic syndrome	15%	30-40%	90%
Serologic correlation with activity of nephritis:			
Antinuclear antibodies*	—	Fair	—
Anti-native DNA antibody	—	Good	—
C3	—	Good	—
C4	—	Good	—
Response to treatment	—	Poor to good	Poor
Prognosis	Good	Fair	Poor
Progression to uremia	10% may progress	Rapid progression in treatment failures	Slow progression

*Conventional lupus screening tests.

ment, being normal with remission and becoming abnormal or remaining abnormal with relapse or poor response to treatment.

Although there are no carefully controlled studies which definitively prove the value of corticosteroid treatment of this renal lesion, the majority of clinicians feel they are of definite value. The histologic changes, however, should be used to guide therapy. In our experience the diffuse proliferative lesion, which is unassociated with significant sclerosis, responds best to aggressive treatment. However, it is folly to pursue this type of treatment protocol when diffuse epithelial proliferation is present (crescents) or when there is substantial sclerosis of the renal parenchyma.

A treatment plan with corticosteroids should be undertaken with as much knowledge as possible of the likelihood of a response and should be based on serologic evidence of active disease, as well as careful histologic study of the renal parenchyma.

Many centers have added cytotoxic drugs such as cyclophosphamide and azathioprine to the treatment regimen. Although their efficacy is as yet unproven, in some patients they appear to produce a response, allowing significant reduction of corticosteroid dosage.

SCLEROSING LESION

The sclerosing lesion is the least common form of nephritis, occurring in approximately 20 per cent of patients. Histologically it is quite similar to the sclerosing membranous change seen in the primary nephrotic syndrome (see Chapter 16). Clinically it is characterized by a high incidence of the nephrotic syndrome, unresponsiveness to corticosteroid treatment, and slow progression to renal failure.

References

1. Baldwin, D. S., Lowenstein, J., Rothfield, N. F., Gallo, G., and McCluskey, R. T.: The clinical course of the proliferative and membranous forms of lupus nephritis. Ann. Intern. Med. 73:929, 1970.
2. Drinkard, J. P., Stanley, T. M., Dornfeld, L., Austin, R. C., Barnett, E. V., Pearson, C. M., Vernier, R. L., Adams, D. A., Latta, H., and Gonick, H. C.: Azathioprine and prednisone in the treatment of adults with lupus nephritis. Medicine 49:411, 1970.
3. Gary, N. E., Maher, J. F., and Schreiner, G. E.: Lupus nephritis. Renal function after prolonged survival. New Eng. J. Med. 276:73, 1967.
4. Muehrcke, R. C., Kark, R. M., Pirani, C. L., and Pollak, V. E.: Lupus nephritis: A clinical and pathologic study based on renal biopsies. Medicine 36:1, 1957.
5. Pollak, V. E., and Pirani, C. L.: Renal histologic findings in systemic lupus erythematosus. Mayo Clin. Proc. 44:630, 1969.
6. Pollak, V. E., Pirani, C. L., and Schwartz, F. D.: The natural history of the renal manifestations of systemic lupus erythematosus. J. Lab. Clin. Med. 63:537, 1964.
7. Rothfield, N. F., McCluskey, R. T., and Baldwin, D. S.: Renal disease in systemic lupus erythematosus. New Eng. J. Med. 269:537, 1963.
8. Zweiman, B., Kornblum, J., Cornog, J., and Hildreth, E. A.: The prognosis of lupus nephritis. Role of clinical-pathologic correlations. Ann. Intern. Med. 69:441, 1968.

Chapter Eighteen

Wegener's Granulomatosis and Polyarteritis Nodosa

Introduction

The clinical diseases associated with vasculitis are varied; Table 18-1 lists syndromes in which it plays a dominant role. Renal involvement in specific diseases, however, including Henoch-Schönlein purpura, systemic lupus erythematosus, and scleroderma, are discussed in other chapters. Of the remainder, only Wegener's granulomatosis and polyarteritis nodosa commonly are associated with significant renal involvement.

Renal biopsy often is helpful in establishing the diagnosis of Wegener's granulomatosis. It is particularly useful in differentiating this disease from Goodpasture's syndrome, which may have a similar clinical presentation. Because the lesion is often characteristic, kidney biopsy for polyarteritis nodosa can be diagnostic as well as prognostic.

TABLE 18-1 Clinical Syndromes Associated with Vasculitis*

1. Polyarteritis nodosa
2. Wegener's granulomatosis
3. Arteritis associated with serum sickness
4. Hypersensitivity angiitis
5. Henoch-Schönlein purpura
6. Allergic granulomatous angiitis
7. Giant cell arteritis, including temporal arteritis
8. Takayasu's arteritis
9. Rheumatoid arteritis
10. Vasculitis associated with systemic lupus erythematosus
11. Vasculitis associated with scleroderma
12. Vasculitis associated with childhood dermatomyositis

*From Classification of rheumatic disease. J.A.M.A., *224*(Suppl. 5):678, 1973.

WEGENER'S GRANULOMATOSIS

Clinical Data

In 1936, Wegener described a syndrome of necrotizing granulomatosis vasculitis of the respiratory tract in addition to glomerulonephritis. Although the etiology of this syndrome is unknown, it is presumed to be a disease mediated by the deposition of immune complexes in the vascular wall; the allergen(s) has (have) not yet been identified.

Additionally, the syndrome is more common in the males than females (2 to 1 ratio), occurring frequently during the fifth decade, although the total age range is large. The patient often presents with complaints related to the upper respiratory tract such as rhinorrhea, sinus pain, and mucosal ulcerations. Cough and hemoptysis are common pulmonary complaints as well. Fever, malaise, and anorexia also can be present when secondary infection of the sinuses occurs or when the disease is fulminant. Furthermore, anemia, leukocytosis, and an elevated erythrocyte sedimentation rate occur frequently. Unlike polyarteritis nodosa, however, eosinophilia is rare. The radiographic pulmonary lesions also are variable, and can be of fleeting duration. The most common finding is nodular lesions in the lower lung fields which may cavitate.

Renal involvement is present in approximately 80 per cent of the cases, although initially it may be asymptomatic. Urinalysis reveals proteinuria, hematuria, and red cell casts. When the kidneys are affected, it can be of a slowly or rapidly progressing variety and generally parallels the severity of involvement in other organ systems. Differing in another way from polyarteritis nodosa, however, hypertension usually is not present until significant impairment of renal function occurs. In addition to the pulmonary and kidney involvement, pericarditis, skin lesions, cranial neuritis, polyarthritis, and polyarthralgia are common. Although the renal lesions are not pathognomonic, the changes may be of aid in confirmation of the diagnosis, especially when the respiratory lesion is mild.

Histology

LIGHT MICROSCOPY. The glomerular histologic lesion in Wegener's granulomatosis is characterized by its irregularity of involvement, both within and among individual glomeruli. There also is considerable variation in the severity of the lesion among patients. In some cases, for example, nearly all glomeruli are affected by a florid, acute inflammatory process, whereas in others the lesion may affect only a small number of segments of glomeruli. In addition, there may be considerable variation in the degree of involvement between glomeruli in a single specimen. The most regular morphologic feature, in fact, is the segmental nature of glomerular involvement, which often also occurs in systemic lupus erythematosus and other vasculitides (Fig. 18-1). The final distinctive feature, however, is the irregularity in the apparent ages of the lesions (Fig. 18-2). Some glomeruli may display features of an acute inflammatory process, whereas others may be partially or completely sclerosed.

The light microscopic characteristics of the inflammatory process include localized proliferation of glomerular cells, often epithelial, which results in the formation of a crescent (Fig. 18-3). A variable number of neutrophils may also be evident in the region. Fibrin frequently is present in the spaces between epithelial cells, and obvious necrosis accompanied by localized thrombosis of the capillaries often is found as well (Fig. 18-1).

The tubules and interstitium are affected as a result of the vascular injury. The changes are therefore nonspecific.

Granulomatosus arteritis, while characteristic of Wegener's granulomatosis, is an uncommon finding.

ELECTRON MICROSCOPY. Electron microscopy can document the presence of deposits in the mesangial regions and occasionally on the epithelial aspect of the glomerular basal lamina. They are few in number, however, and resemble those seen in postinfectious glomerulonephritis, or, less frequently, in early membranous lesions.

IMMUNOFLUORESCENCE. On immunofluorescence, deposits of IgG and C3 have been described in the mesangium, and sometimes along peripheral capillary loops in a granular pattern. Fibrin commonly is found between epithelial cells when crescents are present but there is no diagnostic or prognostic significance in the type, amount, or distribution of deposited serum proteins.

Clinical Course and Prognosis

Prior to the use of antimetabolites, the usual course of Wegener's granulomatosis was rapid deterioration and death in approximately 5 to 12 months; uremia was the most common cause of death. Steroid treatment alone had little effect on mortality, but the addition of antimetabolites (the usual combination being steroids with azathioprine or cyclophosphamide) has improved prognosis considerably. Fauci and Wolff (1973), for example, report prolonged remissions in 16 of 18 patients treated with cyclophosphamide, a great improvement in what formerly was a uniformly fatal illness. After a period of drug therapy, many patients also were able to have treatment withdrawn without subsequent relapse of the disease.

Text continued on page 258

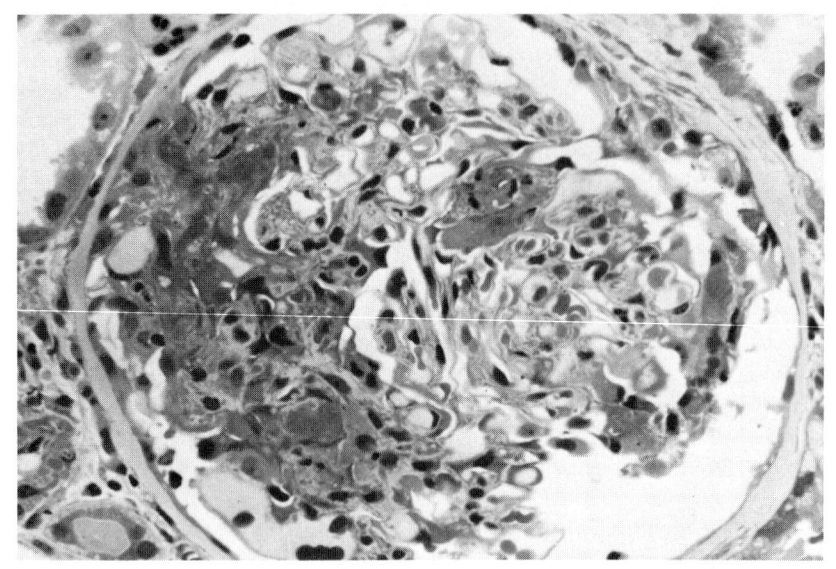

Figure 18-1 Three years prior to admission, the 47 year old female from whom this specimen was taken developed first a hearing loss in the right ear and upper respiratory infection which persisted, and then hearing loss in the left ear. Nasal pharyngeal and tympanic membrane biopsies revealed granulomas. One year prior to admission she developed bilateral diffuse interstitial pulmonary infiltrates which contained many eosinophils. Renal function, which had previously been normal, deteriorated. The creatinine level was 3.74 mg/dl. This glomerulus demonstrated irregular involvement of the tufts. Many capillary loops are patent at the 12 and 7 o'clock positions. However, between eight and 11 the capillary spaces are obliterated by accumulation of protein within the lumen and Bowman's space. The overall cellularity is increased and there are some neutrophils present within the capillary spaces. (H&E, ×300.)

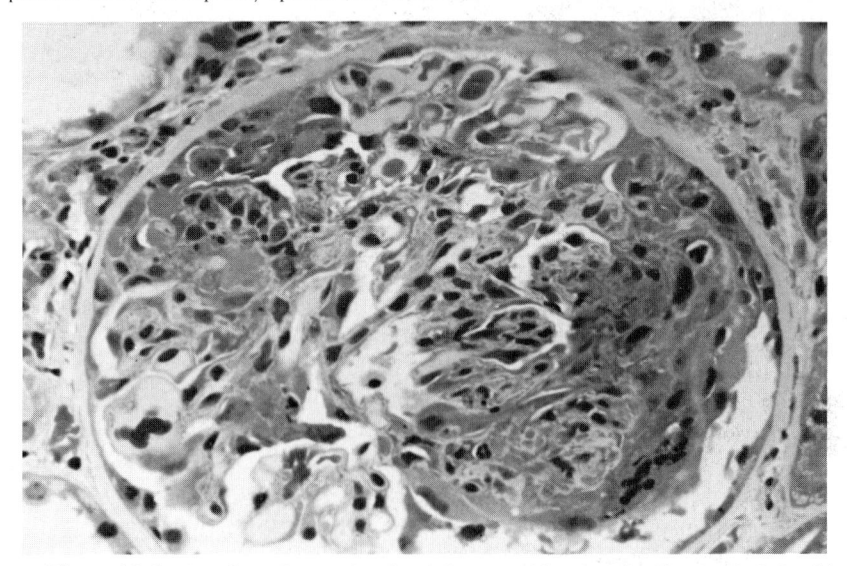

Figure 18-2 Another glomerulus from the same biopsy as in Figure 18-1. In this glomerulus the glomerular capillary loops are markedly compressed in the region of the 2 o'clock to 5 o'clock positions. There is an increase in the amount of extracellular material (basal lamina) in this region. There is also a marked proliferation of epithelial cells in the adjacent Bowman's space. (H&E, × 300.)

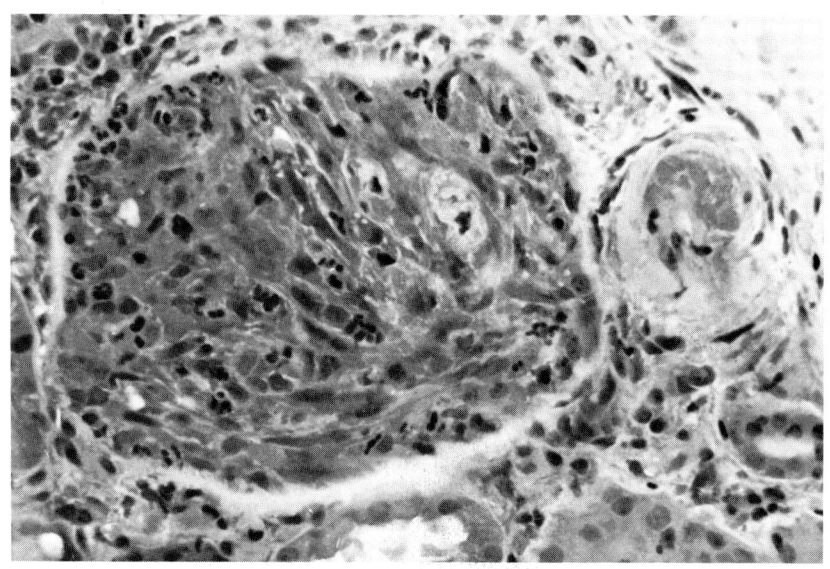

Figure 18-3 The marked variability with which the lesion affects glomeruli is well demonstrated in this patient. This glomerulus is also from the same biopsy as Figures 18-1 and 18-2. Here the glomerular capillary loops are nearly completely obliterated by proliferating epithelial cells in Bowman's space and infiltration by large numbers of neutrophils. A small portion of a glomerular tuft is recognizable between the 2 and 3 o'clock positions as a small knot of unstained extracellular material. Note also that the interstitium is infiltrated with inflammatory cells in the adjacent tissue and that the inflammation extends between tubules (H&E, ×300.)

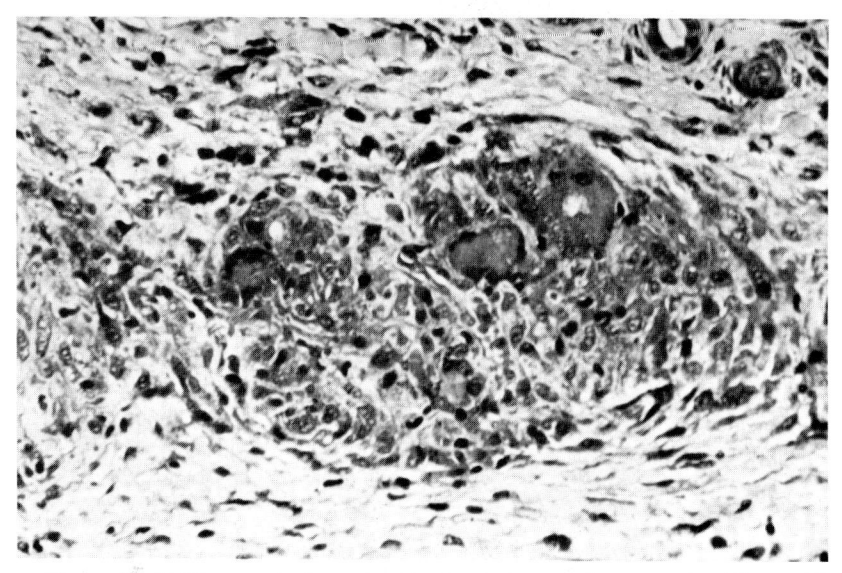

Figure 18-4 The vessels shown in this photomicrograph are nearly obliterated by a dense accumulation of inflammatory cells. Note that in the upper portion of the inflammatory mass there are three multinucleated giant cells. This is a relatively unusual finding in renal biopsies of patients with Wegener's granulomatosis; however, when found the diagnosis is clear. (Trichrome stain, paraffin-embedded material, ×300.)

POLYARTERITIS NODOSA

Clinical Data

The clinical syndrome of polyarteritis nodosa was first described by Kussmaul and Maier in 1886. As with Wegener's granulomatosis, this syndrome is thought to be mediated by the immune system. It is not known, however, whether the hypersensitivity is the result of endogenous or exogenous antigens.

The disease is most common in males (2 to 1 ratio) with a peak age incidence in the fifth to sixth decade. It is insidious in onset and protean in nature, making it difficult to date the onset and distinguish from other systemic illnesses. Frequent presenting complaints include fever, anorexia, and weight loss, which often are associated with arthritis, arthralgias, and skin lesions. Mononeuritis multiplex occurs in over 50 per cent of cases.

Additionally, anemia, leukocytosis, and elevated erythrocyte sedimentation rate are present in most patients, and eosinophilia also can be found in almost 50 per cent of cases. Although abnormal urinary sediment findings are present initially in 75 per cent of cases, only 30 per cent have renal functional impairment. A telescopic urinary sediment which contains the typical elements found in acute, rapidly progressive, and chronic glomerulonephritis are considered typical of this disease, but these changes are not pathognomonic, as they occur in rapidly progressive glomerulonephritis of any etiology. Hypertension also is common in early stages, usually accompanying advancing renal impairment. Finally, the presence of hypertension or renal impairment at initial presentation indicates severe or advanced disease, and thus gives a poor prognosis.

Histology

GENERAL FINDINGS. The renal lesions are of two distinct types: those affecting the large vessels and those affecting primarily the microvasculature, including the glomeruli. In the large vessel variety (classic or nodosa variety) the renal lesion is that of infarction; the intervening glomeruli, tubules, interstitium, and vessels are normal. Renal failure is uncommon. The microvascular type affects the renal vasculature diffusely and uniformly; thus, renal failure is common and occurs early in the course of the disease.

LARGE VESSELS

LIGHT MICROSCOPY
Glomeruli. In this disease the glomerular changes reflect the degree of alteration in large vessels, varying from mild ischemia through complete infarction.

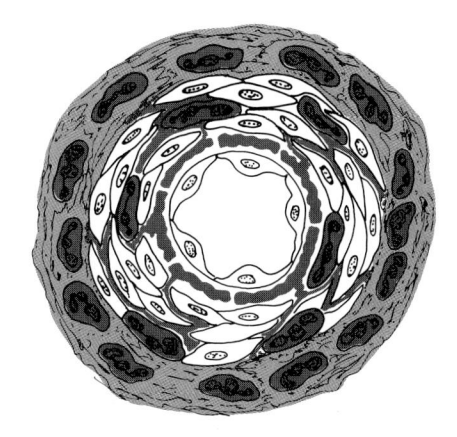

Figure 18-5 Drawing depicting diffuse inflammatory infiltration of the vessel wall.

Tubules and Interstitium. No alterations of note are evident in the tubules and interstitium, except those appearing as a late sequela of ischemia. Obvious necrosis, of course, also is present in infarcted zones.

Vessels. The vascular lesion is distinct and quite florid in polyarteritis nodosa. The process may involve a small segment of a vessel wall, but commonly affects the entire circumference (Figs. 18-5 and 18-6). The lesion results in disruption of the normal structures by

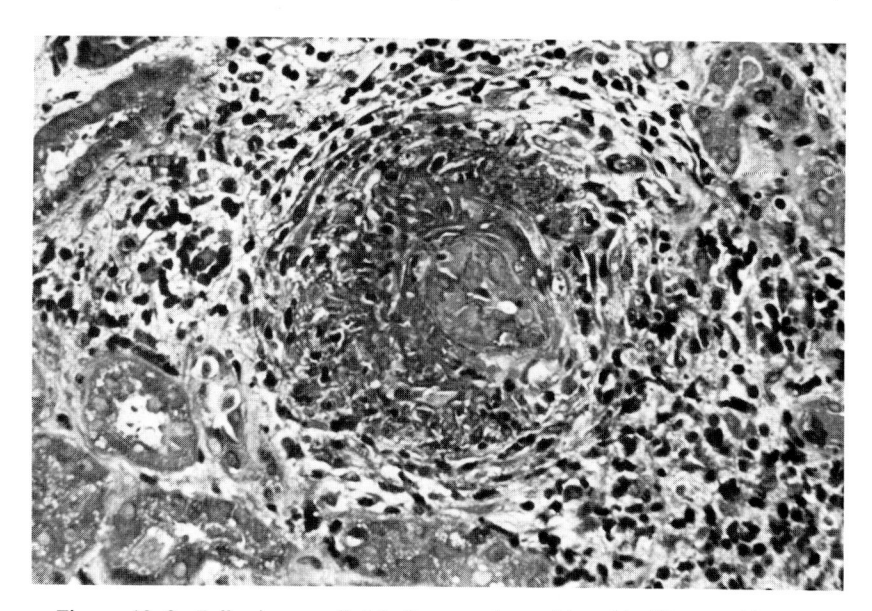

Figure 18-6 Following a cellulitis from an insect bite, this 57 year old man was admitted to a local hospital and found to have a BUN of 60 mg/100, creatinine of 2.3 mg/dl, hematuria and proteinuria, and he was found to be hypertensive, confused, and febrile. Left lower lobe infiltrate was noted by chest x-ray. Urine sediment was quite active. A section of the renal biopsy demonstrated the vascular lesion noted in the photomicrograph, which involved many small arteries and arterioles. Note the dense inflammatory infiltrate in the surrounding tissue, in the adventitia and the media throughout the entire thickness. The vascular space is difficult to identify. The inflammatory cells consist of mononuclear cells as well as neutrophils (H&E, ×300).

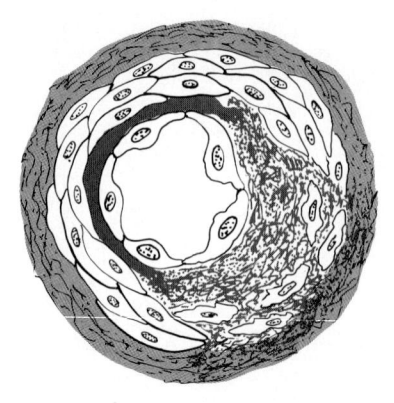

Figure 18-7 Drawing depicting segmental necrosis of the vascular wall.

a homogeneous, eosinophilic material often referred to as fibrinoid. Since the resident cells often are destroyed, the process has been called fibrinoid necrosis (Figs. 18-7 and 18-8). Neutrophils, eosinophils, and lymphocytes, in that order of prevalence, make up the cellular infiltrate. As the injury heals, the plasma proteins and disrupted cells are replaced by connective tissue (Fig. 18-9). The lumen often is occluded partially or completely by this response. However, since the vascular lesion is spotty and affects only a short segment of the artery, the biopsy needle may miss the involved areas of the vessel completely.

ELECTRON MICROSCOPY

No additional information is obtained from electron microscopic examination.

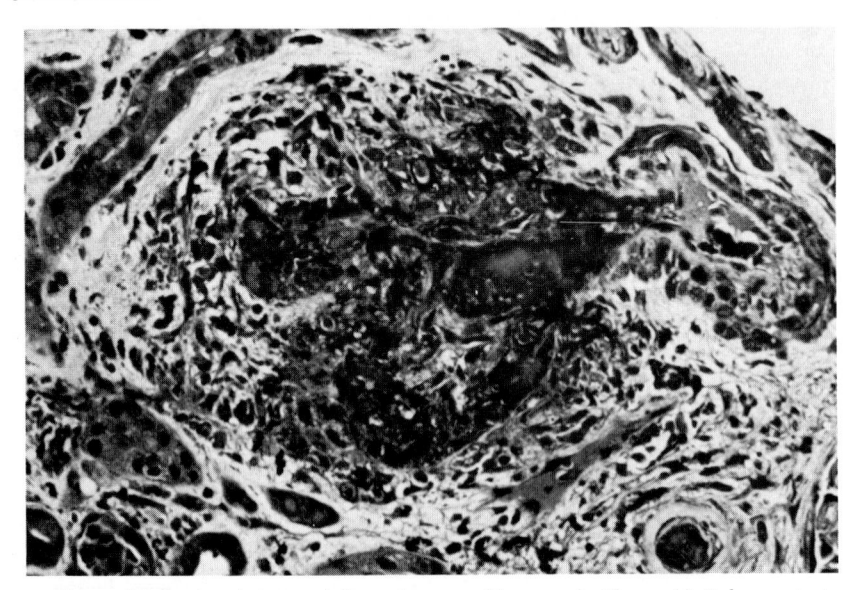

Figure 18-8 Another vessel from the same biopsy as in Figure 18-6 demonstrates the irregularity of the vascular lesion. The vessel segment on the right is nearly normal, whereas that on the left demonstrates diffuse infiltration of the wall by inflammatory cells and thrombosis of the lumen. (Trichrome stain, paraffin-embedded material, ×300.)

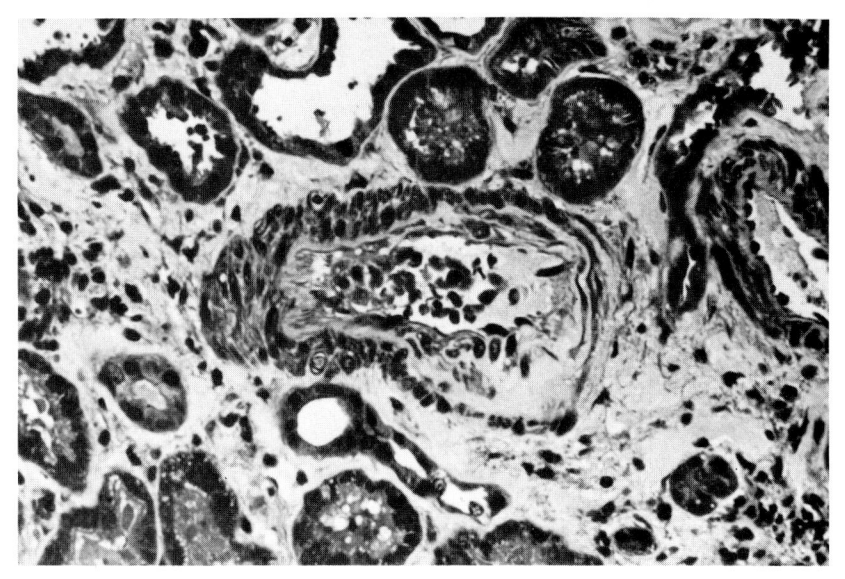

Figure 18-9 Same patient as in Figures 18-6 through 18-8. The patient improved on steroid therapy; however, one month later he developed weakness and nuchal rigidity, and was found to have an intracerebral hemorrhage. He expired 20 hours after admission. On autopsy the vessel lesions in the kidney were all similar to that noted in this photomicrograph. The inflammatory infiltrate had disappeared and multiple areas of scarring involving a significant portion of the vascular wall were seen. (Trichrome stain, paraffin-embedded material, ×300.)

Fluorescence Microscopy

On fluorescence microscopy, immunoglobulins, fibrin, and other plasma proteins are observed to be present throughout the affected vascular wall.

Microvascular Form

Light Microscopy

While arcuate-sized vessels may be involved in the microvascular variety it is more common to see smaller vessels and glomeruli damaged. Similar sized vessels are affected in other organs as well.

Glomeruli. Most often the lesions involve all glomeruli, although the degree of change may vary. Characteristically, fibrin is deposited in capillary loops and the surrounding Bowman's space, with subsequent epithelial proliferation (Fig. 18-10). Crescents also are common, and neutrophils may be present in capillary loops and crescents. In longstanding cases, there are areas of sclerosis within glomeruli and synechiae, which may be plentiful (Fig. 18-11).

Tubules and Interstitium. Interstitium infiltration and edema parallel the degree of epithelial cell proliferation, although no specific tubular changes are evident. In biopsies later in the course of the

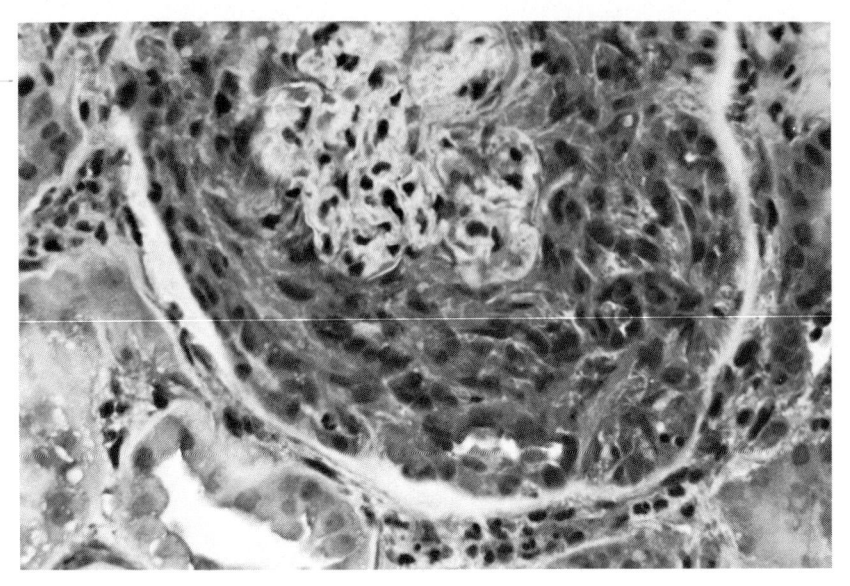

Figure 18–10 Three months prior to admission this 59 year old female developed polyarthritis and Raynaud's phenomenon. Three months later she developed Guillain-Barré syndrome, and reduced renal function was noted. On admission to hospital, serum complement levels were found to be normal, creatinine clearance was 40 ml/min, and saline excess was noted. Blood pressure was normal. The glomerulus pictured here was typical for all 15 noted in the renal biopsy. The glomerular capillary loops are compressed by marked proliferation of the epithelial cells. A small number of neutrophils are noted within the crescent. The large blood vessels were essentially unremarkable. In the arterioles, there was evidence of extravasation of serum proteins into the wall. (H&E, ×300.)

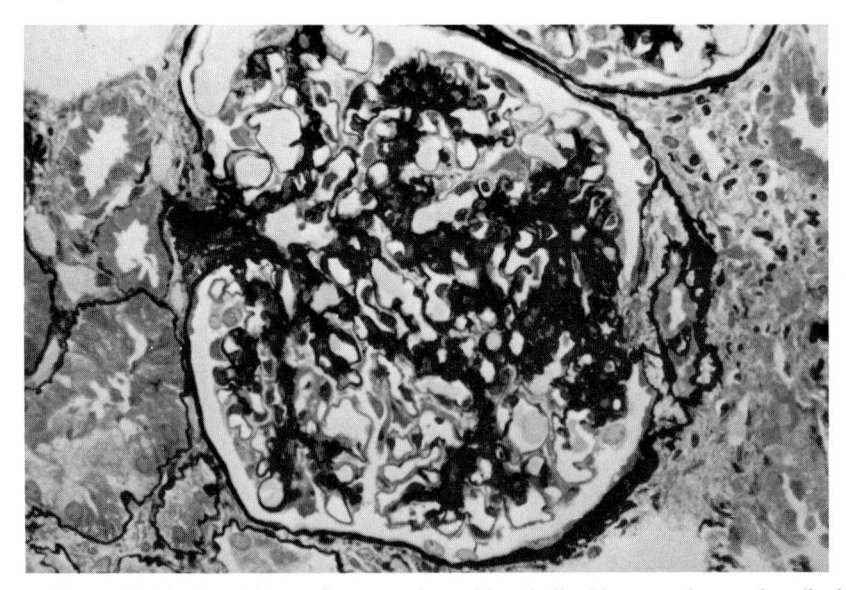

Figure 18–11 Renal biopsy from a patient with a similar history to the one described in Figure 18–10. This patient responded to therapy and one year later a repeat renal biopsy demonstrated that 14 of 16 glomeruli had synechiae similar to the one depicted in this photomicrograph. There is a modest increase in the mesangial matrix in many of the glomerular tufts. However, at the 3 o'clock position is an organized synechia. (Silver methenamine, ×300.)

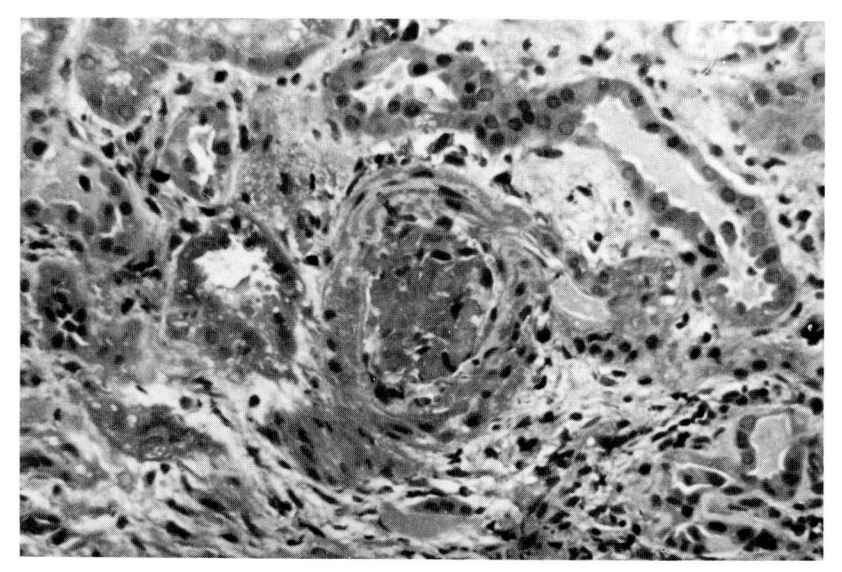

Figure 18-12 An arteriole from the same patient as in Figure 18-10. This is a small artery and one of the arteriole branches can be seen at the 3 o'clock position. The lumen contains a thrombus consisting of an admixture of coagulated protein and inflammatory cells. The endothelium is not apparent. No inflammatory cells are noted within the wall of the artery. (H&E, ×300.)

disease, however, tubular atrophy and interstitial fibrosis accompany the glomerulosclerosis.

Vessels. Small arteries and arterioles frequently are affected. The changes are characterized by deposition of fibrin and other plasma proteins and loss of the normal architecture (fibrinoid necrosis). These lesions are not histologically dissimilar from the large vessel variety but in general are more diffuse. Infiltration by acute inflammatory cells is another trait, and the endothelial cells are swollen and appear to be increased in number as well (Fig. 18-12).

ELECTRON MICROSCOPY

No additional information is obtained by electron microscopy.

FLUORESCENCE MICROSCOPY

As in the large vessel type, plasma proteins, including immunoglobulins, are present in the involved vessels; in the microvascular form, similar deposits can also be seen distributed diffusely throughout the glomeruli.

Clinical Course and Prognosis

Prior to the availability of corticosteroid therapy, deaths from renal failure occurred with high frequency in the first year of the illness. In a series of patients reported by Frohnert and Sheps, for example, the 5 year survival rate of corticosteroid treated patients was 48 per cent as opposed to 13 per cent in untreated patients. Sixty-six per cent of the patients surviving 2 to 5 years, however, required continuous steroid therapy because of the relapsing nature of the illness. Antimetabolites also have been reported to be of benefit in the treatment of these patients.

References

1. Fauci, A. S., and Wolff, S. M.: Wegener's granulomatosis: Studies in eighteen patients and a review of the literature. Medicine 52:535, 1973.
2. Frohnert, P. P., and Sheps, S. G.: Long-term follow-up study of periarteritis nodosa. Amer. J. Med. 43:8, 1967.
3. Goodman, G. C., and Churg, J.: Wegener's granulomatosis. Pathology and review of the literature. Arch. Pathol. 58:533, 1954.
4. Heptinstall, R. H.: Pathology of the Kidney. Boston, Little Brown & Company, 1974.
5. Horn, R. H., Fauci, A. J., Rosenthal, A. J., et al.: Renal biopsy pathology in Wegener's granulomatosis. Am. J. Pathol. 74:423, 1974.
6. Kussmaul, A., and Maier, R.: Veber eine bisher nicht beschriebene eigenthumliche Arterienerkrankung (Periarteritis Nodosa), die nit Morbus Brightii und rapid Fortshreitender allgemeiner Muskell-Ahmung Cinhergeht. Dtsch. Arch. Klin. Med. 1:484, 1866.
7. Rose, G. A., and Spencer, H.: Polyarteritis nodosa. Quart. J. Med. 26:43, 1957.
8. Walton, E. W.: Giant-cell granuloma of the respiratory tract (Wegener's granulomatosis). Brit. Med. J. 2:265, 1958.
9. Wegener, F.: Uber generalisierte, Septische Gefasserkrankungen. Verh. Dtsch. Ges. Path. 01.29:202, 1936.
10. Zeek, P. M.: Periarteritis nodosa and other forms of necrotizing angitis. New Eng. J. Med. 248:765, 1953.

Chapter Nineteen

Henoch-Schönlein Purpura

Introduction

Robert Willan in 1808 was the first to describe a peculiar syndrome in 17 patients consisting of hemorrhage, anasarca, and vivices. Common symptoms in these patients also included arthralgia, abdominal pains, nausea, vomiting, and fever. Willan suspected renal involvement as well, but this was not confirmed until Henoch's finding of hematuria and proteinuria in 1874. Since then, the incidence and severity of renal manifestations have been a subject of controversy, especially following Osler's report in 1904 that 50 per cent of 29 patients had evidence of kidney dysfunction, and in fact, five died of uremia. More recent figures, however, indicate that these early estimates were low; in current studies, urinary sediment changes, which point to renal abnormality, have been evident in 60 per cent of cases during the acute phase of the illness. In addition, reports of persistent urinary abnormalities have been recorded in from as low as 6 per cent to as high as 40 per cent of the patients after varying periods of follow-up. These statistics indicate that renal involvement is an integral part of this syndrome. Renal biopsy, therefore, is helpful in determining the extent of injury and prognosis.

Clinical Data

The clinical data can be demonstrated by examining a recent study of 59 patients hospitalized at the University of Washington Hospitals who had the clinical diagnosis of Henoch-Schönlein purpura. The diagnosis was made using the characteristic clinical criteria, including

Text continued on page 268

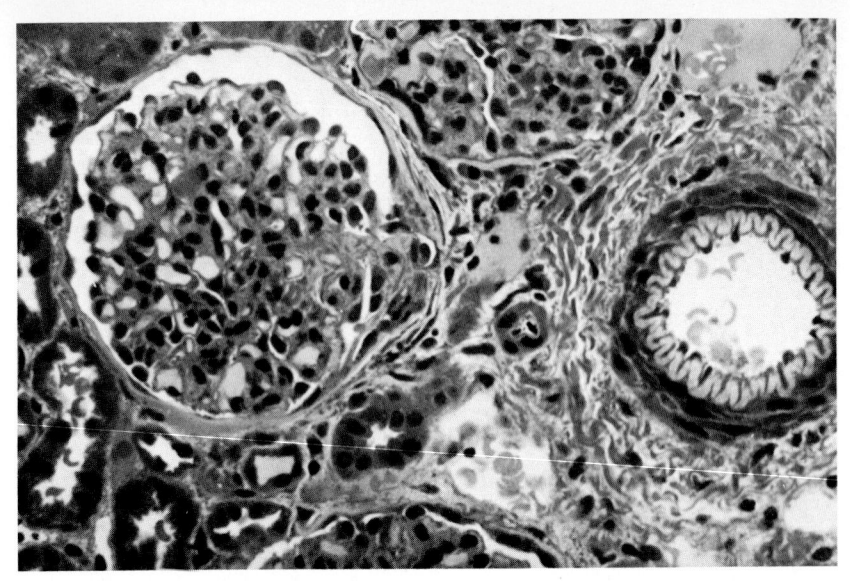

Figure 19-1 Specimen from a 14 year old boy who was admitted following an episode of acute abdominal pain with mild melena. The urine was found to contain multiple red blood cell casts. Protein excretion was 1.4 g/24 hours. The three glomeruli shown are typical of those in this biopsy. The glomerulus at left center has a synechia at the 3 o'clock position and focal hypercellularity in this region. The other two glomeruli also demonstrate localized areas of hypercellularity within individual tufts. IgA deposits were noted in the mesangial regions of all glomeruli. There were, as well, small amounts of IgM and C3. Note that the interstitium, tubules, and vessels are unaffected in this patient. The amount of connective tissue surrounding the vessel is normal for this size. (H&E, ×300.)

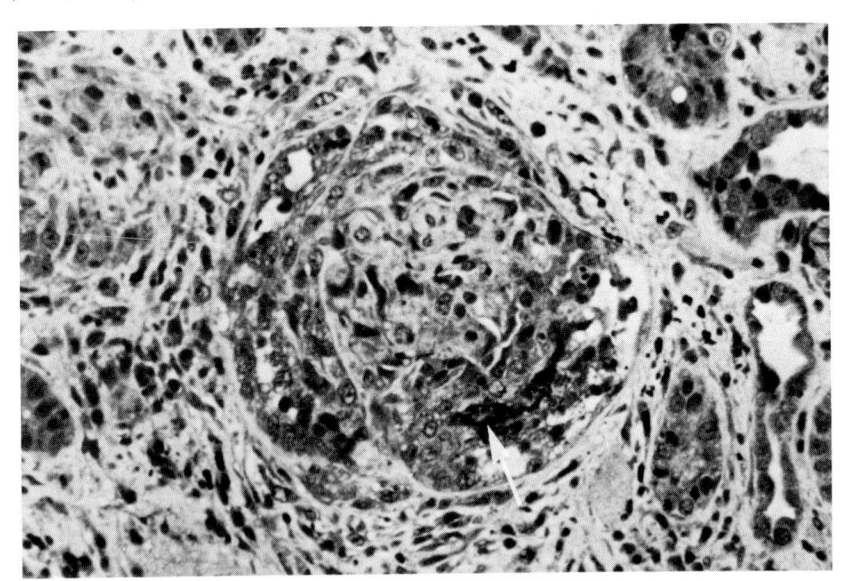

Figure 19-2 On admission, this 12 year old boy had fever, arthralgias, abdominal pain, and a lower abdominal rash. His creatinine level was 2.2 mg/dl, and the urine sediment was quite active. Protein excretion was 3 g/24 hours. This glomerulus is typical of nearly one-third of those in this biopsy. There is marked proliferation of epithelial cells and compression of the glomerular capillaries. Deposits of plasma protein are noted between glomerular epithelial cells from the 3 to the 5 o'clock positions (arrow). Inflammatory cells, primarily neutrophils, also are noted in the epithelial crescent. There also is substantial infiltration of the interstitium by acute inflammatory cells. In this patient the renal disease progressed, and he was placed on hemodialysis within 4 years. He did not respond to several courses of steroids or to cytotoxic drugs. (Trichrome stain, paraffin-embedded tissue, ×300.)

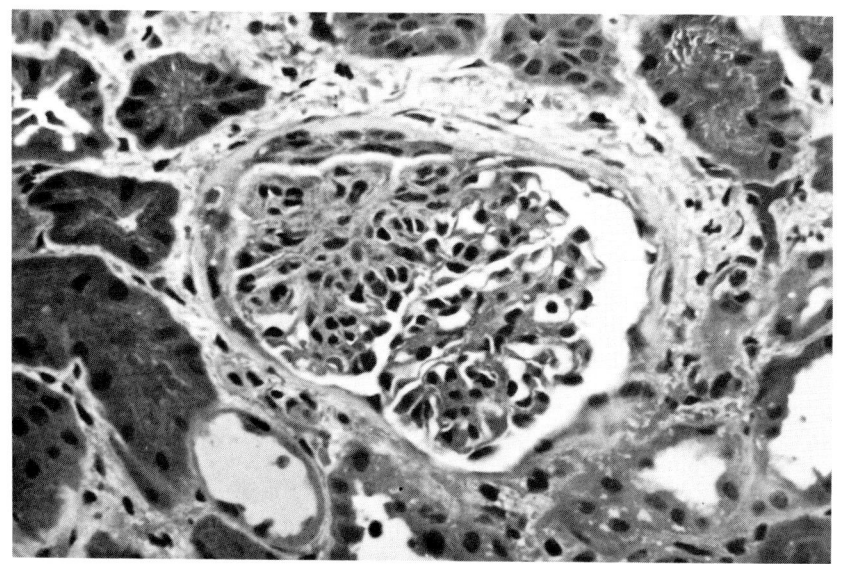

Figure 19-3 Specimen from a 9 year old girl who had an episode considered to be typical of Henoch-Schönlein purpura without evidence of renal function impairment. Over the ensuing 3 years she had multiple episodes of hematuria without proteinuria following acute intercurrent illnesses. Because of persistent hematuria her condition was reevaluated. Renal function remains normal. The glomerulus pictured here is representative of three of 24 glomeruli; the remainder were normal. Nearly one-half is occupied by an increased amount of extracellular material. Synechiae were present in all three affected glomeruli. Note that the surrounding interstitium also contains an increased amount of connective tissue. This feature was localized to the regions of the synechiae. (H&E, ×300.)

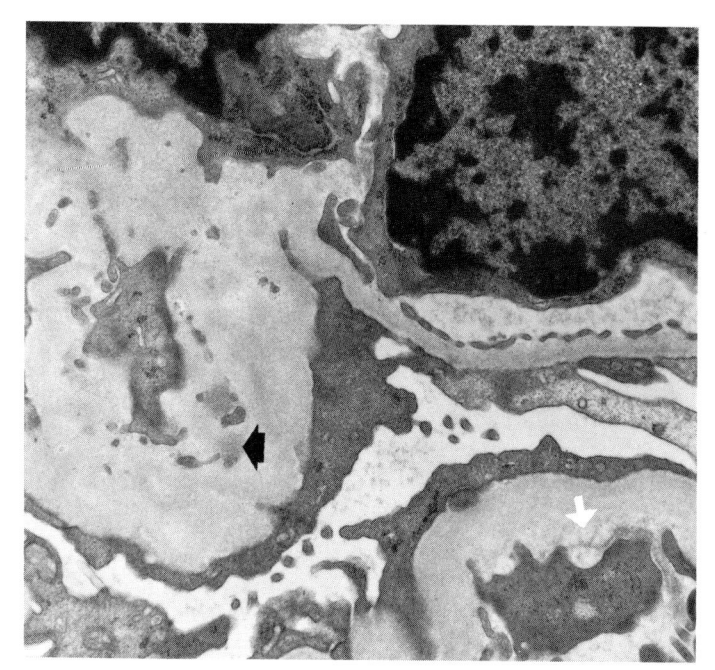

Figure 19-4 Renal biopsy from the same patient as Figure 19-1. In one area, the subendothelial space is noted to be widened (light arrow). There is a small amount of flocculent material in this region. The capillary space above is relatively unremarkable. To the left, the mesangial region is noted to be somewhat expanded. There are areas of increased density in this region, corresponding to the deposition of immunoglobulins noted by fluorescent microscopy (heavy arrow). (×10,000.)

skin rash, abdominal pain, melena, hematuria, joint symptoms, edema, and fever.

The incidence of renal involvement in males was nearly three times that in females for the whole series. Eighty per cent of patients were under 10 years of age and 95 per cent were under 15 years old. Furthermore, all patients had the characteristic skin rash over the lower abdomen and legs, with the next most prevalent finding being arthralgia. Gastrointestinal complaints, peripheral edema, fever, and renal abnormalities also occurred with almost equal frequency, in roughly half the patients. The incidence of renal complications was higher in this group, however, since the study involved hospitalized cases. The data also agree with a study by Allen and associates (1960) on 131 patients who were ill enough to require hospitalization.

Urinary sediment changes vary from microscopic hematuria to a telescopic sediment with marked albuminuria. Evidence of reduced kidney function is uncommon at the onset of the disease and occurs most frequently in those over 15 years of age.

Histology

LIGHT MICROSCOPY. Although not pathognomonic, the renal morphologic alterations of Henoch-Schönlein purpura are quite characteristic. The most common feature is proliferation of intraglomerular cells (mesangial), affecting segments of glomeruli (segmental), and in an irregular distribution among glomeruli (focal) (Fig. 19–1).

In many cases, however, no renal lesions are visible in glomeruli; the only abnormality evident is red cells in the tubular lumina. Once in a while a patient also has marked proliferation of epithelial cells in many glomeruli, deposition of fibrin-fibrinogen antigen in Bowman's space, and an associated tubulo-interstitial lesion of great severity (Fig. 19–2). It is in these cases that renal function is reduced, progressively becoming more depressed. In addition, as the patients with focal proliferative or segmental necrotizing lesions are followed sequentially, the end result often is a localized scar or synechiae (Fig. 19–3).

ELECTRON MICROSCOPY. The most common ultrastructural findings are a mild to moderate increase in mesangial matrix, mesangial deposits and focal thickening of the glomerular capillary loop secondary to endothelial cell swelling and deposition of flocculent material in the subendothelial space (Fig. 19–4).

FLUORESCENCE MICROSCOPY. The characteristic finding by fluorescence microscopy is mesangial IgA deposits affecting most glomeruli. Fibrin-fibrinogen antigen may be present and is particularly prominent in areas of epithelial proliferation.

Clinical Course and Prognosis

Even though renal involvement in Henoch-Schönlein purpura is common, it generally follows a benign course. Although recurrences of this syndrome occur frequently, the vast majority of these patients recover without permanent sequelae. There also is a good correlation between initial renal histology and subsequent clinical course; the presence of severe histologic kidney involvement at the onset suggests a more prolonged course and a persistent abnormal urinary sediment, whereas milder changes are associated with a benign course and quick recovery. The disease also tends to be more serious in older male children. The mean age of patients with severe nephritis in the University of Washington study, for example, was 14 years, 88 per cent being male, in contrast to a mean age of 8 years for the entire group, in which there was a 70 per cent male predominance.

Additionally, many patients have abnormal urinary sediments with normal renal function long after signs and symptoms of disease activity in other organs have abated. Our study, for instance, showed that hematuria persisted through the second year of follow-up; in fact, more than half of these patients had hematuria up to 5 years after the initial evaluation. In general, patients with the most severe renal involvement have the more prolonged abnormalities in urine sediment. The cause of this continued "apparent activity," however, is obscure. Two patients we have followed had focal fibrinoid changes in their glomeruli at a time of stable renal function and no other clinical evidence of the disease. It is possible that the initial disease process caused irreversible but nonprogressive changes. The number of recurrences of this syndrome does not appear to be related to the age of onset, and there is no clinical evidence that recurrences differ in severity from the initial episode. In addition, it is impossible to predict recurrences on the basis of the severity of the initial episode.

Steroid therapy is useful in the treatment of the nonrenal manifestations of the disease, but it is of questionable benefit in the treatment of the renal changes. The data obtained from the University of Washington study suggest that some patients who relapse frequently may benefit from combined steroids and immunosuppressive drugs. In addition, the more severe forms of the nephritis associated with the histologic findings of diffuse epithelial proliferation, which include fibrinoid changes in the vessels and glomeruli, may be amenable to this form of therapy as well.

References

1. Allen, D. M., Diamond, L. K., and Howell, D. A.: Anaphylactoid purpura in children (Henoch-Schönlein syndrome). Am. J. Dis. Child. 99:833, 1960.

2. Ballard, H. S., Eiseinger, R. O., and Gallo, G.: Renal manifestations of the Henoch-Schönlein syndrome in adults. Am. J. Med. *49*:328, 1970.
3. Bergstrand, A., Bergstrand, O. G., and Bucht, H.: Kidney lesions associated with anaphylactoid purpura in children. Acta Pediatr. *49*:57, 1960.
4. Burke, E. C., Mills, S. D., and Stickler, G. B.: Nephritis associated with anaphylactoid purpura in childhood: Clinical observations and prognosis. Staff Meet. Mayo Clin. *35*:641, 1960.
5. Oliver, T. K., Jr., and Barnett, H. L.: Incidence and prognosis of nephritis associated with anaphylactoid (Henoch-Schönlein) purpura of children. Am. J. Dis. Child. *90*:544, 1955.
6. Osler, W.: On the visceral manifestations of the erythema group of skin disease. Am. J. Sci. *127*:1, 1904.
7. Osler, W.: The visceral lesions of purpura and allied conditions. Brit. Med. J. *1*:517, 1914.
8. Roberts, F. B., Slater, R. J., and Laski, B.: The prognosis of Henoch-Schönlein nephritis. Can. Med. Ass. J. *87*:49, 1962.
9. Urizar, R. E., Michael, A., Sisson, S., and Vernier, R. L.: Anaphylactoid purpura. II. Immunofluorescent and electron microscopic studies of the glomerular lesions. Lab. Invest. *19*:437, 1968.
10. Vernier, R. L., Worthen, H. G., Peterson, R. D., et al.: Anaphylactoid purpura. I. Pathology of the skin and kidney and frequency of streptococcal infection. Pediatrics *27*:181, 1961.
11. Wedgewood, R. J. P., and Klaus, M. H.: Anaphylactoid purpura (Henoch-Schönlein syndrome): A long term follow-up study with special reference to renal involvement. Pediatrics *16*:196, 1955.
12. Willan, R.: Cutaneous Disease. London J. Johnson, 1808.

Chapter Twenty

Hemolytic Uremic Syndrome and Thrombotic Thrombocytopenic Purpura

Hemolytic uremic syndrome and thrombotic thrombocytopenic purpura are related closely and may share a common etiology, or at least a common pathogenesis. Because of this, they will be discussed together in this chapter. They differ primarily only in the age of presentation and in organ system involvement. Table 20-1 summarizes similarities and differences.

HEMOLYTIC UREMIC SYNDROME

Clinical Data

The hemolytic uremic syndrome is a disease of childhood, occurring with greatest frequency in infants under the age of 1 year, with no

TABLE 20-1 Clinical Characteristics of the Hemolytic Uremic Syndrome and Thrombotic Thrombocytopenic Purpura

	Hemolytic Uremic Syndrome	Thrombotic Thrombocytopenic Purpura
Age	Children	Young adults
Sex	Females = Males	Females > Males
Organ Involvement		
Renal	Severe	Moderate
Neurologic	Rare	Common
Hemorrhagic	Occasional	Common
Other systems	Rare	Common
Prognosis	Fair	Poor

sex predilection. The disease is further characterized by acute renal failure, thrombocytopenia, and hemolytic anemia, which develop a few days after the onset of gastrointestinal symptoms (vomiting, diarrhea, or abdominal pain) in a previously well child. Pallor, lethargy, hepatomegaly, and hypertension also are common accompaniments. Additionally, a blood smear shows the classic signs of fragmentation hemolysis with burr cells, schistocytes, and anisocytosis. The platelet count usually is depressed, and platelet survival time is found to be shortened when studied during the first 2 weeks of the illness, indicating rapid platelet destruction. Although fibrin degradation products can be found in the urine and serum, turnover studies indicate that major consumption of clotting factors does not occur in this syndrome. Hematuria and proteinuria are found universally on presentation, and renal function impairment often is present as well.

Histology

GENERAL FINDINGS. The major abnormalities lie in the vascular tree. There is a good correlation between the degree of injury, size of the blood vessel involved, and the clinical course. Those patients with mild, short-lived renal dysfunction generally have abnormalities restricted to the endothelial regions of glomerular capillaries. More prolonged oliguria is associated with lesions which extend past the endothelium and involve the media of arteries. Finally, irreversible renal failure is associated with severe injury of the vascular wall, thrombosis of large vessels, and cortical infarction (necrosis). The findings in the tubules and interstitium follow those in the vessels, appearing to be secondary to ischemia or local capillary endothelial cell injury.

GLOMERULI

The most consistent early change is endothelial cell swelling. This may be difficult to appreciate in paraffin-embedded tissue, but in plastic-embedded biopsies the peripheral capillary loops appear to have a thickened wall (Figs. 20-1 and 20-2). The more severely affected capillaries contain inflammatory cells and an increased number of red blood cells. The few remaining capillary loops appear to be dilated (Fig. 20-3). Finally, in severely affected patients many glomeruli are infarcted (Fig. 20-4) The capillaries are filled with red blood cells and serum protein, and cellular detail is lost. Epithelial cell proliferation (crescents) and fibrin deposition between the cells may be seen in this situation.

Residual glomerular changes are difficult to detect when the initial course was brief and the only visible injury was endothelial cell swelling. The only change is minor wrinkling of the peripheral basal lamina near the mesangial region, a change which can best be appreciated on silver-stained sections. Following more severe injury, obsolescent glomeruli may occasionally be seen as the glomerular lesions seem to resolve nearly completely save for the basal lamina wrinkling mentioned above.

TUBULES AND INTERSTITIUM

The tubules often contain hyaline casts, red blood cells, and granular debris. The proximal tubule epithelium reflects the ischemic injury, containing many cytoplasmic granules or vacuoles, or both, as well as occasional mitotic figures (Fig. 20–5). The lumen appears large since the cytoplasm is thinned. The changes are reversible except in those instances where there is infarction of the cortex—so-called cortical necrosis.

The interstitial changes are primarily edema and a minimal infiltration by inflammatory cells (Fig. 20–6). When the vascular injury is severe, red blood cells appear free in the interstitium in large numbers. As with the tubular injury, these changes are reversible if vascular flow is restored.

VESSELS

The biopsies all show swelling of endothelial cell cytoplasm. In more severely affected vessels there is disruption of the smooth endothelial lining by infiltrating mononuclear and neutrophilic inflammatory cells (Fig. 20–6). Red blood cell fragments and serum proteins also are seen in these areas. The most pronounced change is complete disruption of the vascular architecture and occlusion of the lumen by a thrombus (Fig. 20–7). The size of the vessel involved and the degree of involvement correlates well with the lesions in other vessels and renal structures distal to the site of injury. It follows, therefore, that large vessel disease has the poorest prognosis for overall renal damage and dysfunction.

The vascular lesions heal completely in the majority of patients who recover renal function. However, when oliguria is prolonged, the vessels may be significantly altered. The changes are both endothelial and medial. The endothelial layer consists of enlarged cells surrounding a small lumen. The subendothelial space is widened by multilayers of cells and extracellular material. Finally, the media appears to be thinned and the extracellular matrix between smooth muscle cells is increased (Fig. 20–8).

ELECTRON MICROSCOPY. The glomerular changes vary considerably but generally parallel those seen by light microscopy. Endothelial cell changes include a prominent cytoplasm and the development of many surface projections (Fig. 20–9). The cytoplasmic fenestrations are

Text continued on page 279

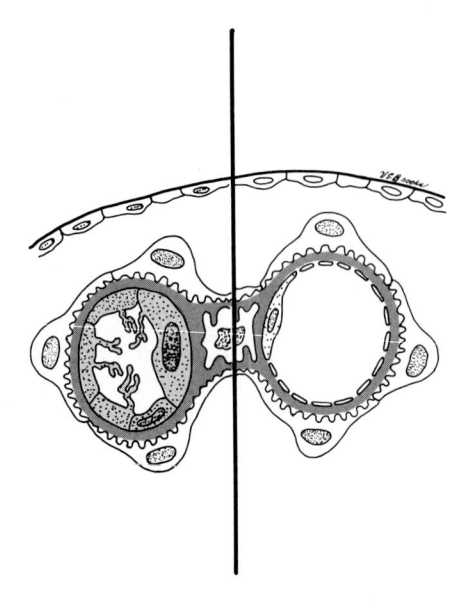

Figure 20-1 Schematic representation of endothelial cell swelling.

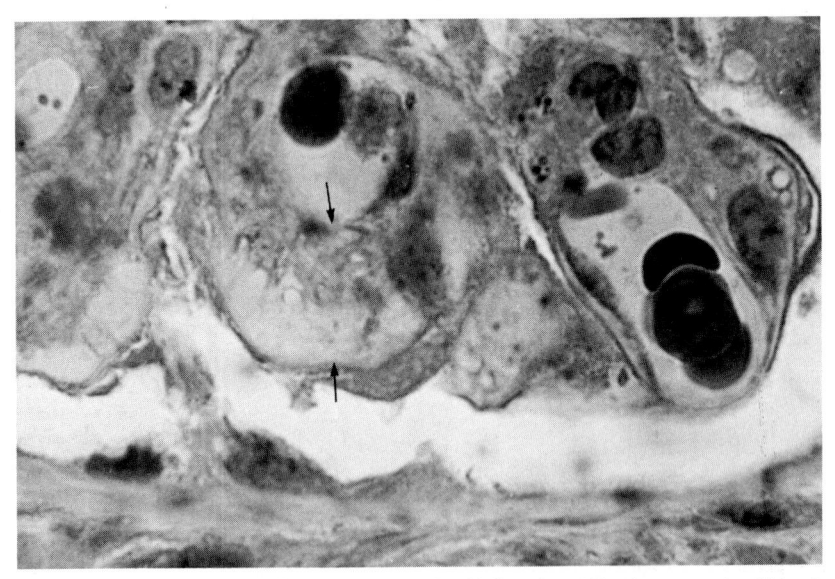

Figure 20-2 Specimen from a 14 month old female. Following a week of bloody diarrhea, this patient was admitted with mild fever and no other pertinent clinical findings. The initial platelet count was 53,000, hematocrit 24% and BUN 27 mg/dl. Urine sediment demonstrated red cells but no casts. Renal biopsy revealed a diffuse lesion, as in the photomicrograph above. The endothelial cell cytoplasm is diffusely swollen, resulting in a markedly diminished size of the capillary (arrow). Inflammatory cells are not seen in this area. (H&E, × 1200.)

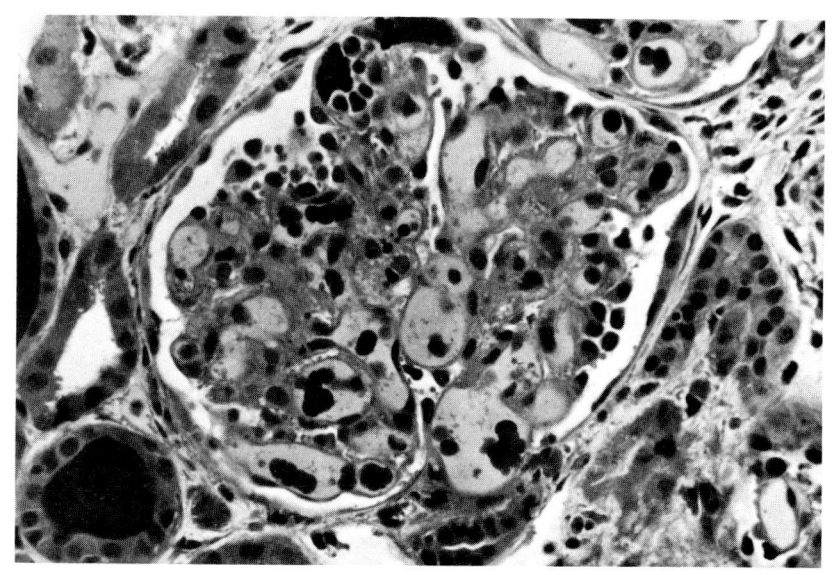

Figure 20-3 Same patient as in Figure 20-2. The diffuseness of the lesion can be more readily appreciated in this photomicrograph. The capillary spaces alternate between being quite small and difficult to appreciate and being very large, dilated, and filled with red blood cells. Note the red blood cell casts in the tubule at the 7 o'clock position. (H&E, ×300.)

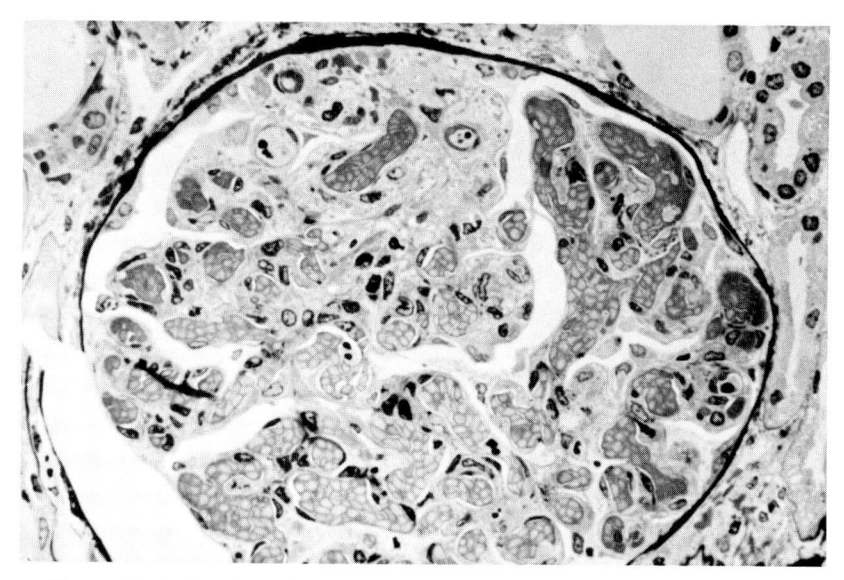

Figure 20-4 Specimen from a 38 year old woman who was admitted to hospital because of a 3 month history of cough, malaise, and myalgia. On admission, the creatinine level was 8.0 mg/dl, she was hypertensive, and the urine contained many red cells and a few casts. Hematocrit was 28 mg/100 ml, and platelet count was 80,000. Renal biopsy demonstrated areas of near infarction alternating will less ischemic areas. The glomerulus pictured here resided in a zone of severe ischemia. Note that the capillary loops are filled with red blood cells. The glomerular details are difficult to visualize. (Silver methenamine, ×300.)

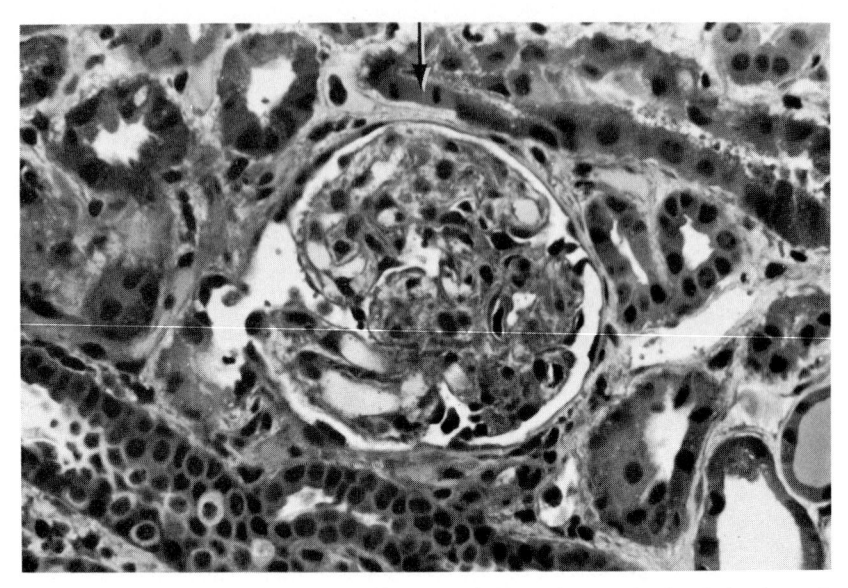

Figure 20-5 The tubules are often remarkable. The proximal tubule above the glomerulus demonstrates a mitotic figure (arrow) and a very granular luminal border in place of a normal brush border. Elsewhere the tubular epithelium is noted to be thin. Casts such as is seen at the 4 o'clock position in this photomicrograph were common in the biopsy. (H&E, ×300.)

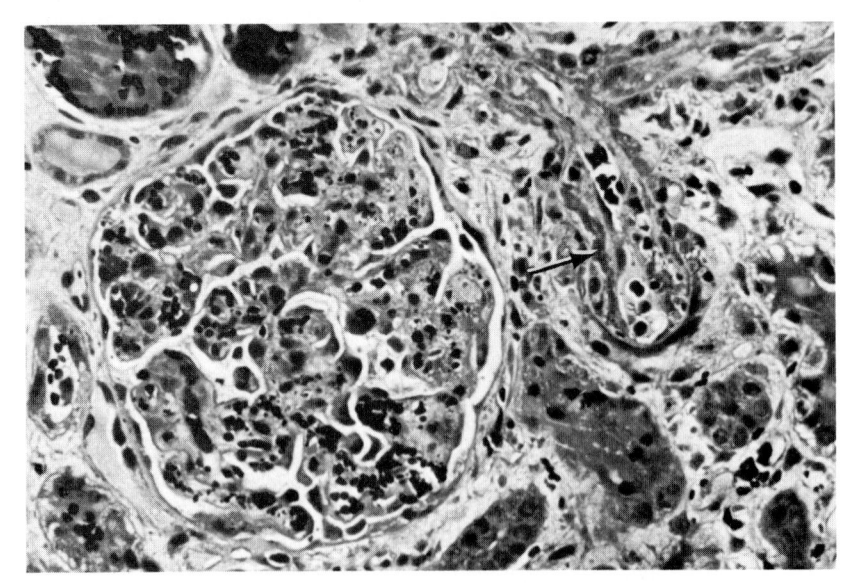

Figure 20-6 An area from the biopsy of the same patient as in Figure 20-4. Marked interstitial widening due to both edema and infiltration by inflammatory cells is apparent in this photomicrograph. The vessel to the right of the glomerulus is severely affected. The lumen is patent. The wall is disrupted by the presence of both inflammatory cells and a protein coagulum (arrow). This appears to be limited to the subintimal region (H&E, × 300.)

HEMOLYTIC UREMIC SYNDROME 277

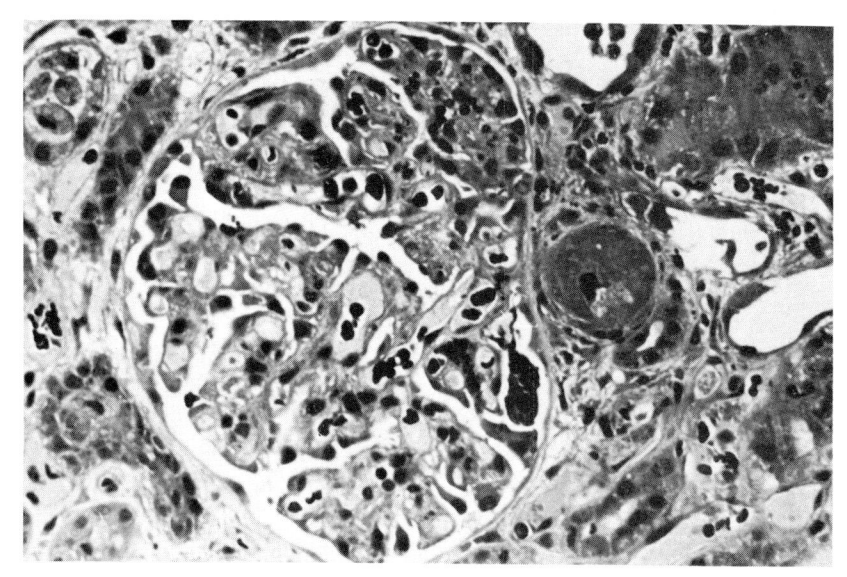

Figure 20-7 The afferent arteriole of this glomerulus from the same patient as in Figure 20-6 is completely occluded by a thrombus. The surrounding interstitium is edematous and contains inflammatory cells. Note that the glomerulus shows markedly decreased capillary spaces as well as loss of cellular detail. (H&E, ×300.)

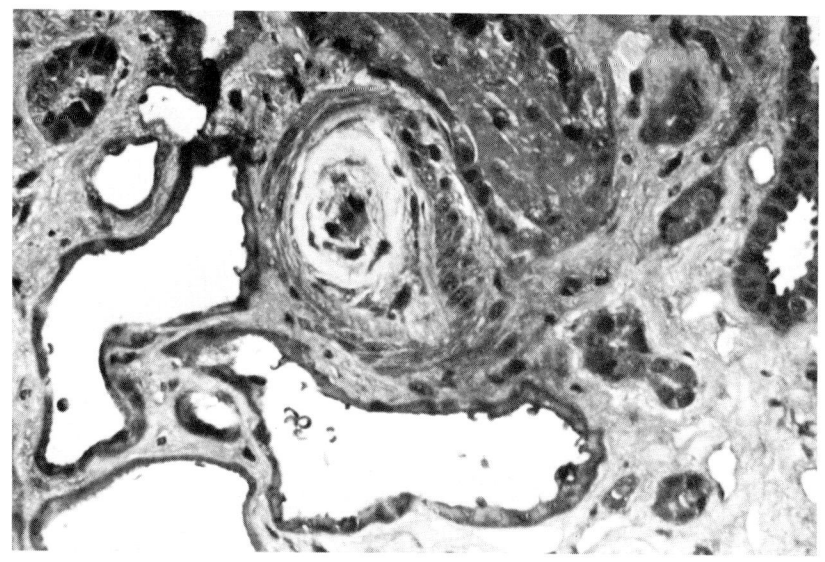

Figure 20-8 Specimen from an 11 month old female who developed the hemolytic uremia syndrome and was totally anuric for 3 weeks. She slowly regained renal function and the serum creatinine level stabilized at 2.4 mg/dl. The major histologic finding in the vessels is demonstrated in this small artery. There is a marked increase in the amount of extracellular material between cells of the intima and media. Note that there is also an increase in interstitial connective tissue. (H&E, ×300.)

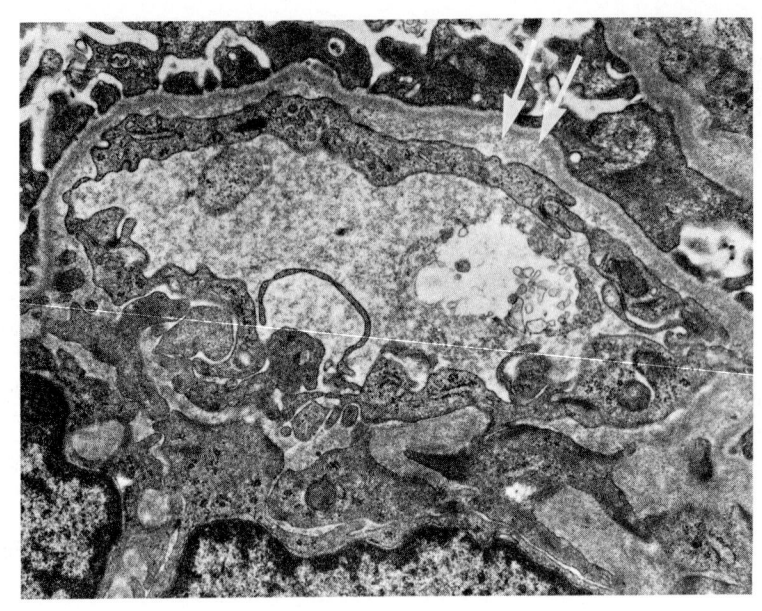

Figure 20-9 An electron micrograph of the same patient as in Figures 20-2 and 20-3, demonstrating thickening of the endothelial cell layer and an increased number of villi on the capillary surface. There is widening of the subendothelial space. In this region an electron-lucent, flocculent material (arrow) can be seen. (×1500.)

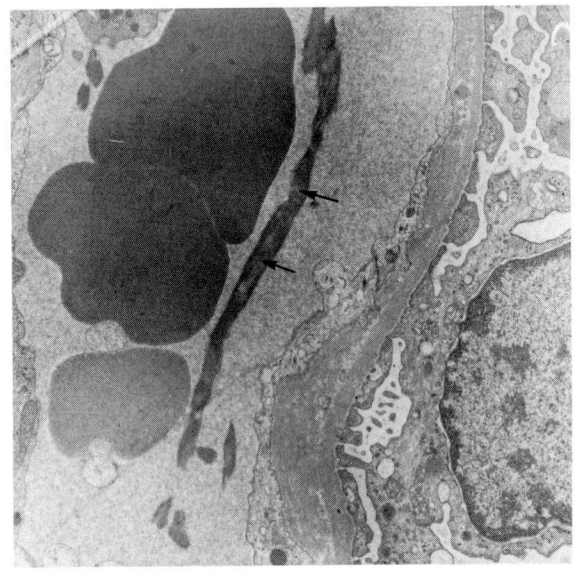

Figure 20-10 In some areas of the biopsy, the amount of subendothelial flocculent material was accentuated, as can be seen in this micrograph. The lumen also contained occasional profiles of fibrillar material resembling fibrin (arrow). (×6300.)

largely effaced and the cytoplasm contains many more organelles than usual. The subendothelial space is expanded and contains variable amounts of a flocculent, electron-dense material (Fig. 20–10). Occasionally there may be seen profiles of polymerized fibrin within capillary loops. The subendothelial expansion is pronounced in these cases.

FLUORESCENCE MICROSCOPY. No specific deposits are noted, except that fibrin-fibrinogen antigen is present in peripheral capillary loops and in affected blood vessels when extensive vascular injury is present.

Clinical Course and Prognosis

The clinical features are remarkably consistent in children with hemolytic uremic syndrome. Initially, the patients appear well and then are stricken suddenly with transient, severe gastrointestinal symptoms, usually including vomiting, diarrhea, and abdominal pain. In some there also is concurrent fever. Subsequently, thrombocytopenia, hemolytic anemia, and acute renal insufficiency appear. Thrombocytopenia results from platelet destruction and is accompanied by minimal changes in fibrinogen turnover and fibrin degradation products. The finding of selective platelet consumption is indicative of abnormal vascular surface-related, thrombotic consumption, which contrasts with the continued platelet and fibrinogen consumption that occurs with intravascular coagulation. Finally platelet and red cell destruction decreases spontaneously after 2 to 3 weeks, regardless of the therapy given.

These children's renal failure also invariably is acute. In the University of Washington study, for instance, approximately half the patients had oliguria, and 22 per cent required dialysis. Renal function improved within 1 month in most patients, whereas approximately 10 per cent have permanent renal dysfunction. Glucocorticoids or heparin treatments appear to have no advantage, however, over a program of careful management of fluid and electrolyte balance and early dialysis.

In summary, when prolonged oliguria, anuria, and/or hypertension are present concurrently, on light microscopy of the renal biopsy the vessels show severe lesions. Some are partially or completely occluded or necrotic, and some have inflammatory cells in the walls. The absence of hypertension and a shortened period of oliguria, or both, is associated with normal vessels by light microscopy and has a good prognosis. Although serial biopsies are not available to analyze the evolution of the vascular lesions, it is probable that these acute changes are followed by partial or complete recanalization of the vessels, leading to the observed clinical improvement.

THROMBOTIC THROMBOCYTOPENIC PURPURA

Clinical Data

Thrombotic thrombocytopenic purpura presents in much the same fashion as the hemolytic uremic syndrome. Whereas the hemolytic uremic syndrome affects primarily the blood and the kidneys, thrombotic thrombocytopenic purpura shows a predilection for multiple organ involvement, including severe renal dysfunction, in over half the cases. This syndrome occurs most commonly in young adults, with a higher incidence in women. In addition, the disease has a higher incidence during pregnancy and the postpartum period. Neurologic complications are the most frequent presenting symptoms, often eventually causing death. The disease is fulminant as well, with death occurring in 78 per cent of the cases within 3 months. Unlike the hemolytic uremic syndrome, however, renal failure occurs late in the illness.

The hematologic findings are similar to those described under the

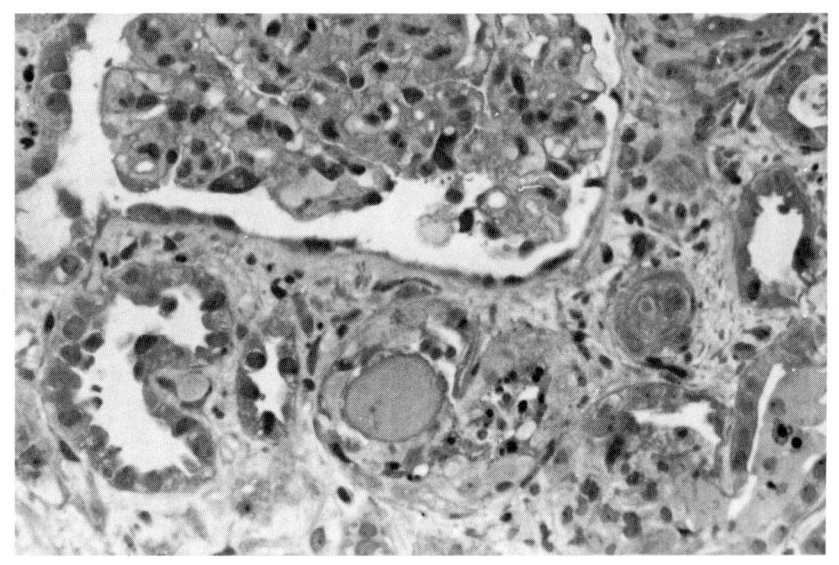

Figure 20–11 Three days prior to admission, this 53 year old woman developed nausea, vomiting, and diarrhea. On admission, the hematocrit was 22%, platelet count was 20,000, creatinine level was 18 mg/dl, and blood pressure was normal. CNS symptoms included hallucinations and paranoid delusions. Following high doses of steroid therapy, her symptoms stabilized and 4 weeks later a renal biopsy was obtained. There is a sharp diminution in the size of the capillary spaces, and the peripheral capillary loops appear to have thickened walls. This histologic picture is quite similar to that of the hemolytic uremic syndrome. The small vessel noted at the 3 o'clock position is nearly completely occluded by what appears to be endothelial cells. Note that the interstitium is markedly widened and contains inflammatory cells. The tubule near the center of the micrograph shows desquamation of the epithelial cells, and the lumen is filled with granular and hyaline debris. Many tubules are similarly affected. (H&E, ×300.)

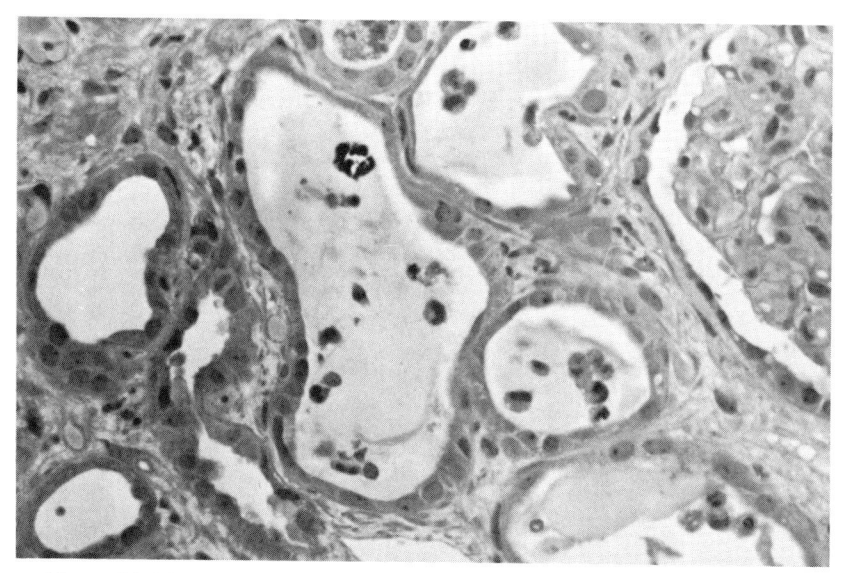

Figure 20-12 Marked flattening of tubular epithelial cells can be seen in this photomicrograph. Neutrophils as well as tubular epithelial cells may be found in the lumen. Here again the interstitium is seen to be edematous and filled with inflammatory cells. (H&E, ×300.)

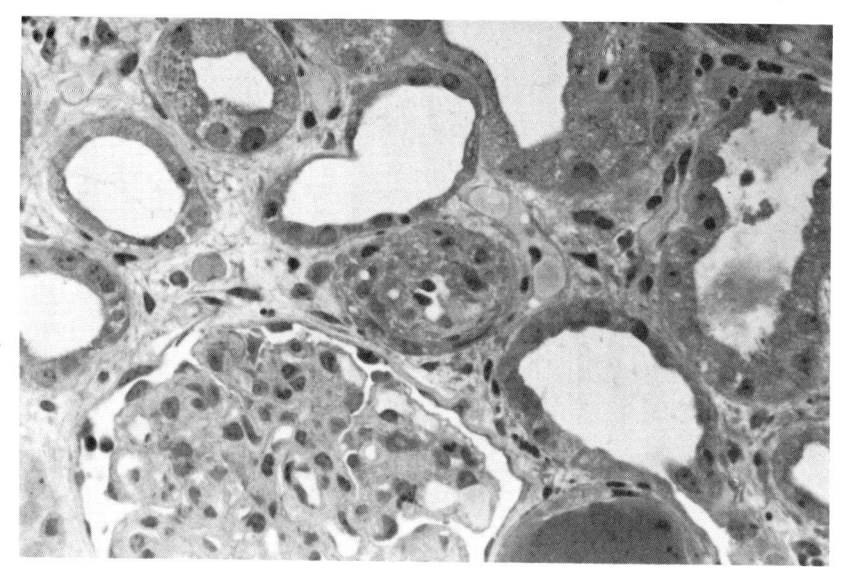

Figure 20-13 This vessel, from the same patient as in Figure 20-11, is representative of those in the rest of the biopsy. The media is definable and appears to be relatively unaffected. There is an increase in the number of cells in the subintimal region, and there appears to be deposition of serum proteins in this region as well. The interstitium is edematous and contains inflammatory cells, as noted in Figure 20-11. (H&E, ×300.)

hemolytic uremic syndrome, although hemorrhagic complications are more common in thrombotic thrombocytopenic purpura. There also is pronounced formation of platelet thrombi, and secondary activation of the coagulation system is more common.

In addition, the acute nature of these symptoms and the prominent hemostatic abnormalities are so characteristic of the illness that the diagnosis usually is clear from laboratory and clinical data. Renal biopsy, however, is helpful in assessing the degree of damage after the acute attack, as well as in determining the prognosis for those patients with persistent renal abnormalities.

Histology

The histologic changes in thrombotic thrombocytopenic purpura are similar to those noted in the hemolytic uremic syndrome, except that thrombi are seen more frequently in the junction between the afferent arteriole and the glomerulus.

GLOMERULI

Glomeruli are affected irregularly, but in those in which a thrombus can be identified, distal segments of the glomeruli are infarcted (Fig. 20–11). In less affected glomeruli, endothelial swelling may be the only abnormality.

TUBULES AND INTERSTITIUM

No characteristic lesions are apparent in the tubules and interstitium (Fig. 20–12), although infarcts may be visible in patchy distribution secondary to the vascular injury.

VESSELS

In cases of thrombotic thrombocytopenic purpura, the vessels also may show lesions that are identical to those evident in the hemolytic uremic syndrome, although large vessels usually are affected (Figs. 20-11 and 20–13) more prominently. Endothelial proliferation may be more pronounced than in the hemolytic uremic syndrome.

ELECTRON MICROSCOPY. On electron microscopy, the glomerular and vascular lesions are indistinguishable from those noted in the hemolytic uremic syndrome.

FLUORESCENCE MICROSCOPY. Deposits of fibrin-fibrinogen antigen are evident in the areas appearing to be thrombi by light microscopy. Immunoglobulin deposition is inconsistent and unhelpful.

Clinical Course and Prognosis

Unlike the hemolytic uremic syndrome, whose clinical course is associated with survival of the majority of children, with no renal impairment or only mild dysfunction when careful supportive management is applied, thrombotic thrombocytopenic purpura is almost universally fatal. More recently, survivors have been reported occasionally.

Furthermore, although the illness has been considered a disease of disseminated intravascular coagulation for years, recent studies and experimental evidence, as previously described, have demonstrated that the diffuse platelet thrombi were the underlying lesion, whereas the blood clotting system was involved only secondarily. Unfortunately attempts to treat this injury with steroids, dextran, heparin, or splenectomy have not had a consistent effect on the clinical course and outcome. In our experience the use of anti-thrombogenic drugs has shown encouraging results when used early in the course of the disease.

References

1. Amorosi, E. L., and Ultmann, J. E: Thrombotic thrombocytopenic purpura: Report of sixteen cases and review of the literature. Medicine 45:139, 1966.
2. Gianantonio, C., Vitacco, M., Mendilaharzu, J., and Rutty, A.: The hemolytic-uremic syndrome. J. Pediatr. 64:478, 1964.
3. Harker, L. A., and Slichter, S. J.: Platelet and fibrinogen consumption in man. New Eng. J. Med. 287:999, 1972.
4. Jaffe, E. A., Wachman, R. L., and Merskey, C.: Thrombotic thrombocytopenic purpura: Coagulation parameters in twelve patients. Blood 42:499, 1973.
5. Lieberman, E.: Hemolytic-uremic syndrome. J. Pediatr. 80:1, 1972.
6. Riella, M. C., Hickman, R. O., Striker, G. E., Slichter, S. J., Harker, L., and Quadracci, L. J.: The renal microangiopathy of the hemolytic-uremic syndrome in childhood. Proc. Clin. Dialysis Transpl. Forum 4:112, 1974.

Chapter Twenty-One

Diabetic Glomerulosclerosis

Introduction

A wide variety of lesions may occur in diabetic patients, but the most characteristic is an increase in extracellular material in the form of thickened basal laminae or nodules in the glomerular mesangium. In 1936 Kimmelstiel and Wilson first identified the association of diabetes mellitus, renal disease, proteinuria, and the characteristic nodular lesion (Kimmelstiel-Wilson syndrome). In 1944, Laipply and his associates recognized that the basal lamina in the peripheral glomerular capillary loops also may be thickened, and more recently it has become clear that similar changes occur in nearly every organ system with a basal lamina.

Clinical Data

The classic clinical findings described for diabetic nephropathy are edema, proteinuria, and hypertension. In general, they correlate relatively well with the presence of glomerulosclerosis. However, the clinical findings also can be caused by arterionephrosclerosis, which has a higher incidence in diabetics.

The majority of juvenile-onset diabetics develop nephropathy. The duration of the diabetic state tends to correlate with its onset, occurring approximately 17 years after the initial diagnosis of juvenile-onset diabetes and somewhat later in adult-onset diabetes. In addition, only 30 per cent of the latter group develop overt clinical nephropathy.

Proteinuria usually is the first sign of nephropathy, followed by the gradual appearance of hypertension and edema. Retinopathy is almost always present with nephropathy, although the opposite is not true.

Renal biopsy is of limited value in the clinical evaluation of renal disease in diabetic patients. Since the presence of proteinuria correlates well with the nephropathy, only atypical clinical presentations which may indicate the presence of a second disease require renal biopsy.

Histologic Findings

Light Microscopic Changes

Glomeruli. The glomerular changes are primarily those of sclerosis and accumulations of proteinaceous material (insudation) in the extracellular spaces. The sclerotic lesions have been subdivided into two categories: (1) a nodular lesion, and (2) a diffuse increase in the amount of extracellular material. Additionally, glomeruli may show only ischemic changes as a consequence of severe vascular disease, especially in adult-onset diabetes.

The Nodular Lesion. Fifty per cent of patients with diabetic nephropathy have this lesion. As originally described by Kimmelstiel and Wilson, it consists of a rounded, homogeneous, eosinophilic area in the central portion of a lobule or lobules (Fig. 21–1). Patent capillaries

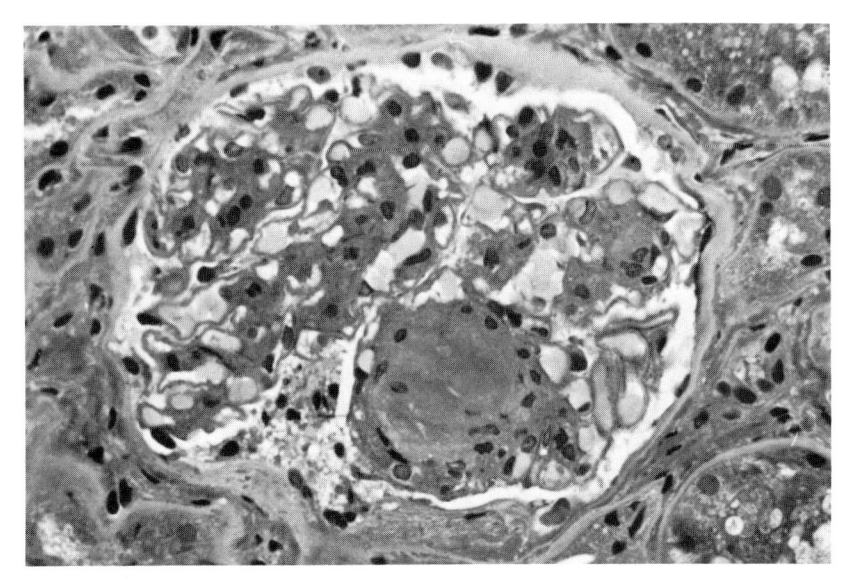

Figure 21-1 Specimen from a 33 year old man with juvenile onset diabetes mellitus who developed proteinuria one year ago. Serum creatinine is 1.9 mg/dl; 24-hour urine protein, 7.5 g. Five of 22 glomeruli demonstrate the nodular increase in extracellular material noted between the 5 and 6 o'clock positions in this glomerulus. Elsewhere the mesangial matrix is increased, and there appears to be an increased number of cells in the mesangial region. The peripheral capillary loops appear to be thickened, as does Bowman's capsule. Note the vacuolization of the epithelial cells in the surrounding tubules consistent with heavy proteinuria. (H&E, ×300.)

often are visible around the margin of a lobule. These nodules frequently occur in the peripheral portions of the glomerulus, opposite to the vascular pole. The exact number of nodules within and among glomeruli varies considerably and does not appear to be related to changes elsewhere. The nodules also are PAS positive, and on silver staining they show more or less concentric laminations (Fig. 21-2). This is in contrast to patients who have other varieties of mesangial sclerosis, in which the thickened areas have an irregular, disordered array of "fibrils." In addition, the glomerular basal lamina in diabetic patients usually is thickened, but this change may be difficult to appreciate on light microscopy and often is overemphasized on electron microscopy.

The Diffuse Sclerotic Lesion. Seventy-five per cent of diabetics with nephropathy have a diffuse increase in mesangial matrix and thickening of the glomerular basal lamina. The basal laminal changes are not usually as prominent or as regular as the mesangial changes (Figs. 21-3 and 21-4).

Nodules can be present without substantial thickening of the lamina, but an expanded basal lamina rarely occurs without nodules. Additionally, in those cases in which there is diffuse thickening with nodules, there also may be an apparent hypercellularity in the mesangial regions (Fig. 21-1). Whether there is any validity in so distinguishing these diffuse and nodular lesions is unclear, however, since there appears to be no clinical, laboratory, or prognostic significance to the changes.

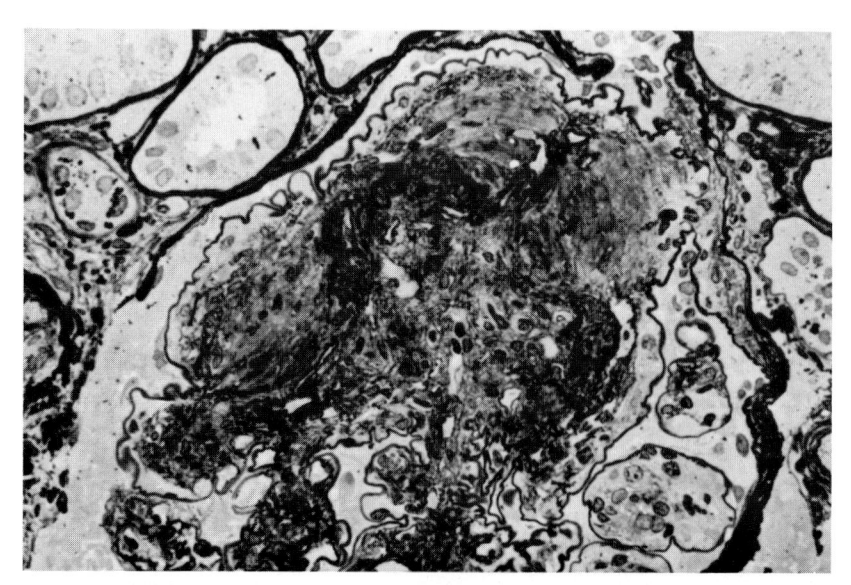

Figure 21-2 Silver staining of these nodular areas from the same patient as in Figure 21-1 demonstrates the halo of capillary loops around the nodular zone and the laminated appearance of the sclerotic material. (Silver methenamine, ×300.)

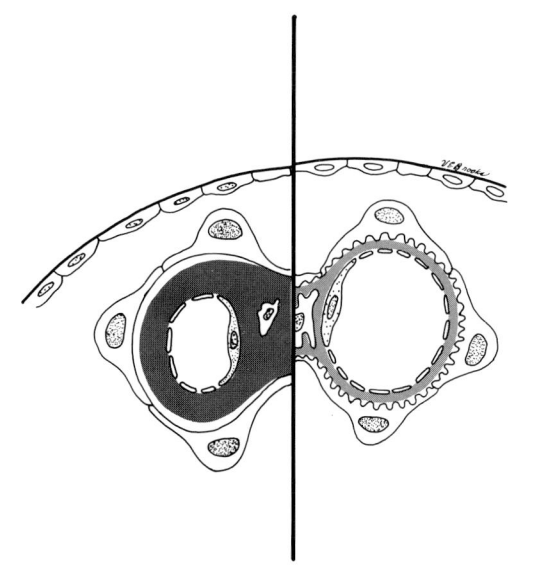

Figure 21-3 Schematic drawing demonstrating diffuse increase in GBL and mesangial matrix.

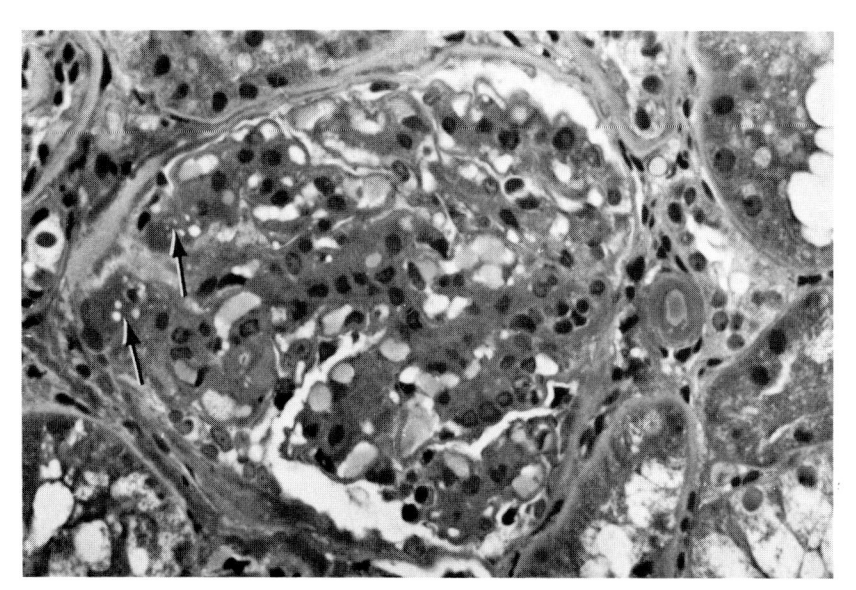

Figure 21-4 The same patient as in Figure 21-1. The prominence of the mesangial cellularity varies among patients and among mesangial regions within the same glomerulus. Adhesion of peripheral capillary loops to Bowman's capsule is a relatively frequent finding. In these zones, the capillary spaces appear to be filled with a proteinaceous material, "the insudative lesion" (arrow). The afferent arteriole at the 3 o'clock position contains a homogeneous "collar" of extracellular material. The endothelial and medial cells are not readily seen in this preparation. (H&E, ×300.)

The Insudative Lesion. This lesion is an eosinophilic homogeneous structure lying within the glomerular basal lamina at the periphery of a lobule (Figs. 21-4 and 21-5). Such lesions may be single or multiple. The vascular space in these areas is absent. In addition, although they generally have a hyaline appearance, they may be foamy and contain lipid. The insudative lesions have been shown by electron microscopy to be accumulations of proteinaceous material containing lipid and cellular debris located in extracellular sites. The same characteristics and composition also are evident in vascular and glomerular zones. Apparently cell proteins accumulate in areas of ischemia or injury, as do fragments of dead cells, which are then localized in these extracellular "pockets." Although this material is PAS positive, it does not stain with silver stains. It had been given multiple names in the past, including "hyalin," "fibrin caps," and "capsular drops." The insudative lesion does not represent an increase in the amount of normal extracellular material (sclerosis), however, since it is primarily an accumulation of plasma components and cell debris.

TUBULES. As in other conditions associated with proteinuria, the tubular epithelial cells often are vacuolated and contain lipid. The most characteristic change, however, is thickening of the tubular basal lamina, which often has a "hair on end" appearance (Fig. 21-6). It frequently seems as if this thickening occurs considerably before interstitial fibrosis is evident, and it often parallels glomerular basal lamina thickening and mesangial sclerosis.

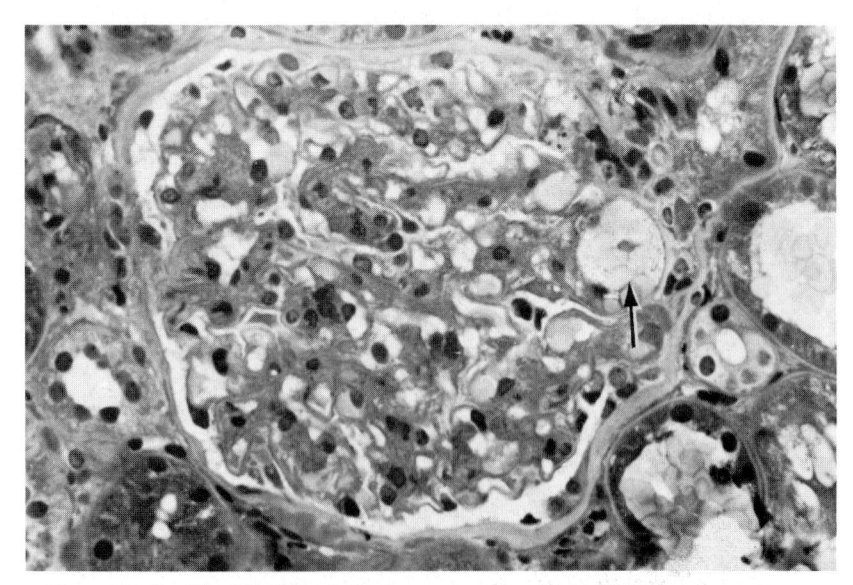

Figure 21-5. The insudative lesion in another glomerulus; it may appear to be somewhat more granular and vacuolated (arrows). (H&E, ×300.)

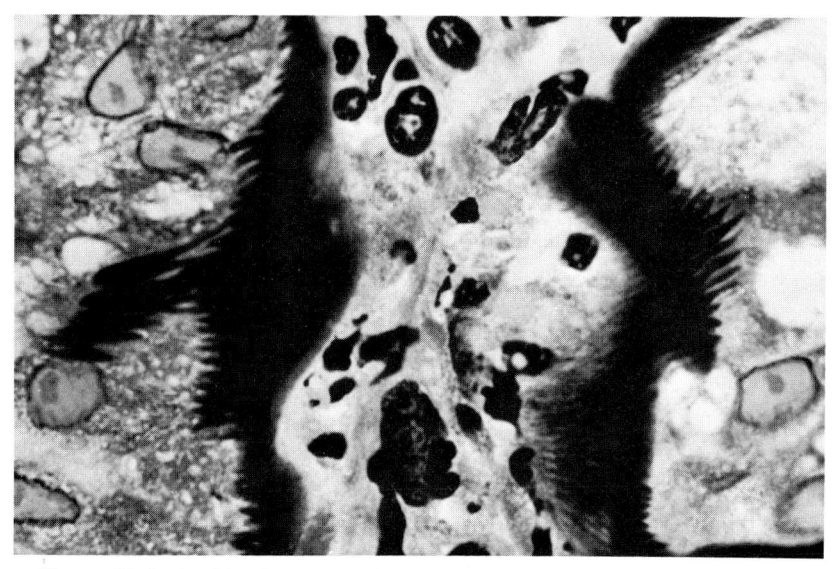

Figure 21-6 In this photograph, the tubular basal lamina are thickened throughout. Characteristic of this lesion in diabetes mellitus is an irregularity on both the tubular and capillary luminal side consisting of spikes of basal lamina material. (Silver methenamine, ×300.)

VESSELS. Approximately 85 per cent of patients with diabetic nephropathy have vascular lesions. Hyaline deposits and insudation commonly occur in both the larger and the smaller vessels in renal biopsy specimens (Fig. 21-7, 21-8, and 21-9). The hyaline deposits also usually are present in both the afferent and efferent glomerular arterioles (Fig. 21-4). Vascular changes may exist in the absence of abnormalities in other compartments. When glomerular changes occur, however, vascular changes are always present.

INTERSTITIUM. The interstitium is prominently affected by a variable and often marked increase in connective tissue (Fig. 21-10). The changes also tend to be diffuse and reflect alterations in the vascular compartment. The frequent presence of chronic inflammatory cells has led many to infer that chronic bacterial infection is present; however, this has not been confirmed by bacteriologic cultures of urine and kidney tissues, and it probably represents a reaction to degenerating tubules.

ELECTRON MICROSCOPY

Electron microscopy adds little information to that already noted, except to substantiate the impression that the mesangial matrix is increased in amount earlier than indicated by light microscopic studies alone. Second, the increased numbers of mesangial cells early in the disease and their close proximity to the extracellular material support

Text continued on page 292

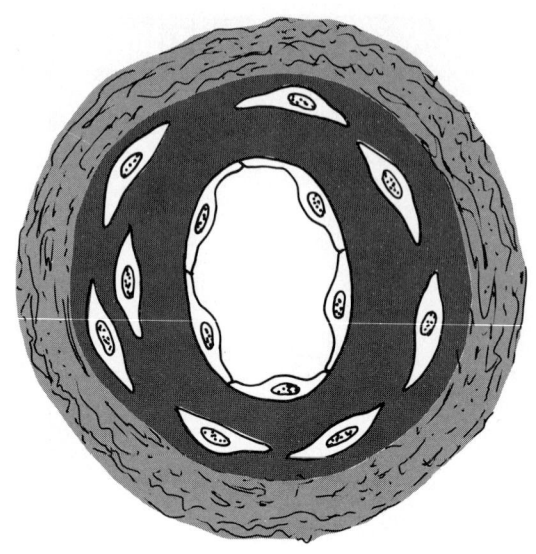

Figure 21-7 Schematic drawing showing a marked increase in subendothelial connective tissue.

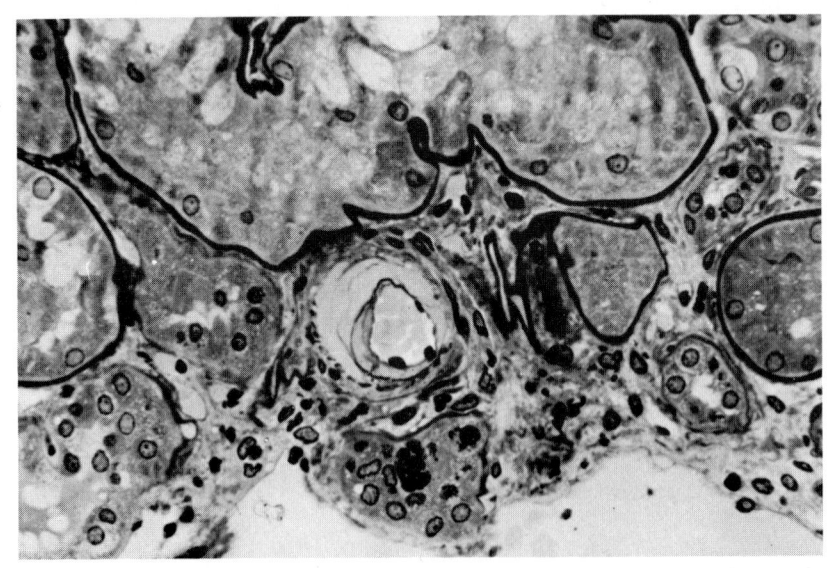

Figure 21-8 Section of biopsy specimen from the same patient as in Figure 21-1, showing subintimal and medial deposits a homogeneous mass which may affect many vessels, arteries, small arteries, and arterioles in the kidneys of diabetic patients. The cells appear to be displaced to the periphery of such deposits. (Silver methenamine, ×300.)

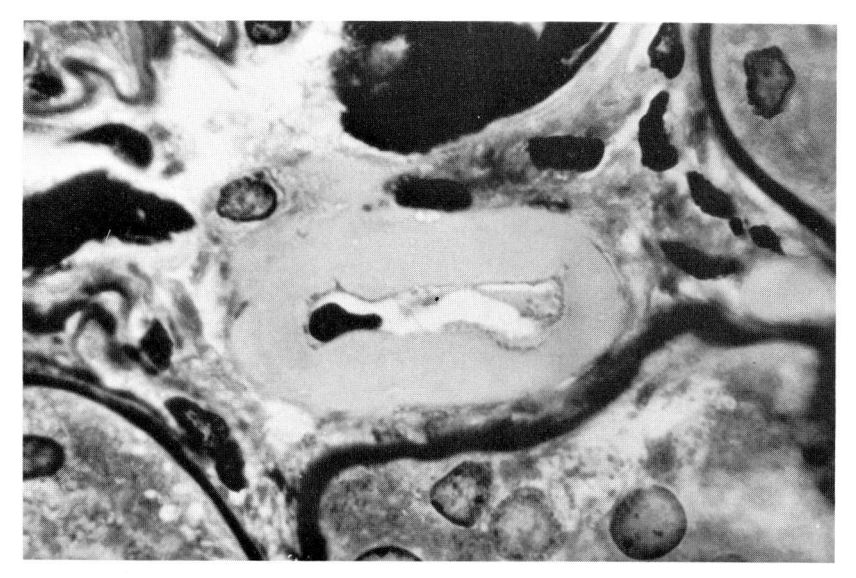

Figure 21-9 At higher magnification than in Figure 21-8, a small arteriole is seen to contain a large mass of homogeneous material. The endothelial cell layer is visible as a thin dark line at the luminal surface. The medial cells are not apparent. (Silver methenamine, ×1200.)

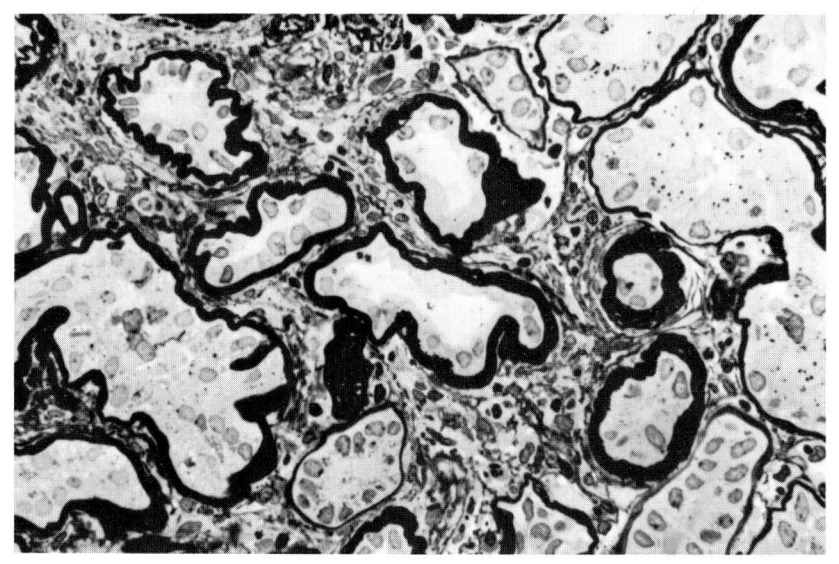

Figure 21-10 The interstitium contains an increased amount of connective tissue, as well as scattered inflammatory cells. Note that in the areas of interstitial fibrosis the basal lamina of the tubules is also thickened. (Silver methenamine, ×300.)

the belief that the mesangial cells are involved substantially in the production of an excess amount of mesangial matrix.

FLUORESCENCE MICROSCOPY

An unexpected finding is linear fluorescence of glomerular basal lamina in approximately 50 per cent of cases of diabetic nephropathy. Deposits of IgG are present most commonly, but complement, other immunoglobulins, and plasma proteins such as albumin can be found in a similar pattern, suggesting that their presence is mediated by a nonimmune mechanism. There is no correlation between presence of these and any of the light or electron microscopic findings. In addition, granular deposits of Ig and complement are present in the glomerular basal lamina and mesangial areas in almost all cases. The significance of this finding also is unknown.

Clinical Course and Prognosis

No correlation has been found between degree of change in the glomeruli and the clinical course or laboratory findings in terms of the level of proteinuria or glycosuria. Glomerular changes may be pronounced without a change in renal function. For instance, a few patients have been described with the nodular form of the nephropathy who had neither proteinuria nor decrease in renal function.

The reason for deterioration in kidney function in patients with diabetes mellitus is not clear; some progress more slowly, others more rapidly. The major indication that renal failure is imminent seems to be the nephrotic syndrome. For example, when protein excretion exceeds 3g per 24 hours, deterioration of renal function is common, occurring in about 2 years in most patients. This probably is a better prognosticator than either the age of onset or the duration of the disease. In one report, for instance, there was an 81 per cent mortality rate in patients with continuing proteinuria over a period of 12 years, in contrast to 39 per cent in a control group who did not have proteinuria.

In other forms of nephrotic syndrome associated with progressive renal failure, such as the sclerosing lesion of primary nephrotic syndrome (Chapter 16), protein excretion tends to decrease with progressive loss of renal function. In diabetic nephropathy, however, the heavy proteinuria continues even when the creatinine clearance has fallen below 10 per cent of normal.

Uremia is the cause of death in 5 per cent of diabetics; more importantly, it is the cause of death in 20 per cent of diabetic patients under 40 years of age. Unfortunately, no effective measures have been found to prevent progression of the nephropathy. Recently, however, patients have become acceptable candidates for chronic dialysis and transplantation. The diabetic lesion has been shown to recur in transplanted kidneys, but its significance is as yet unmeasured, since the lesions were quite minimal when studied.

References

1. Kimmelstiel, P., Osawa, G., and Beres, J.: Glomerular basement membrane in diabetics. Am. J. Clin. Path. 45:21, 1966.
2. Kimmelstiel, P., and Wilson, C.: Intercapillary lesions in glomeruli of kidney. Am. J. Pathol. 12:83, 1936.
3. Kussman, M. J., Goldstein, H. H., and Gleason, R. E.: The clinical course of diabetic nephropathy. J.A.M.A. 236:1861, 1976.
4. Laipply, T. C., Eitzen, O., and Dutra, F. R.: Intercapillary glomerulosclerosis. Arch. Intern. Med. 74:354, 1944.
5. Salinas-Madrigal, L., Pirani, C. L., and Pollak, V. E.: Glomerular and vascular "insudative" lesions of diabetic nephropathy. Electron microscopic observations. Am. J. Pathol. 59:369, 1970.
6. Salomon, M. I.: Diabetic nephropathy: Clinicopathologic correlation. A study based on renal biopsies. Metabolism 12:687, 1963.
7. Salomon, M. I., and Zak, F. G.: The kidney in diabetes mellitus. Geriatrics 21:156, 1966.
8. Thomsen, A. C.: The kidney in diabetes mellitus. Copenhagen, Munksgaard, 1965.
9. Watkins, P. J., Blainey, J. D., Brewer, D. B., Fitzgerald, M. G., Malins, J. M., O'Sullivan, D. J., and Pinto, J. A.: The natural history of diabetic renal disease. Quart. J. Med. 41:437, 1972.
10. Westberg, N. G., and Michael, A. F.: Immunohistopathology of diabetic glomerulosclerosis. Diabetes 21:163, 1972.

Chapter Twenty-Two

Progressive Systemic Sclerosis (Scleroderma)

Introduction

Systemic sclerosis, or scleroderma, is a rare disease of unknown etiology. It is characterized by widespread alterations of connective and vascular tissues. Frequently, the initial symptoms are edema and Raynaud's phenomenon, followed by thickening and induration of the skin on fingers and face, later involving the trunk and lower extremities as well. Visceral changes include blood vessel lesions and varying degrees of fibrosis in the lungs, intestines, heart, and kidneys. The location and extent of visceral involvement are major determinants of prognosis, and the usual relentless course has led to the term "progressive systemic sclerosis."

Clinical Data

Scleroderma affects females more frequently than males (4:1), whites more often than blacks (4:1), and has its greatest incidence in adults (ages 30 to 60). The diagnosis of this disease is made from the typical symptom complex and physical findings. Occasionally it is necessary to confirm the diagnosis by skin biopsy. There are no diagnostic laboratory findings other than the characteristic histologic lesions.

Although clinical renal involvement in scleroderma has been noted since 1892, it was the report of Moore and Sheehan in 1952 that stimulated increased interest in renal lesion. Two recent long-term studies suggest that significant renal involvement occurs in nearly 45 per cent of these patients.

When evidence of kidney dysfunction is found, it usually is seen within 3 years of the onset of clinical symptoms of systemic sclerosis. The most consistent signs of renal involvement are proteinuria (35 per cent of cases), hypertension (25 per cent of cases), and azotemia (20 per cent of cases).

Histology

The primary changes in the blood vessels and those in other compartments are reflective of the severity of the vascular lesion and the rapidity of its development. It is not possible to predict the histologic findings on the basis of blood pressure level or changes in other organ systems. The majority of patients do not develop the rapidly progressing form of the vascular disease, and in these it is difficult to distinguish the vessel changes from those resulting from other forms of slowly progressive vascular disease. The slowly progressive form is discussed in Chapter 14 and will not be considered further here.

GLOMERULI. The glomerular changes are variable, reflecting either local endothelial injury or ischemia, even to the point of infarction as a result of progressive occlusion of the vascular supply (Fig. 22–1). When local endothelial damage is the most prominent change, the glomeruli are enlarged and the capillary spaces are reduced by swollen endothelial cells (Fig. 22–2). In paraffin-embedded tissues, this may give the false impression that there is a thickened basal lamina if silver or PAS stains are not used.

The changes of moderate ischemia are those of wrinkled and collapsed glomerular basal laminae, whereas complete infarction with loss of nuclear detail appears in those patients with thrombosis in the larger blood vessels.

TUBULES AND INTERSTITIUM. The tubular and interstitial changes reflect the vascular lesions as well. In those with vascular thrombosis, segmental infarcts with tubular necrosis, interstitial edema, and interstitial hemorrhage may be seen (Fig. 22–3). Those with more slowly progressing vascular change may be associated with tubular atrophy, interstitial fibrosis, and a scattering of mononuclear inflammatory cells (Fig. 22–4).

VESSELS. The most characteristic changes are seen in the interlobular arteries, although those in distal branches may be equally prominent. In general, the distal lesions cannot be differentiated from those found in malignant hypertension. The interlobular artery changes are conspicuous in both the adventitial and the intimal regions, the media being less affected. The adventitial lesion is one of dense fibrosis extending into the surrounding interstitium. The intimal findings are the most florid, consisting of a loosely arranged concentric array of elongated cells, between which is an abundant amount of pale extracellular material containing an acid mucopolysaccharide (Fig. 22–5).

Text continued on page 298

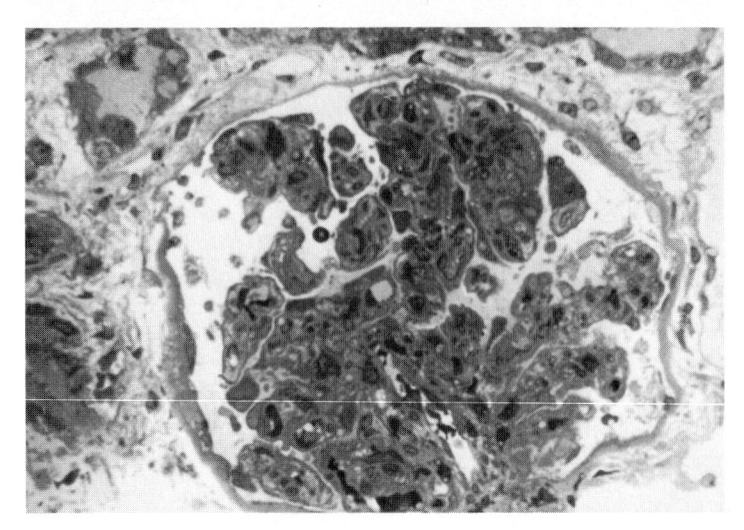

Figure 22–1 Biopsy from a 54 year old woman with a 10 year history of arthritis arthralgia and Raynaud's phenomenon. One month earlier her blood pressure was 225/130, and a serum creatinine level of 3.6 mg/dl was found. On admission, she was obtunded, and the only skin changes were slight shininess of the dorsal upper hands near the tips of the fingers. The glomerulus is quite remarkable in that the capillary spaces are nearly completely obliterated by what appears to be an increased number of cells, as well as increase in the amount of cytoplasm. The capillary loops, rather than appearing expanded, are somewhat contracted, and the refractile peripheral basal lamina can be seen to be wrinkled and "shriveled." The interstitium is widened by both the increase in connective tissue and the appearance of edema. (H&E, × 300.)

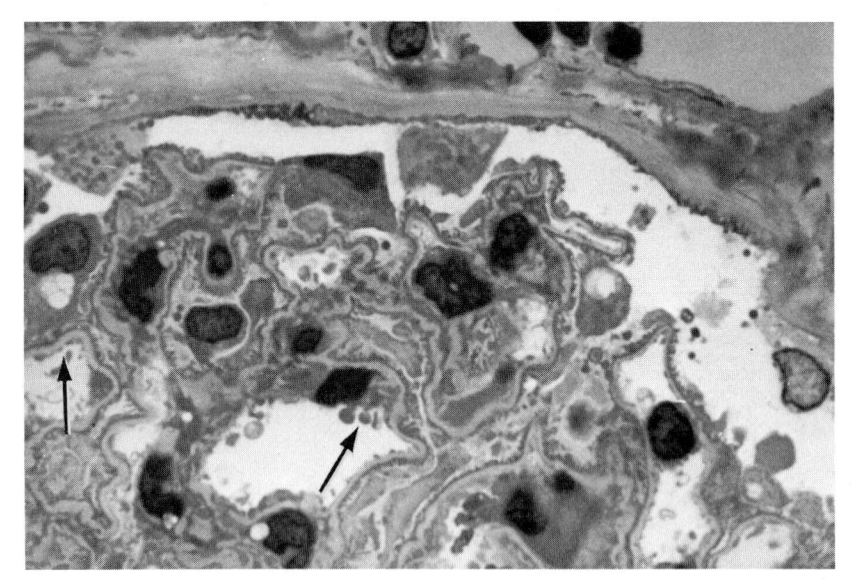

Figure 22–2. Twenty years ago this 49 year old man developed cold, painful hands. Twelve years later a sympathectomy was performed because of nonhealing ulcers of the toes and fingers, eventually resulting in gangrene of the right foot and necessitating below the knee amputation. On admission, he was noted to have sclerodactylia telangiectasia, but a normal blood pressure. Laboratory data revealed normal renal function, negative urinalysis results, normal serum complement, no cryoglobulins, and negative antinuclear factor. Renal biopsy demonstrated a relatively diffuse endothelial cell swelling in the glomeruli similar to that noted in this photomicrograph. The endothelial cell layer is visible in nearly every capillary loop and is quite thickened. The surface villiform projections can be seen in a number of areas (arrows). The lucent basal lamina is wrinkled in many areas, and most peripheral capillary loops do not appear to be fully distended. (H & E, × 1200.)

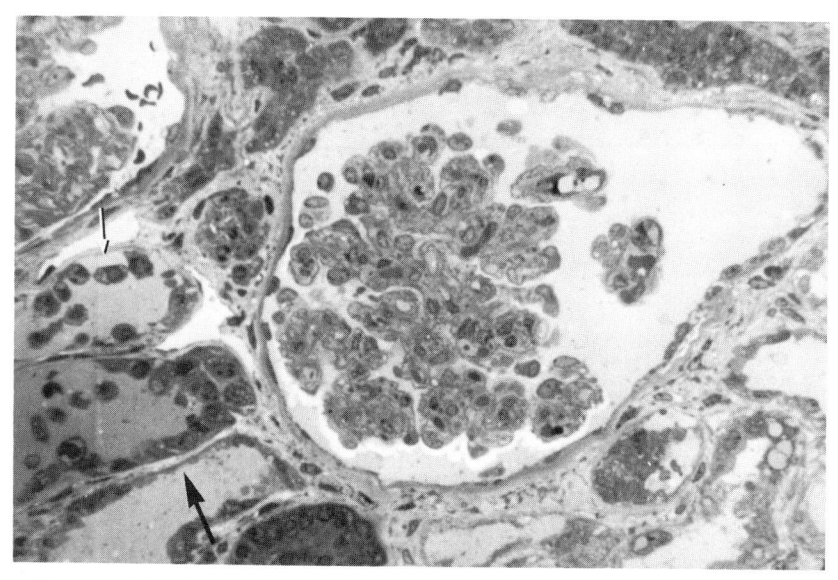

Figure 22-3. Same patient as in Figure 22-1. The tubular epithelial cells in many areas can be seen to be separated from the basal lamina and to lie within the lumen (light arrow). Elsewhere the epithelial lining is seen to be thin and irregular (heavy arrow). The interstitium is widened due to both edema and an increase in the amount of connective tissue. (H & E, × 300.)

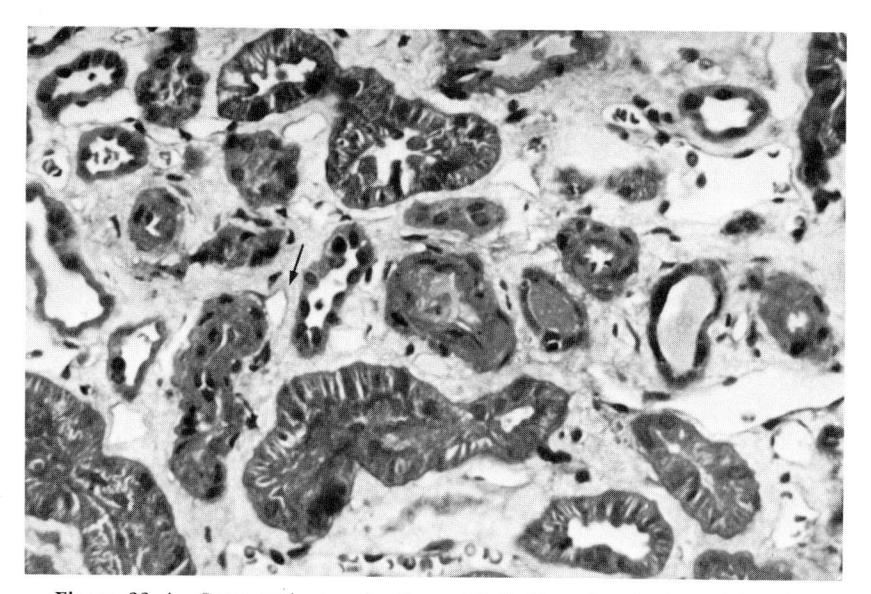

Figure 22-4. Same patient as in Figure 22-2. Note that the interstitium here is considerably increased over the normal. In many areas the capillaries surround only a relatively small portion of the perimeter of the tubules (arrow). There is an increase in the amount of interstitial connective tissue and some edema as well. (H & E, × 300.)

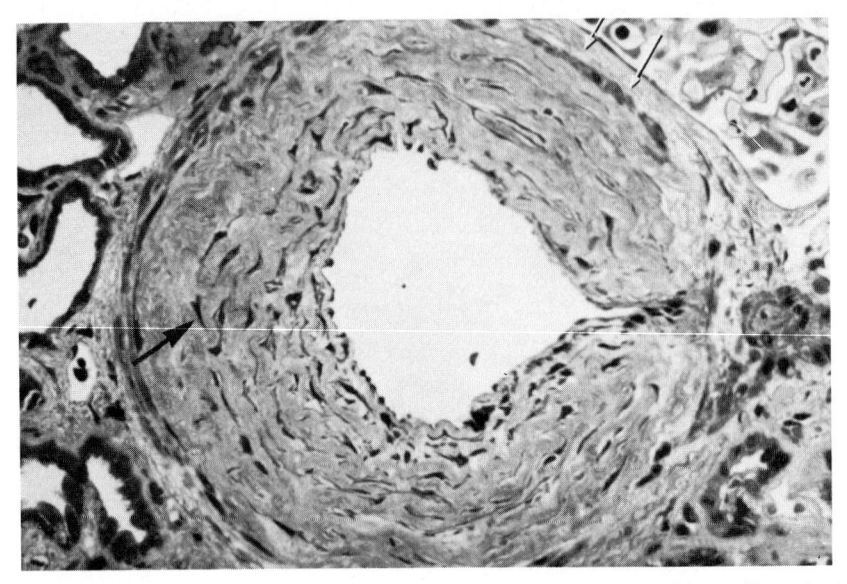

Figure 22-5. Same patient as in Figures 22-2 and 22-4. In this medium sized vessel, which has a branch exiting at approximately the 3 o'clock position, the media consists of only a few small, irregular remnants of smooth muscle cells (light arrows). On the luminal side of the cells there are concentric rows of lamellae of connective tissue, between which are interspersed elongated stellate cells (heavy arrow). Note that the lumen is considerably compromised by this "intimal proliferation." (H&E, × 300.)

The histologic appearance of this material has given rise to the term "mucoid" (or "mucinous") degeneration. The internal elastic lamina remains intact and the end result is a marked narrowing of the lumen, sometimes to the point of apparently complete obstruction. Thrombosis also may be observed.

The smaller arteries and arterioles are also conspicuously affected. As noted above, the changes cannot be differentiated from those found in malignant hypertension. In systemic sclerosis, however, they are seen equally often in the absence of hypertension. The changes consist of intimal proliferation, leakage of plasma proteins into the media (so-called fibrinoid necrosis), and, occasionally, thrombosis of the lumen (Figure 22-6). The afferent arterioles are similarly affected, but in this case the plasma protein leak is more prominent than the intimal proliferation (Fig. 22-7).

Clinical Course and Prognosis

The presence of renal vascular lesions in systemic sclerosis signifies a poor prognosis. Whereas Cannon and his associates (1974) found that only 10 per cent of 116 patients without overt signs of renal disease died during a 20 year follow-up period, 60 per cent of the 94 patients with demonstrable renal disease died during the same period. In addi-

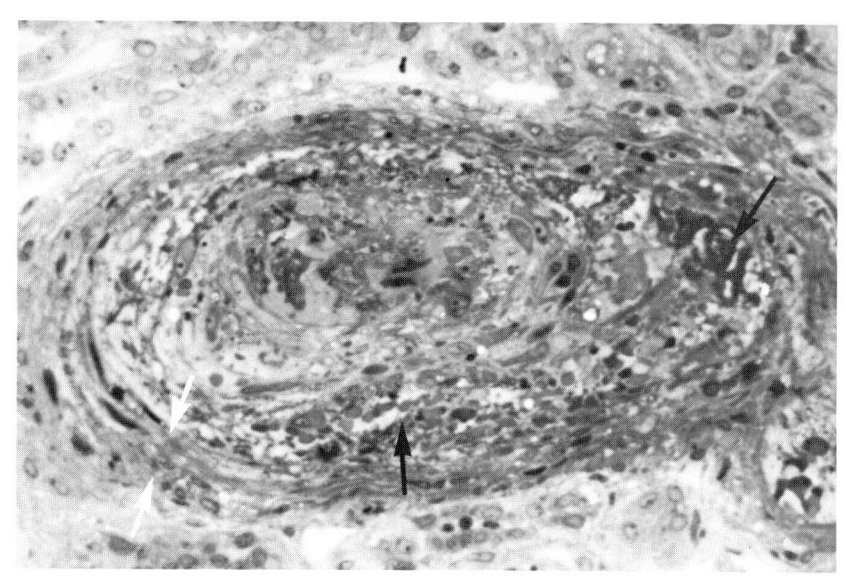

Figure 22-6. Same patient as in Figure 22-1. In this small arteriole the media (light arrows) represents a relatively small amount of the total thickness of the vascular wall. The lumen is quite small. The endothelial cells are detached from their basal lamina and lie within the vascular lumen, which is filled with protein and degenerating cells. At the upper right (heavy arrow) is a collection of serum proteins. Red blood cells are present in the vascular wall (dark arrow at lower center). These changes have been called "fibrinoid necrosis." (H&E, × 300.)

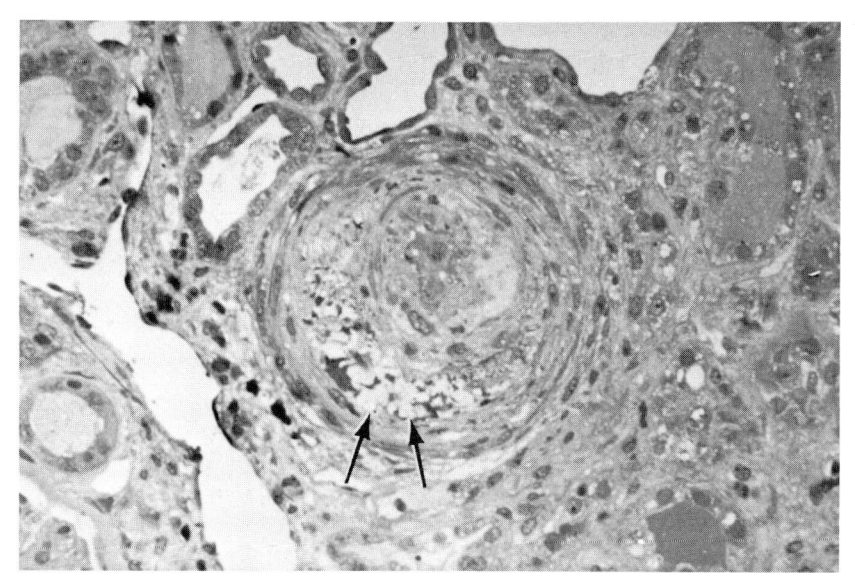

Figure 22-7. Same patient as in Figure 22-6. In the smaller arterioles, cellular proliferation is not as common as in larger vessels. Between the 6 and 10 o'clock positions, the proliferating cells between the media and the vascular lumen are displaced by deposits of serum protein and cellular debris (arrows). The vascular lumen is displaced to one side of the structure and is difficult to discern in this preparation. (H & E, × 300.)

tion, of all the patients who died of systemic sclerosis in this series, 82 per cent had renal involvement.

Although malignant hypertension has been thought to be a common sequela of renal vascular change, it occurs in only 30 per cent of patients who have the characteristic histologic vascular lesion. However, the presence of severe hypertension signifies an extremely poor prognosis, with death occurring in the majority of patients within a year of onset. The most common course is one of mild but persistent hypertension, which terminates abruptly with uremia after a period of years. Two factors probably act alone or in concert to produce hypertension and renal failure: first, vasoconstriction of renal cortical vessels, and second, intimal proliferation in the interlobular arteries. These changes may stimulate the release of renin and the generation of angiotensin, producing additional vasoconstriction, perpetuating and exacerbating the problem, and ultimately leading to complete occlusion of the involved vasculature. Since these changes tend to be irreversible, they lead to the proteinuria, azotemia, and rapidly progressive renal failure observed in systemic sclerosis.

Unfortunately, current treatment of scleroderma is unsatisfactory. Certain drugs appear to offer modest improvement of the skin manifestations, but none have been useful in treating visceral lesions. In addition, steroids have been tried without benefit, and might also be harmful in patients with renal failure. Because of the correlation between hypertension and vascular disease, however, it seems appropriate to control hypertension when it appears, and patients treated in this manner could possibly obtain a prolongation of renal function as well. Although this disorder is considered a systemic one, there is at present no contraindication to using dialysis or transplantation when end-stage renal failure occurs. When selecting patients for dialysis or transplantation, however, it is important that no extensive heart or lung disease be present and that peripheral blood vessels be accessible and in good condition for arteriovenous shunts.

References

1. Cannon, P. J., Hassar, M., Case, D. B., Casarella, W. J., Sommers, S. C., and LeRoy, E. C.: The relationship of hypertension and renal failure in scleroderma (progressive systemic sclerosis) to structural and functional abnormalities of the renal cortical circulation. Medicine 53:1, 1974.
2. Goetz, R. H.: The pathology of progressive systemic sclerosis (generalized scleroderma): with special reference to changes in the viscera. Clin. Proc. 4:337, 1945.
3. Medsger, T. A., Jr., Masi, A. T., Rodnan, G. P., Benedek, T. G., and Robinson, H.: Survival with systemic sclerosis (scleroderma). Ann. Intern. Med. 75:369, 1971.
4. Moore, H. C., and Sheehan, H. L.: The kidney of scleroderma. Lancet 1:68, 1952.
5. Osler, W.: The Principles and Practice of Medicine. New York, D. Appleton & Co., 1892.
6. Rodnan, G. P.: The natural history of progressive systemic sclerosis (diffuse scleroderma). Bull. Rheum. Dis. 13:301, 1963.

Chapter Twenty-Three

Amyloidosis

Introduction

   Amyloidosis is the term used for diseases characterized by the accumulation of an extracellular, eosinophilic, hyaline substance distributed irregularly and in varying degrees throughout virtually all organs of the body. Much effort has been spent in devising a suitable classification for this disorder. Until recently, the diagnosis of amyloidosis was rarely made during the lifetime of the patient. For this reason, most of the older classifications depend upon the distribution of amyloid in various organs and upon the tinctorial properties of the deposit. More recently, however, investigators have preferred to consider amyloidosis in terms of a clinical classification, such as presence or absence of other diseases, or genetic associations, rather than in terms of the tissue distribution and tinctorial properties, until more can be known about these at a molecular level. For example, amyloidosis occurring as a complication of certain chronic diseases (osteomyelitis, tuberculosis, leprosy, rheumatoid arthritis, myeloma) is referred to as *secondary* amyloidosis. In contrast, the finding of amyloid in previously healthy individuals without coexistent or antecedent illness is called *primary* amyloidosis. In addition, *heredofamilial* forms of the disease, such as primary familial amyloidosis with polyneuropathy, familial Mediterranean fever with amyloidosis, familial amyloid nephropathy, and so forth, have been described.

   The prevalence of amyloidosis in the population at large, or even in high-risk patients such as those with rheumatoid arthritis, is not known. Amyloidosis in certain selected age groups is quite frequent. For example, amyloid was found in brain, pancreas, and heart tissues in 90 per cent of patients over the age of 60 years who died with senile dementia. In patients with familial Mediterranean fever, evidence of amyloidosis has been obtained in 40 per cent of those studied. The frequency of amyloidosis from histologic evidence at autopsy is about 0.5 per cent, with the majority of cases occurring in patients with rheumatoid arthritis and myeloma. Amyloid nephropathy is present at necropsy in approximately 20 per cent of these cases.

Clinical Data

Renal damage is the most common and most serious manifestation of amyloidosis, being the major cause of death in most series. Despite this, renal amyloid may be present and asymptomatic for many years, and progression of the disease is not inevitable. Severe renal insufficiency leading to death from uremia results from extensive replacement of renal tissue by amyloid accumulations. Hence, uremia as the presenting manifestation of renal amyloidosis is relatively uncommon.

Routine blood examination reveals no specific abnormalities. However, in a series of 100 patients with amyloidosis studied by Isobe and Osserman (1974), abnormal quantities of monoclonal immunoglobulins, Bence Jones proteins, or both, were usually found when appropriate studies were done.

Hematuria and pyuria are seen infrequently. Hyaline and granular casts are relatively common, particularly in patients exhibiting marked proteinuria. Proteinuria is the most common laboratory finding and a reliable indicator of renal involvement. The occurrence of proteinuria in association with chronic suppurative disease, inflammatory diseases (such as rheumatoid arthritis), or heredofamilial disease (such as Mediterranean fever) should always raise the suspicion of renal amyloidosis. Proteinuria may be quite massive and reach the nephrotic range either initially or later. Clinical reports suggest that 60 per cent of patients with amyloidosis become nephrotic during the course of their illness. In biopsy diagnoses in patients presenting with the nephrotic syndrome, on the other hand, the frequency of unsuspected amyloid in different series ranged from 5 to 12 per cent. Radiographically, the amyloid kidney is classically described as being enlarged; however, it is not unusual to find normal sized or even small kidneys. Small amyloidotic kidneys are always associated with advanced renal insufficiency, and the evolution of relatively large or normal sized kidneys to shrunken ones may occur within a surprisingly brief time.

The diagnosis can be established with certainty only by histologic examination. The value of liver and renal biopsy, as well as rectal biopsy, has been well demonstrated. Renal biopsy appears to be safe, in contrast to several reported hemorrhages following liver biopsy in the presence of amyloidosis.

The incidence of renal vein thrombosis with renal amyloid appears to be rather high in cases which present with the clinical picture of rapidly progressive uremia or the sudden onset of the nephrotic syndrome. However, there is a higher incidence of renal vein thrombosis in the presence of the nephrotic syndrome from other types of glomerulopathy, making this relationship nonspecific.

Histology

GLOMERULI. The glomeruli are diffusely affected, but the degree of involvement varies among glomeruli and within different segments of individual glomeruli. The most readily apparent change is an increase in the amount of extracellular material of a type which presents a smooth, homogeneous appearance often referred to as "glassy" or "hyaline" (Fig. 23–1 and 23–2). In some cases the deposits of amyloid may be so extensive as to mimic the changes seen in diabetes mellitus or other forms of chronic sclerosing glomerulonephritis. The material is PAS positive and shows characteristic dichroic birefringence following congo red staining. Cellular proliferation is not a common feature. Silver staining of methacrylate-embedded tissue reveals that the mesangial regions and peripheral capillary loops often are punctuated or "perforated" by spike-like projections of argyrophilic material which appears to be continuous from the subendothelial to the subepithelial aspect of the basal lamina (Figs. 23–3 and 23–4). This is a nearly characteristic feature for amyloid.

TUBULES AND INTERSTITIUM. There are no specific tubular changes. Vacuolation of epithclial cells as a consequence of proteinuria may occur. In patients with advanced disease there may be extensive changes of interstitial fibrosis and tubular atrophy. In these cases, amyloid often may be identified in the interstitium (Fig. 23–5).

VESSELS. The deposits of amyloid in vessels, when present, lie between the cells of the media and often extend into the adventitia (Fig. 23–5).

Electron Microscopy

Observations at this level contribute little additional information. The amyloid fibrils are nonbranching structures ranging in diameter from 8 to 10 nanometers (nm) and up to 1 micrometer (μm) in length (Fig. 23–6). The fibrils tend to be arranged in a random fashion, resembling the straws in a haystack. As is also apparent by light microscopy, the fibrils often appear to extend through the basal lamina and indent the epithelial cells. They also are seen in the mesangial regions of glomeruli and in the media and subendothelial areas of vessels, including interstitial capillaries.

Text continued on page 307

304 AMYLOIDOSIS

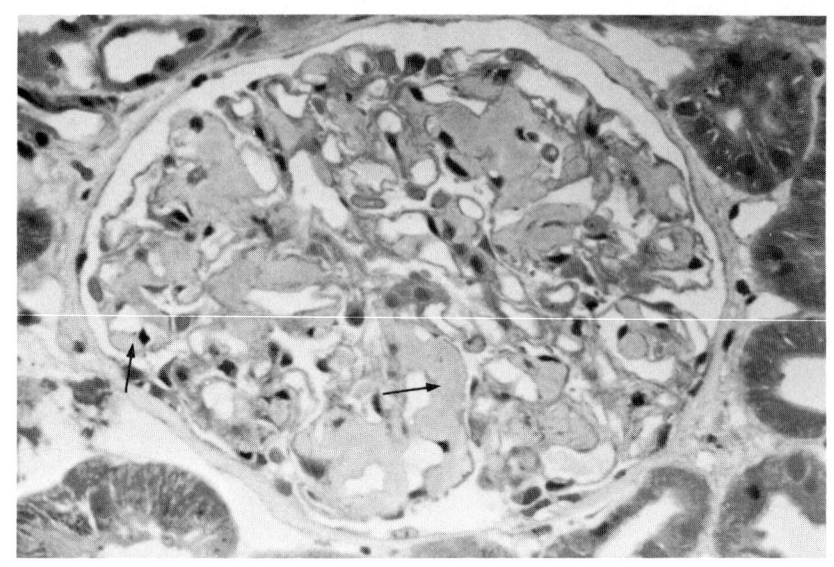

Figure 23-1. Specimen from a 77 year old woman who had noted the onset of edema four months earlier. She was found to have a normal blood pressure, 4+ pitting edema of both extremities, and no other significant physical findings. Her urine contained 8 gm of protein/24 hr. Other pertinent findings were a serum albumin level of 1.5 gm/dl, a serum cholesterol level of 600 mg/dl, and normal renal function. On renal biopsy all glomeruli had the appearance noted here. The mesangial regions and some peripheral capillary loops show nodular and irregular masses of a homogeneous, poorly staining material displacing the normal structures (arrows). The peripheral capillary loops are patent. The number of cells is not remarkable. (H&E, × 300.)

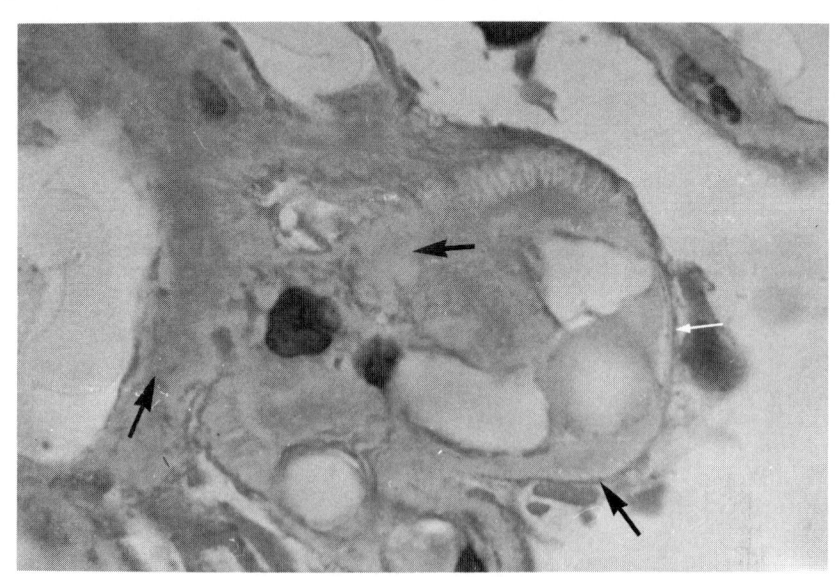

Figure 23-2. At higher magnification than in Figure 23-1, the basal lamina can be seen to be a thin line of pale-staining material at the periphery of the capillary loops (light arrow). Scattered throughout the photomicrograph is a more dense material, generally lying beneath the peripheral basal lamina and in the mesangial matrix (heavy arrows), which is the amyloid substance. The capillary spaces are reduced in size and irregular in shape owing to the deposition of material. (H&E, × 1200.)

Amyloidosis 305

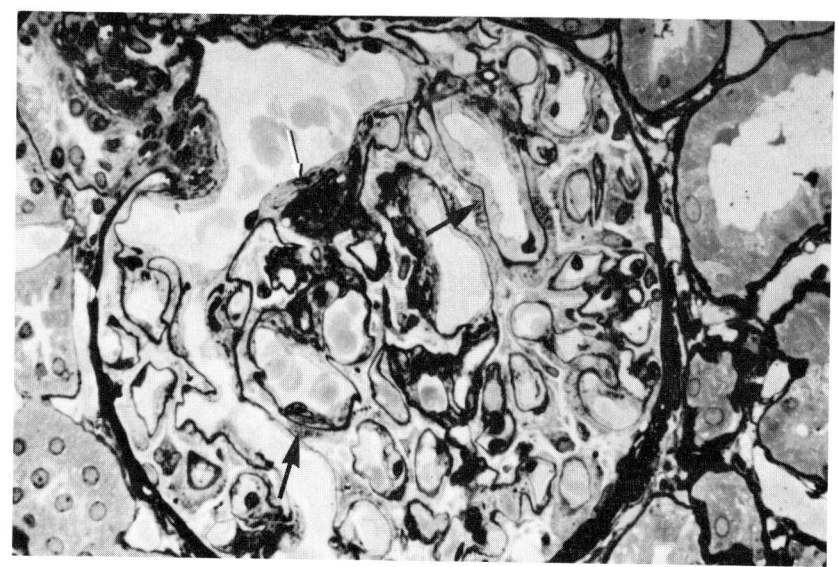

Figure 23–3. The amyloid is not stained with methenamine silver. The large mesangial areas are readily apparent (light arrow). Noted also on a number of peripheral capillary loops is a dense collection of elongated "picket fence" deposits, stained structures between which are deposits of amyloid (heavy arrows). (Silver methenamine, × 600.)

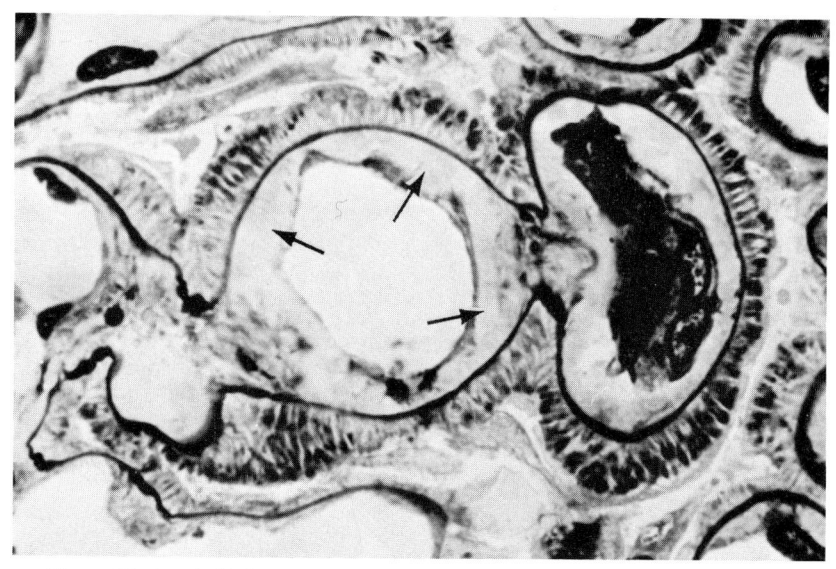

Figure 23–4. At higher magnification, the subendothelial deposits of amyloid (light arrow) are readily apparent. A thin layer of endothelial cells can be seen on the luminal side and the dark-staining basal lamina is visible on its external aspect. Well illustrated here is the subepithelial deposition of amyloid interspersed with spikes of material which stains similarly to the basal lamina. (Silver methenamine, × 1200.)

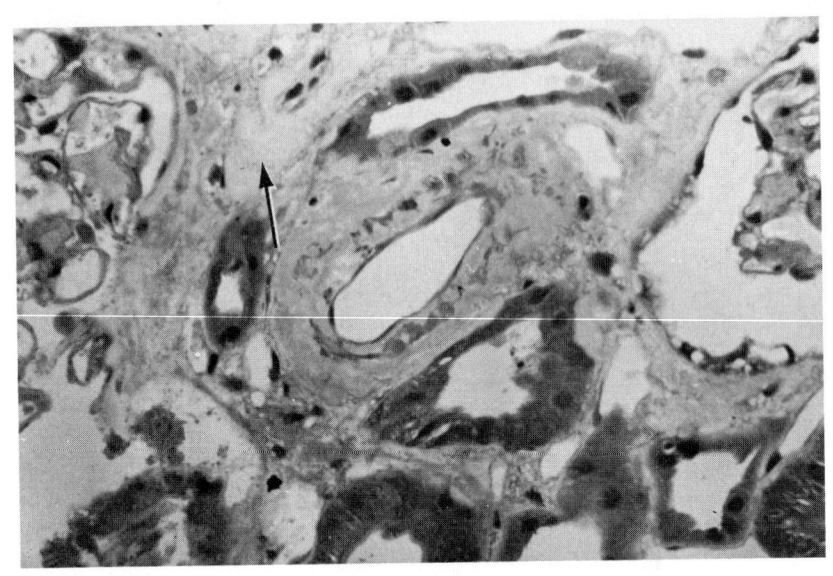

Figure 23-5. Homogeneous eosinophilic masses of amyloid material can be seen both within the interstitium (arrow) and lying within the wall of the vessels. In the latter the smooth muscle cells are seen to be displaced from one another and to be distorted by the amyloid deposit. (H&E, × 600.)

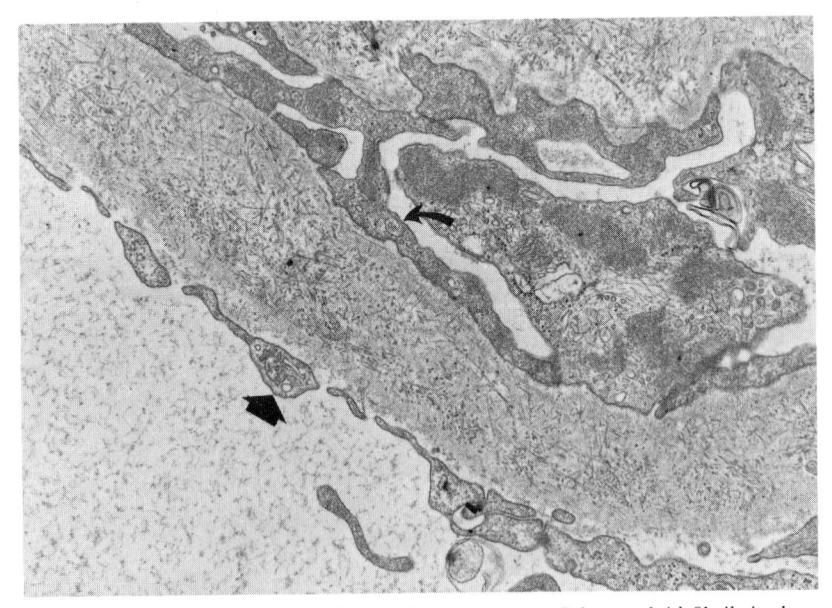

Figure 23-6. The electron microscopic appearance of the amyloid fibrils is characteristic in that there appears to be a tangled array of straight, thin fibrils which resemble in their distribution a game of "pick-up sticks." In this photomicrograph the fibrils are distributed throughout the basal lamina. Neither the endothelial cells (arrowhead) nor epithelial cells (curved arrow) are remarkable. (× 10,000.)

Fluorescence Microscopy

There are no characteristic patterns of protein deposition by fluorescence microscopy.

Clinical Course

Much information about the clinical course of amyloidosis has been obtained through the study of patients with heredofamilial forms of the disease. In a review of familial Mediterranean fever, Sohar and his associates (1967) obtained a detailed picture of the natural history of renal involvement by amyloid deposition. In virtually every patient, death was the result of the renal involvement. The frequency of amyloidosis in their group was 28 per cent. The clinical course of the nephropathy was divided into four stages of variable duration: (1) the preclinical stage, (2) proteinuria, (3) nephrotic syndrome, and (4) uremia. The preclinical stage is not well studied but has been clearly documented when renal biopsies revealed amyloid in vessels of the kidney in the complete absence of symptoms. How long such a state can exist is unknown, but in one instance it lasted 6 years. Of 30 patients with proteinuria, 19 had mild proteinuria for periods ranging between 2 and 10 years. In the remaining 11 patients, the nephrotic syndrome occurred after a variable period of time. The time span between the appearance of proteinuria and the onset of the nephrotic syndrome ranged from 2 to 9 years. In virtually every instance, progressive azotemia followed the onset of the nephrotic syndrome within 1 to 2 years. Thus, although proteinuria may be present for a decade or more, the appearance of the nephrotic syndrome usually heralds the beginning of the terminal phase of the illness, and, in general, end-stage renal failure occurs about 2 years after the nephrotic syndrome first appears.

Although there is no specific treatment for renal amyloidosis, the patient's life span may be quite long if the amyloidosis is associated with a systemic disease which can be treated adequately. Patients with biopsy-proved amyloid renal disease have been reported to be alive after 23 years. The nephrotic syndrome is resistant to steroid treatment but occasionally spontaneous remission may occur without apparent alteration in the amount or appearance of the renal amyloid. For the most part, treatment is supportive and may include dialysis or transplantation in suitable candidates.

References

1. Brandt, K., Cathcart, E. S., and Cohen, A. S.: A clinical analysis of the course and prognosis of forty-two patients with amyloidosis. Am. J. Med. 44:955, 1968.

2. Cohen, A. S.: Amyloidosis. New Eng. J. Med. *266*:522, 574, 628, 1967.
3. Cohen, A. S., Bricetti, A. B., Harrington, J. R., et al.: Renal transplantation in two cases of amyloidosis. Lancet *2*;513, 1971.
4. Glenner, G. G., and Terry, W. D.: Characterization of amyloid. Ann. Rev. Med. *25*:131, 1974.
5. Isobe, T., and Osserman, E. F.: Patterns of amyloidosis and their association with plasma-cell dyscrasia, monoclonal immunoglobulins and Bence-Jones proteins. New Eng. J. Med. *290*:473, 1974.
6. Sohar, E., Gafni, J., Pras, M., and Heller, H.: Familial Mediterranean fever: A survey of 470 cases and review of the literature. Amer. J. Med. *43*:227, 1967.

Chapter Twenty-Four

Multiple Myeloma

Introduction

Among the plasma cell dyscrasias, several clinical patterns are recognized, which may be classified as follows: (1) multiple myeloma, (2) Waldenström's macroglobulinemia, (3) heavy-chain disease, and (4) monoclonal gammopathy of unknown significance. Multiple myeloma is the only one of these dyscrasias which is consistently associated with significant renal disease.

Multiple myeloma is a neoplastic disease of plasma cells manifested primarily by widespread skeletal destruction and frequently accompanied by anemia, hypercalcemia, renal failure, and increased susceptibility to infection. It constitutes a prototype of a monoclonal gammopathy, with an increased production of a specific immunoglobulin molecule or its subunits, or both, by a single clone of plasma cells. In addition, there is decreased production of the other "active" immunoglobulins.

Clinical Data

Myeloma rarely develops before the fourth decade. Onset and early course are usually insidious, accompanied by progressive weakness, loss of appetite and weight, and gastrointestinal symptoms. The classic diagnostic triad of back pain, anemia, and renal disease can all be related to the expanding mass of plasma cells in the bone marrow.

Since 1949, when Sir Henry Bence Jones described a unique protein (now classified as a light-chain polypeptide) in the urine of a patient with multiple myeloma, the relationship between the abnormal protein and the renal disease has been the object of study. The clinical features of renal disease are the result of a number of interrelated features. Tubular damage appears to be related to the filtration of large quantities of light-chain proteins, a portion of which is actively reabsorbed by the proximal tubules.

Other factors of importance in the genesis of renal failure include hypercalcemia and hyperuricemia. Hypercalcemia appears to result from bony destruction, whereas hyperuricemia is due to rapid cell turnover, frequently aggravated by therapy. In addition, amyloid deposits are found in about 10 per cent of autopsy cases of multiple myeloma. Although it is generally thought that the amyloid deposits may be related to the abnormal protein produced in myeloma, immunofluorescent studies have failed to demonstrate the deposition of light-chain proteins in the kidney. It is not uncommon for myeloma to present as an apparently isolated nephropathy with minimal extrarenal signs. Immunoelectrophoresis of serum and urine proteins is important in the detection of this monoclonal gammopathy.

Usually, there is no hematuria or only minimal microscopic hematuria. Proteinuria is common and occurs in 60 to 80 per cent of patients first diagnosed as having myeloma and in all patients with demonstrable nephropathy. In most cases, Bence Jones protein can be demonstrated in the urine, although occasionally proteinuria is seen in the absence of these light-chain proteins. The amount of urinary protein varies; it generally is greater than 1 g daily, often being in the nephrotic range (greater than $2g/m^2/day$). In contrast to other nephropathies, even with this degree of excessive proteinuria, edema, hypoalbuminemia, and hyperlipidemia are uncommon. The rarity of these latter features may be due to the fact that there usually is only a very slight urinary loss of albumin. When the full-blown nephrotic syndrome has been noted in patients with myeloma nephropathy, amyloidosis is frequently found.

Acute renal failure is an occasional feature of myeloma. It often appears at an early stage of the disease and may be the presenting feature. In some cases, it occurs immediately following excretory urography and is thought to result from the fluid restriction required in preparation for this procedure or from the precipitation of light-chain proteins in the lumina caused by the contrast media.

Histology

In the earlier literature amyloid deposition was frequently listed as a common feature in kidneys of patients with multiple myeloma. In fact, it appears that only from 6 to 15 per cent of such patients actually have demonstrable amyloid in renal structures (see Chapter 23). When present, it tends to be located in the adventitia of blood vessels, in the renal interstitium arranged around the basal lamina of the tubules, and in the glomeruli.

GLOMERULI. The glomeruli most often appear normal or reflect the degree of vascular change expected in the patient as a consequence of age.

TUBULES AND INTERSTITIUM. The main histologic change in myeloma is found in the tubular interstitial area. This is related to the apparent toxicity of the light chain of immunoglobulin for renal tubular epithelial cells or damage resulting from the formation of casts. The presence of large numbers of casts in the distal tubules and collecting ducts is typical, and they have been shown by microdissection to extend for a considerable distance within a tubule. They have a characteristic homogeneous, waxy or hard texture (Fig. 24-1) and are differentiated from other casts by the presence of epithelial cell proliferation around the cast, which assumes the form of giant cells in some areas (Fig. 24-2). When the number of casts is large, there may be a marked associated interstitial reaction consisting of edema and dense infiltration by lymphocytes and plasma cells (Fig. 24-3).

VESSELS. No changes, other than those expected as a result of arteriosclerosis, are found. When amyloid accompanies the disease, it may be seen in the media or adventitia of vessels, particularly those of interlobular size or larger.

Electron Microscopy

The number of published studies of electron microscopic observations in multiple myeloma is quite small. In kappa chain myeloma a finely granular, homogeneous subendothelial deposit has been seen.

Fluorescence Microscopy

Glomeruli most often contain no deposits of immunoglobulins. In fact, the most consistent finding is that of kappa or lambda chains of immunoglobulin in casts and in the tubular epithelial cells around them.

Clinical Course and Prognosis

The prognosis of the disease is unfavorable, as few patients survive longer than 3 years. The clinical status of the patient at the time of diagnosis probably provides the best index of prognosis. Initiation of therapy as early as possible extends survival and prolongs the useful,

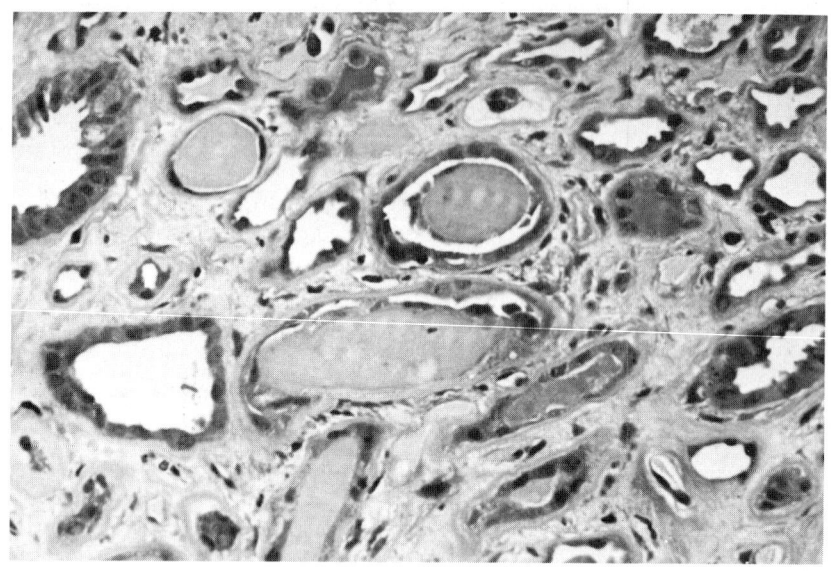

Figure 24-1. Increasing angina pectoris brought this 67 year old man to the hospital. On admission, he was found to be in renal failure. The urine output was 2000 ml/day, but he was unable to maximally concentrate the urine, and the serum creatinine was 19.5 mg/dl. An extensive work-up revealed a monoclonal spike on immunoelectrophoresis and "kappa" light chains in the urine. Renal biopsy showed severe tubulointerstitial disease. Most tubules contained casts similar to that noted in the central portion of this photomicrograph. They have a "hard" appearance — i.e., the margins are sharp and they appear to have multiple lamellae. The interstitium is expanded and contains a small number of inflammatory cells scattered throughout. Multiple tubular profiles are seen in which the epithelium is atrophied. (H&E, paraffin-embedded tissue, × 300.)

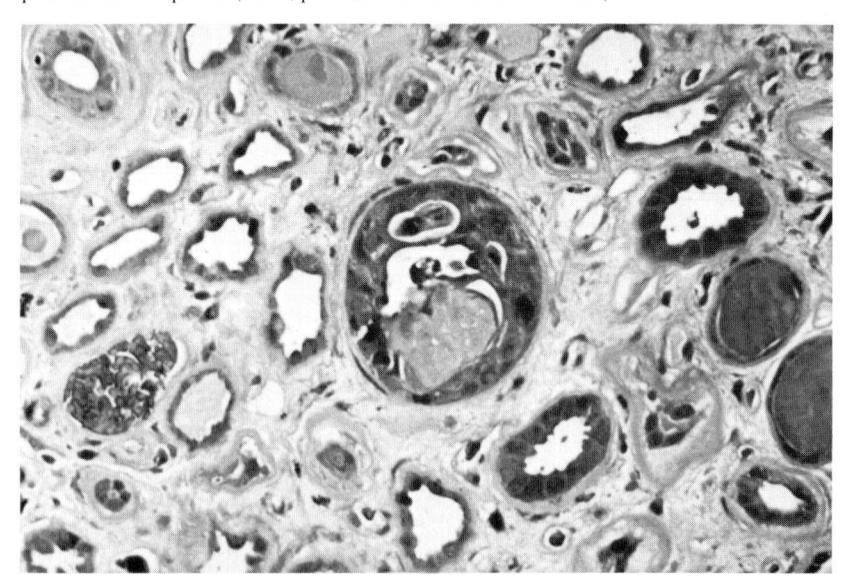

Figure 24-2. The characteristic tubular change in multiple myeloma is the presence of multinucleated epithelial cells surrounding the hard, waxy casts. These are found primarily in the medulla, but they also can be present in the cortical rays. Again note the multiple profiles of atrophied tubules. (H&E, paraffin-embedded tissue, × 300.)

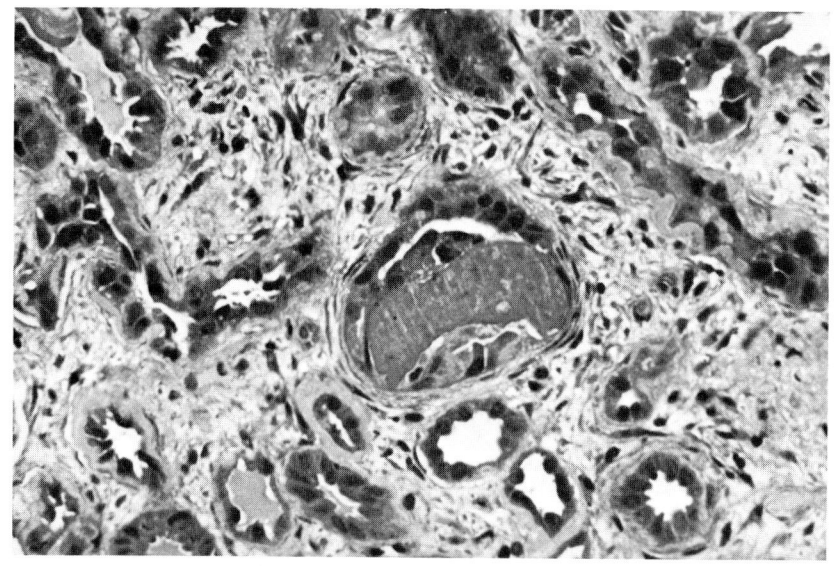

Figure 24-3. In multiple areas the interstitium may contain an increased number of inflammatory cells and interstitial cells. This is frequently most marked in zones where the casts shown in Figure 24-3 are abundant. (H&E, paraffin-embedded tissue, × 300.)

comfortable life of the patient. The important therapeutic measures are chemotherapy to reduce the neoplastic cell population, radiation to control local lesions, maintenance of adequate hydration, and as much ambulation as possible. Although it is doubtful that any of these therapeutic modalities will successfully reverse renal damage, occasionally a striking improvement in renal function is seen. Hypercalcemia may be the most striking manifestation of myeloma, and because of the potential nephrotoxicity, should be treated promptly. To prevent hyperuricemia following treatment with cytotoxic agents, pretreatment with allopurinol should be given.

In addition to chemotherapeutic agents, symptomatic treatment of uremia may be required. Although it is unlikely that transplantation would be useful in most patients with this systemic disorder, hemodialysis may be helpful when the primary presentation of the disease is far advanced renal failure, and when the primary illness is controlled.

References

1. Bence, Jones, H.: On a new substance occurring in the urine of a patient with "mollities ossium." Phil Tr. Roy. Soc. Lond., 1948, p. 55.
2. Maldonado, J. E., Velosa, J. A., Kyle, R. A., Wagoner, R. D., Holley, K. E., and Salassa, R. M.: Fanconi syndrome in adults: A manifestation of a latent form of myeloma. Amer. J. Med. 58:354, 1975.

3. Martinez-Maldonado, M., Yium, J., Suki, W. N., and Ednoyan, G.: Renal complications in multiple myeloma: Pathophysiology and some aspects of clinical management. J. Chron. Dis. *24*:221, 1971.
4. Ooi, B. S., Pesce, A. J., Pollak, V. E., and Mandalenakis, N.: Multiple myeloma with massive proteinuria and terminal renal failure. Amer. J. Med. *52*:538, 1972.
5. Osserman, E. F., and Farhangi, M.: Plasma cell myeloma. *In* Williams, W. J., Bentler, E., Ersley, A. J., and Rundles, R. W. (eds.): Hematology. New York, McGraw-Hill, 1972.
6. Stone, M. J., and Frenkel, E. P.: The clinical spectrum of light chain myeloma. Amer. J. Med. *58*:601, 1975.

Chapter Twenty-Five

Renal Disease of Pregnancy

The pregnant state is associated with a number of renal syndromes, but only one, toxemia, is unique to pregnancy. Severe toxemia is relatively rare, and other pregnancy-related syndromes, such as tubulointerstitial disease of acute onset (Chapter 10) and thrombotic thrombocytopenic purpura (Chapter 20), are more common causes of renal failure. In addition, patients may have preexisting renal disease or while pregnant may develop a renal disease that is totally independent of the gravid state but complicated by it.

Ferris (1975) divides acute renal failure in pregnancy into two groups: (1) that occurring early in pregnancy, which most often is caused by septic abortion, and (2) that occurring in the third trimester, most often in association with toxemia or an obstetric complication. The clinical and histologic data in the nontoxemic syndromes are not dissimilar to those described in Chapters 10 and 20; the remainder of this chapter will therefore be devoted to discussing the toxemic states.

Clinical Data

Toxemia of pregnancy is a syndrome of unknown etiology characterized by the development of edema, hypertension, and proteinuria. It occurs most commonly in primipara during the third trimester but may occur earlier when the pregnancy is complicated by hydatidiform mole, preexisting renal disease, or hypertension.

The onset of toxemia is often insidious, and although occasionally the patient is asymptomatic, she usually notes the appearance of edema, headaches, visual disturbances, and anxiety.

Hypertension is moderate, with systolic levels usually below 200 mm Hg. Funduscopic examination reveals spasm of the retinal arterioles and retinal sheen. Hyperreflexia indicates the presence of encephalopathy, which may lead to generalized convulsions.

Serum urate concentrations are elevated in toxemia, and the level tends to correlate with the severity of the illness. Proteinuria usually occurs following the onset of hypertension but rarely reaches nephrotic ranges (> 2 g/m^2/24 hr). Other than proteinuria, the urinalysis is normal, which is a useful point in distinguishing this disease from other renal syndromes.

Renal biopsy is reserved for those patients in whom the clinical and laboratory evaluations are not characteristic of toxemia and other syndromes are suggested.

Histology

GENERAL FINDINGS. The renal lesions in this syndrome represent a spectrum of vascular injury. Generally, patients in mild preeclampsia reflect minimal clinical signs, whereas severe toxemia is associated with diffuse, severe vascular change.

LIGHT MICROSCOPY. The changes in the glomeruli are diffuse and regular. Glomeruli are large, and the vascular spaces are reduced in size and number. There appears to be an obliteration of these spaces by an expanded mesangial region and swelling of the endothelial cells (Figs. 25-1, 25-2, and 25-3). Although the glomeruli are not diffusely hypercellular, focal areas of endothelial proliferation may be apparent. Inflammatory cells are characteristically absent. The mesangial matrix and glomerular basal lamina as judged by silver staining are severely altered (Figs. 25-4 and 25-5). The mesangial region is expanded and distorted by deposits. The basal lamina contains subendothelial deposits.

Text continued on page 320

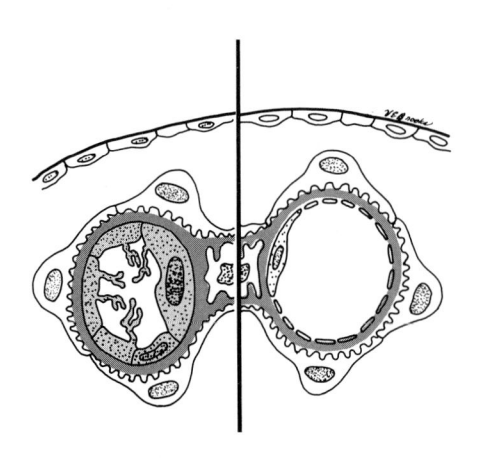

Figure 25-1 Diagrammatic representation of endothelial cell swelling.

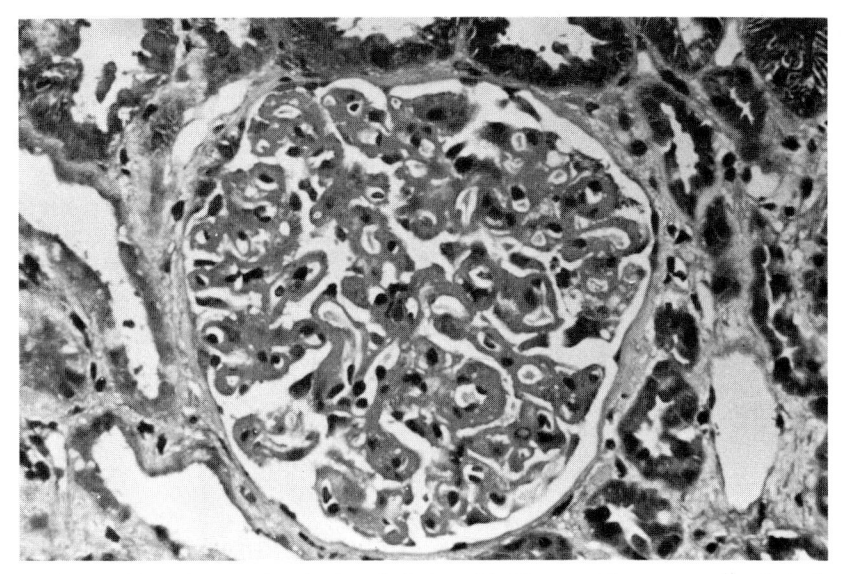

Figure 25-2 One week prior to admission, this 20 year old pregnant female in the second trimester developed a mild upper respiratory infection followed by a marked pedal edema, which quickly progressed to anasarca. On admission, her blood pressure was 240/140, she had retinal arteriolar narrowing, ascites, and peripheral edema, and 24-hour urine protein was 13 g/24 hr. All glomeruli demonstrated the above lesion. The peripheral capillary loops appeared to have very thickened walls. The vascular spaces are diminished. There does not appear to be an increase in the number of cells. The interstitial spaces seem to be widened by edema. (H&E, paraffin-embedded tissue, ×300.)

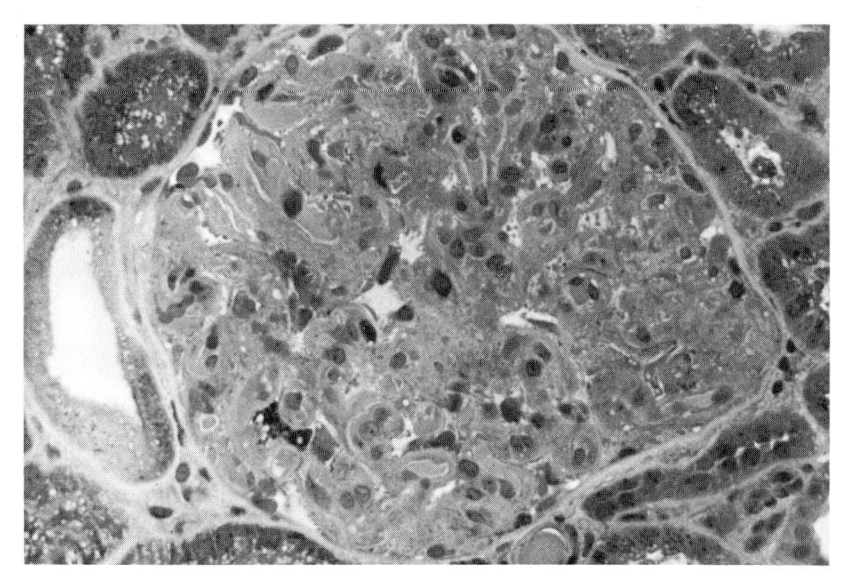

Figure 25-3 This 20 year old woman, during her seventh month of pregnancy, developed hypertension, nephrotic syndrome, and peripheral edema. Following admission to hospital, the hypertension was easily controlled and CNS symptoms did not appear. The glomeruli all showed a similar change. The capillary spaces were markedly decreased, and the peripheral capillary wall appears thickened. In this glutaraldehyde-fixed specimen, cellular detail is more clear than in Figure 25-2, where formalin was the fixative used. The number of cells in this patient's glomeruli are slightly increased. (H&E, ×300.)

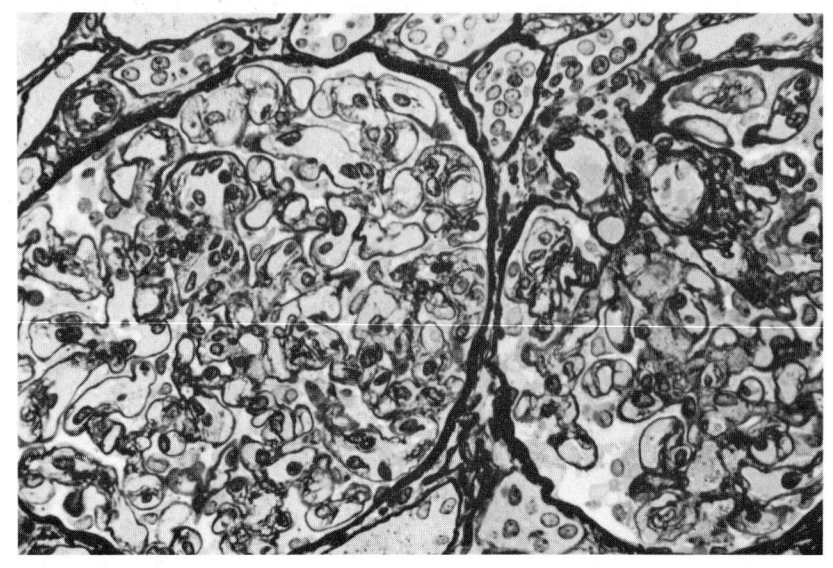

Figure 25-4 Silver staining of the specimen depicted in Figure 25-3 demonstrates that the amount of extracellular material is not increased and that the peripheral basal lamina has a normal contour. (Silver methenamine, ×300.)

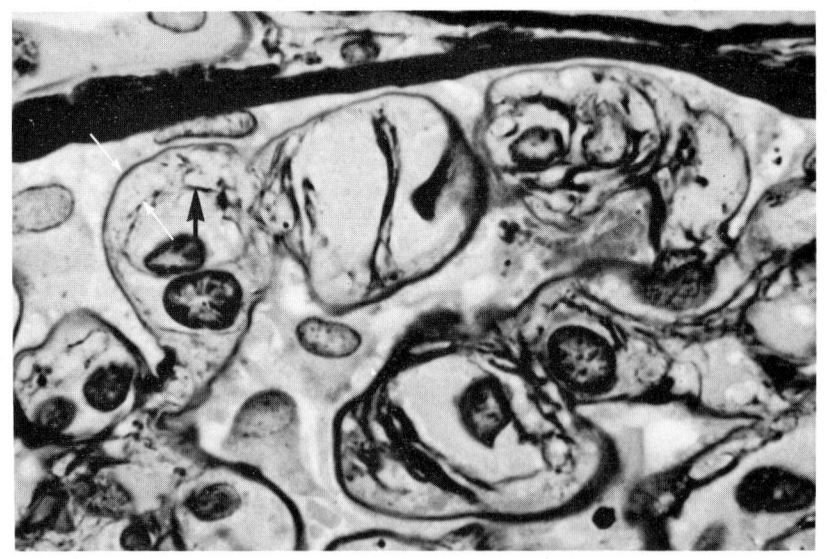

Figure 25-5 At high power the basal lamina is seen to be abnormal. The subendothelial space (arrows) is widened, and the vascular spaces are severely compromised. The endothelial cell layer is outlined on luminal aspect by silver positive material (heavy arrow). Although the peripheral basal lamina appears intact, there are multiple irregular silver-positive densities lying in the subendothelial material. The mesangial matrix is increased in amount and irregular in contour. (Silver methenamine, ×1200.)

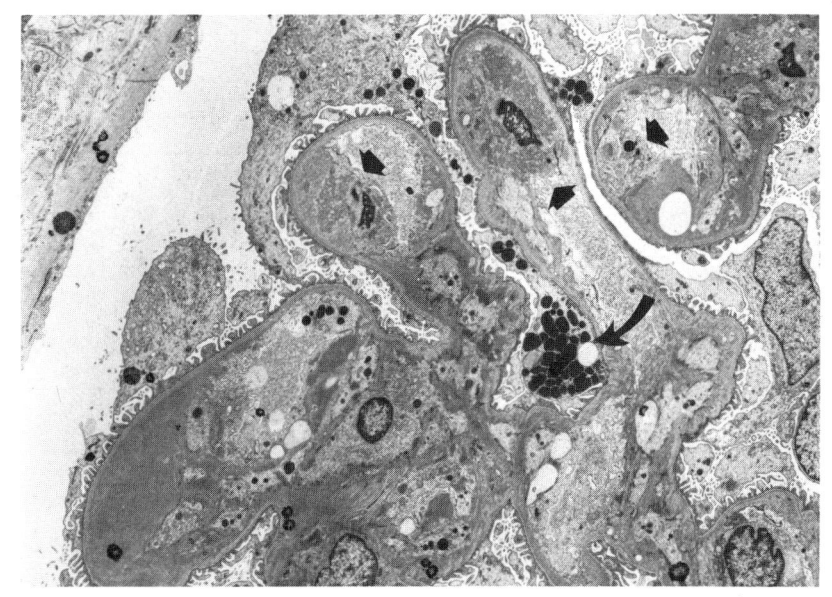

Figure 25-6 The endothelial cell cytoplasm is prominent (arrowheads). Subendothelial deposits of granular material also can be seen. The epithelial cells frequently contain lysosomes (curved arrow). (×2000.)

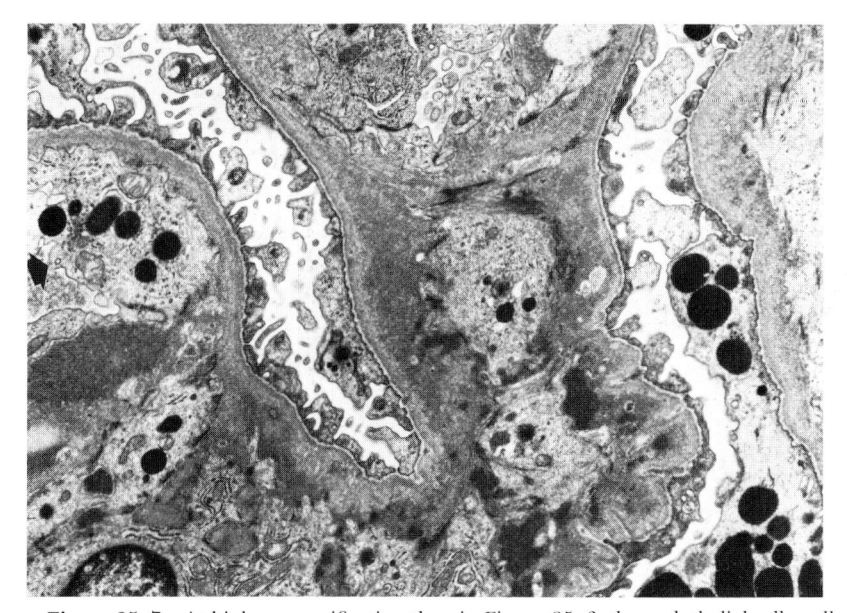

Figure 25-7 At higher magnification than in Figure 25-6, the endothelial cell swelling is quite apparent (arrowhead). The subendothelial densities are irregular in distribution and staining characteristics. The epithelial cell morphology is relatively unaltered save for the previously noted lysosomes. The mesangial cells have pale cytoplasm but are otherwise unremarkable. (×4000.)

Vascular changes beyond endothelial swelling are usually not apparent, unless severe hypertension or diffuse intravascular coagulation supervenes.

The tubules may show an increased number of lysosomes containing protein in the proximal segments. Casts are often seen in the distal tubules and collecting ducts.

ELECTRON MICROSCOPY. The major changes are seen to be in the endothelial cells, which are swollen and vacuolated (Fig. 25-6). There often appears to be an expansion of the lamina rara interna by a slightly granular electron-dense material lying immediately adjacent to the swollen endothelial cells (Fig. 25-7). On occasion the mesangial cells also appear to be swollen. Deposits of material which resembles fibrin often may be seen lying within capillary spaces.

FLUORESCENCE MICROSCOPY. The major reported change has been a relatively uniform and diffuse deposition of fibrin-fibrinogen antigens along peripheral capillary loops as well as in mesangial regions.

Clinical Course and Prognosis

The treatment of toxemia is a subject of much controversy at the present time. Bed rest and careful monitoring of blood pressure, urine output, protein excretion, and fetal development are routine. Salt restriction and diuretic therapy, although used at many medical centers, are considered to be harmful in others.

Signs of central nervous system irritability are best treated with magnesium sulfate, which, however, has little effect on blood pressure. More potent antihypertensive therapy may be necessary if bed rest and salt restriction are unsuccessful in modifying this syndrome.

The prognosis in toxemia is quite good. However, there is a 10 per cent mortality rate when seizures are present, mainly due to intracerebral bleeding. The syndrome usually reverts following delivery, and often induction of labor is necessary. However, this decision must take into account the fetal viability.

References

1. Ferris, T. F.: *In* Burrow, G. N., and Ferris, T. F. (eds.): Medical Complications During Pregnancy. Philadelphia, W. B. Saunders Co., 1975.
2. Kincaid-Smith, P., Fairley, K. F., and Bullen, M.: Kidney disease and pregnancy. Med. J. Austral. 2:1155, 1967.
3. Lindheimer, M. D., and Katz, A. I.: The kidney in pregnancy. New Eng. J. Med. 283:1095, 1970.
4. Schwartz, L. J.: Hypertension and renal disease in pregnancy. Med. Clin. North Am. 55:47, 1971.

Section VI
TRANSPLANTATION

Chapter Twenty-Six

Transplant Rejection and Recurrence of the Original Disease

Over the past 15 years, renal transplantation has progressed from an experimental procedure to an acceptable alternative to chronic dialysis therapy for the treatment of chronic renal failure. It is, in fact, the first choice in many medical centers. Recent figures show that recipients of kidneys from living, related donors have a 75 per cent 2 year graft survival rate, whereas recipients of cadaver kidneys do less well, with an average graft survival of 50 per cent at 2 years. If a graft functions for 2 years, there is a good chance for long-term survival.

The reasons for the variability of graft success can be explained only partially by the degree of antigenic match or mismatch and variations in specific immunosuppressive therapy. Other factors, such as the immune response of a recipient to the graft or variation in individual response to drug therapy, undoubtedly account for some of the observed inconsistencies. Greater understanding of these factors will permit more scientific selection of methods of immunosuppressive therapy and modalities of overall management. In addition, without question some patients are managed best by dialysis and others do best with transplantation; however, neither clinical assays nor other documented parameters exist on which to base this decision.

In the individual patient the diagnosis of the transplant rejection syndrome is often difficult, since there is a good deal of overlap with other causes of renal failure, as, for example, urinary obstruction, large vessel occlusion, or recurrence of the original disease. The diagnosis of the rejection syndrome depends on several clinical and laboratory parameters, including the patient's overall response to anti-rejection therapy. The difficulty in making the diagnosis renders renal histology particularly useful in determining the types of rejection as well as in excluding other causes of renal functional deterioration.

The causes of rejection remain unclear, for the most part. Therefore, we have chosen to use a purely descriptive classification based on time of onset and prognosis—i.e., using the terms immediate, early, and late to describe time of onset, and reversible and irreversible to denote prognosis (Table 26-1).

IMMEDIATE, IRREVERSIBLE REJECTION SYNDROME

The immune mechanism for the immediate, irreversible rejection syndrome has been well studied. The rejection occurs after transplantation of a kidney into a recipient who has circulating antibodies against the renal antigens, causing immediate, irreversible, so-called hyperacute rejection of the organ.

Clinical Data

Immediate rejection often is obvious when the vascular anastomoses are opened. After a few moments, the kidney, instead of pulsating and remaining a pink color, becomes swollen, pulseless, and cyanotic. Urine output, if it had been established, also ceases quickly. Occasionally, however, the onset of rejection may be delayed for some hours, making the diagnosis more difficult, since arterial or venous thrombosis can present in a similar fashion, but for the most part, the diagnosis is obvious at the time of surgery, and the graft is immediately removed. Renal histology in these cases can confirm the presence of diffuse immunologic injury and help differentiate this response from other causes of acute graft failure, such as tubular injury.

Histology

The most prominent feature in this syndrome is rapid accumulation of platelets and neutrophils within glomerular capillary loops (Fig. 26-1). Shortly thereafter, thrombosis of the entire capillary vascular tree also occurs (Fig. 26-2). Although they are not often seen unless the onset of the reaction is delayed, marked interstitial edema and infiltration also occur, followed by tubular necrosis (Fig. 26-3).

Electron microscopy of glomeruli demonstrates accumulation of platelets and fibrin within glomerular capillary loops, endothelial injury, and a large number of neutrophils. In addition, fibrin-fibrinogen antigen can be demonstrated by fluorescence microscopy. However, there is no specific type or distribution of immunoglobulins or complement, and therefore it is not helpful in establishing the diagnosis or prognosis.

TABLE 26-1 Characteristics of Rejection Syndromes

Types of Rejection	Onset	Etiology	Response to Treatment	Histology	Clinical Syndrome
Immediate Irreversible	At time of surgery	Preformed cytotoxic antibodies	Unresponsive	Infarction	Renal nonfunction or immediate cessation of function
Early Reversible	5 days to 6 months posttransplant	Unknown—probably cell-mediated immunity	Good	Interstitial infiltrate and edema	↑ Serum creatinine; ↓ urine volume; hypertension; variable constitutional symptoms
Early Irreversible	First month	Unknown—may represent previous sensitization and recall immunologic response	Rarely reversible	Vascular damage interstitial hemorrhage, tubular injury	Oliguria→anuria; fever, graft tenderness; hypertension
Late Irreversible	After 6 months	Unknown	Unresponsive	Increase in connective tissue in all compartments	Slowly progressive loss of function; hypertension

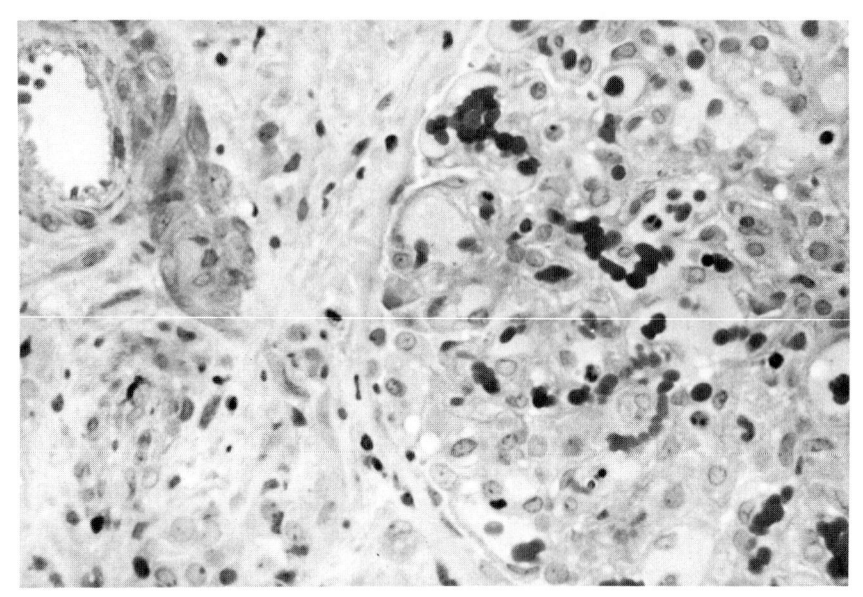

Figure 26-1 Specimen from a 21 year old male who had received a renal graft from a relative, which initially had good blood flow but within a few minutes was noted to be purplish in color and flaccid. The renal biopsy demonstrates an increased number of red cells within capillary spaces and a large number of neutrophils in the same zone. Elsewhere in the renal biopsy no changes were apparent. (H&E, ×300.)

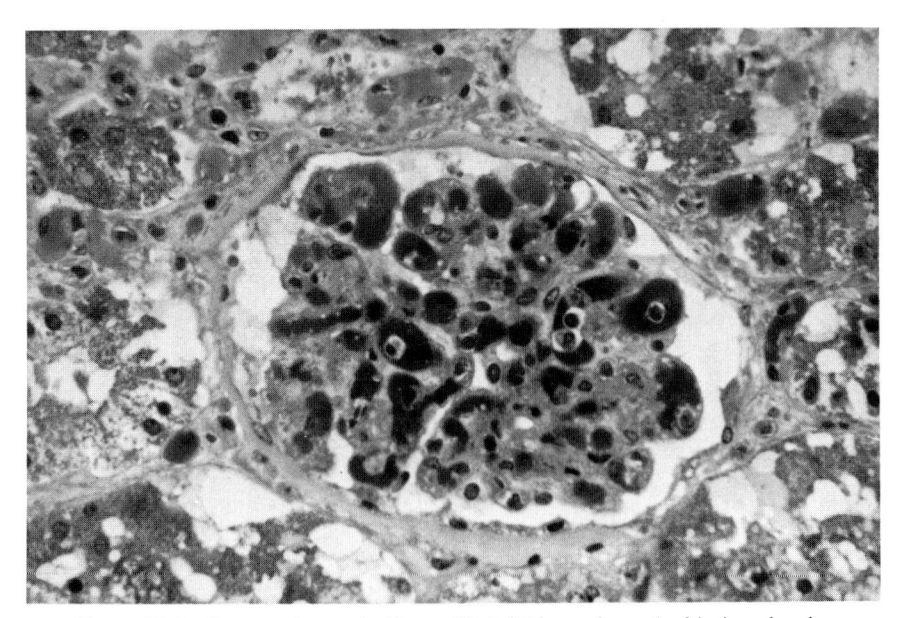

Figure 26-2 Same patient as in Figure 26-1, 72 hours later. At this time the glomerular capillary loops are filled with red blood cells, and the architecture is distorted. The surrounding tubules are undergoing necrosis. (H&E, × 300.)

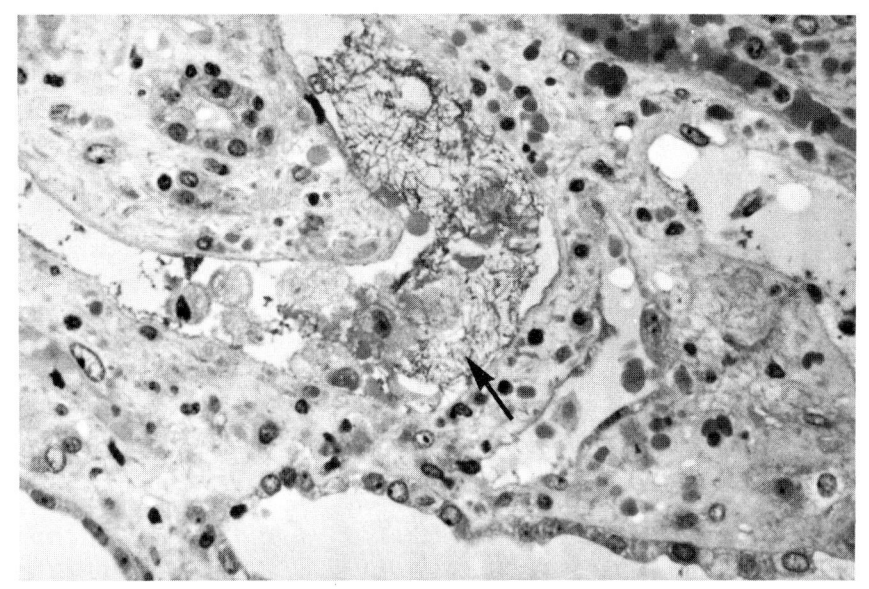

Figure 26-3 Same patient as in Figures 26-1 and 26-2. The interstitium is filled with edema fluid and inflammatory cells. Epithelial cells and fibrin are present within a tubule (arrow). (H&E, ×300.)

Clinical Course and Prognosis

Preventing presensitization of the host, or avoiding transplantation of a kidney to a presensitized host, essentially eliminates this problem. Blood transfusions in the pretransplantation period should be avoided because of a danger of developing preformed cytotoxic antibodies. Although the majority of patients with chronic uremia are significantly anemic, few require blood transfusions to remain asymptomatic. When blood must be given, packed red cells from which white blood cells have been removed should be used, in order to decrease the possibility of sensitization.

The majority of immediate rejection episodes can be predicted by a positive, white blood cell crossmatch in which recipient serum is cytotoxic for donor white blood cells. Unfortunately, because the levels of circulating antibody may fluctuate in some patients, preformed cytotoxic antibodies may be missed. Testing serum from multiple time periods, however, can insure against this.

EARLY, REVERSIBLE REJECTION SYNDROME

This is the most frequently seen form of rejection. Although the exact nature of the injury is unknown, experimental studies suggest the primacy of the cellular immune response.

Clinical Data

The early rejection syndrome often takes place in the first three months, but it can be seen at any time in the posttransplant period.

The first physiologic abnormality to occur is sudden reduction of renal blood flow, followed by diminished urine volume and sodium retention, which become clinically apparent as oliguria, fluid retention, and hypertension. If the episode is particularly severe, graft tenderness, fever, and other constitutional symptoms also may become evident.

There is no single reliable test for the rejection. As with most clinical problems, however, a group of laboratory tests is available. Each contributes to the accuracy of diagnosis, but none is sufficient individually to make a secure judgment. The most dependable indicator appears to be a change in the level of serum creatinine. Proteinuria, lymphocyturia, and decreased urinary sodium concentration are often present. Radioisotopic techniques will show the reduced renal blood flow and help rule out urinary obstruction. A variety of immunologic tests have been developed that demonstrate cellular or humoral immunity of the recipient to the graft. These tests, however, are technically difficult and expensive, and are not used routinely in most centers.

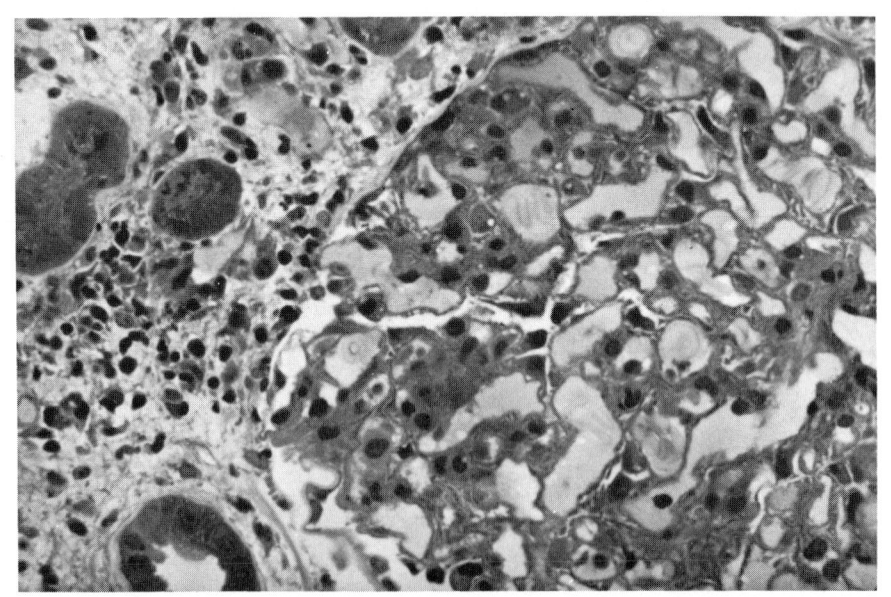

Figure 26–4 Specimen from a 26 year old female, whose original disease was chronic proliferative glomerulonephritis, and who had received a renal transplant from a relative 3 weeks prior to biopsy. Renal function, which initially was good, rapidly deteriorated over 3 days. The major histologic abnormality in the glomeruli is prominence of the endothelial-mesangial regions and decreased capillary spaces. (H&E, ×300.)

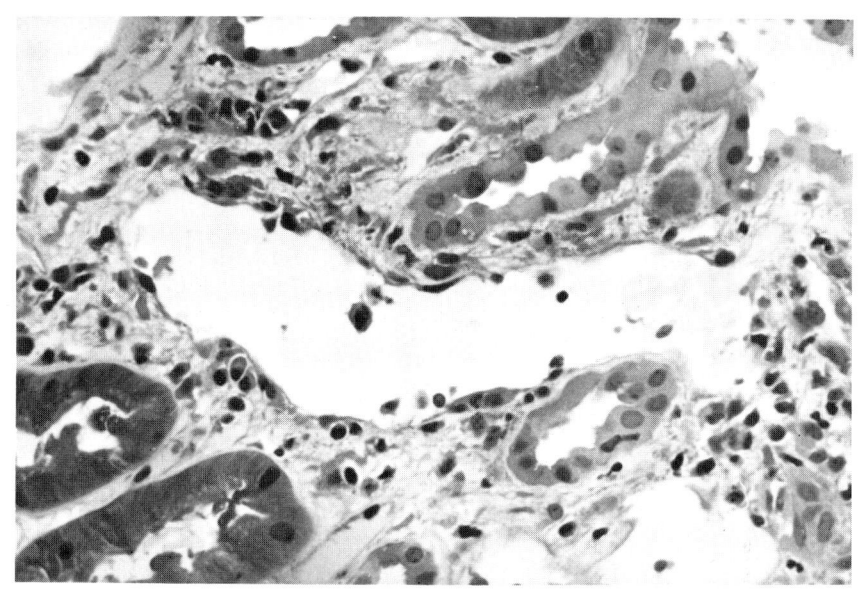

Transplant Rejection and Recurrence of Disease 329

Figure 26–5 Same patient as in Figure 26–4. Surrounding the vein, in the center, is a collection of inflammatory cells consisting mainly of large lymphocytes and plasma cells. Elsewhere the interstitium is relatively unremarkable. (H&E, ×300.)

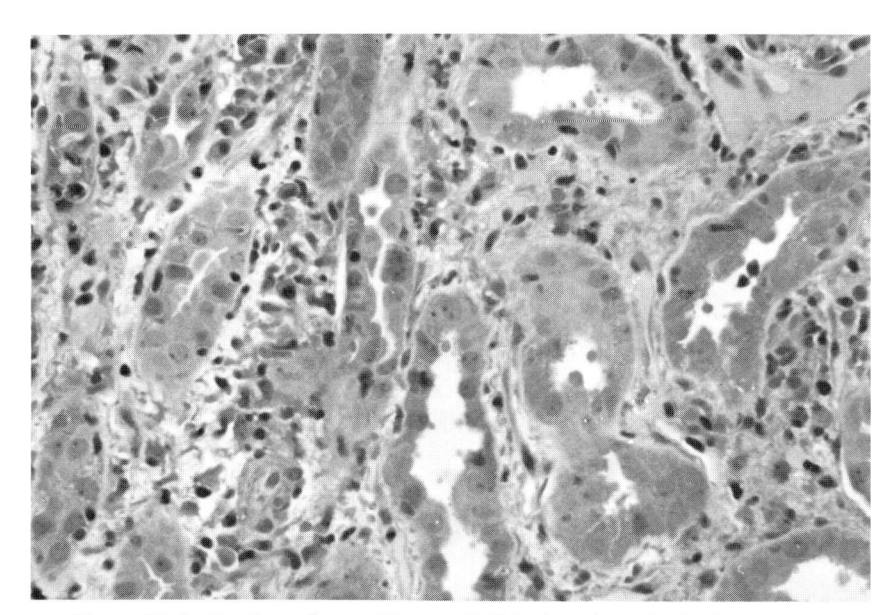

Figure 26–6 Specimen from a 25 year old diabetic patient who had received a graft from a living related donor. For the first 14 days renal function remained normal. Serum creatinine then rose progressively over 3 days to 3.1 mg/dl. The interstitium is profusely infiltrated with inflammatory cells consisting of plasma cells, large lymphocytes, and neutrophils. There is considerable edema fluid resulting in widely separated tubules. Inflammatory cells also are noted within the tubular epithelial cell layer. (H&E, ×300.)

Histology

GLOMERULI. The glomeruli are variably affected. In most instances the only light microscopic change is that the vascular spaces may appear to be moderately narrowed (Fig. 26-4). Electron microscopy further reveals that this change is the result of endothelial swelling.

INTERSTITIUM. The interstitial changes reflect the severity of the rejection process. The characteristic features vary from focal perivenous collections of lymphocytes (Fig. 26-5) to marked diffuse interstitial infiltration and edema, resulting in wide separation of the tubules (Fig. 26-6). The amount, distribution, and type of infiltrate also is highly variable; it may be dense and pleomorphic. The cells consist primarily of lymphocytes and plasma cells, but small numbers of neutrophils are common as well.

TUBULES. Tubular changes are often inconspicuous. However, small lymphocytes commonly are seen between epithelial cells when there is substantial interstitial infiltrate (Fig. 26-7). For the most part, tubular injury parallels interstitial changes and may vary in intensity between patients with similar clinical findings. It also varies between areas within the kidney.

VESSELS. In the vessels, there may be substantial difference between the lesion seen in recipients of organs from cadavers and that

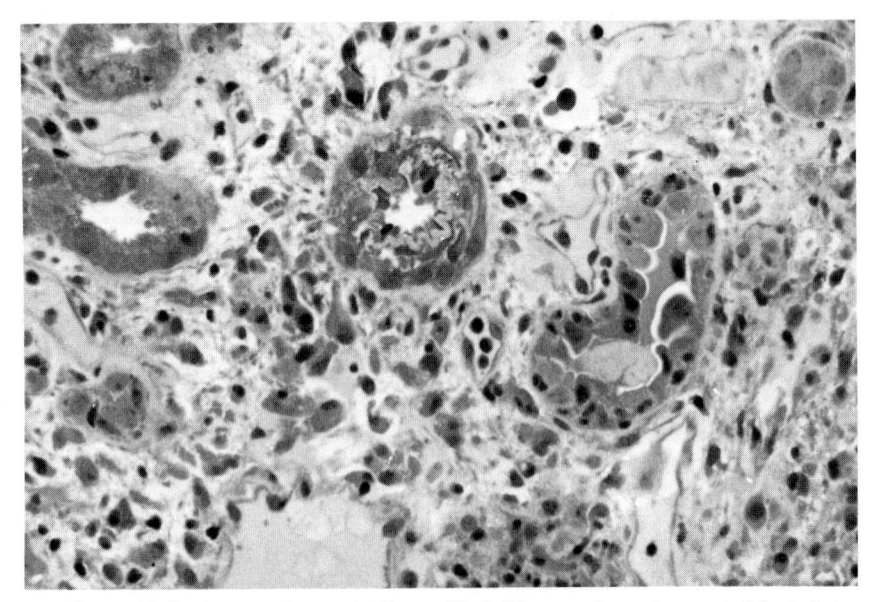

Figure 26-7 Same patient as in Figure 26-6. The severity and extent of the inflammatory filtrate are again obvious. In this region the tubule to the right of the vessel is heavily infiltrated by inflammatory cells. (H&E, ×300.)

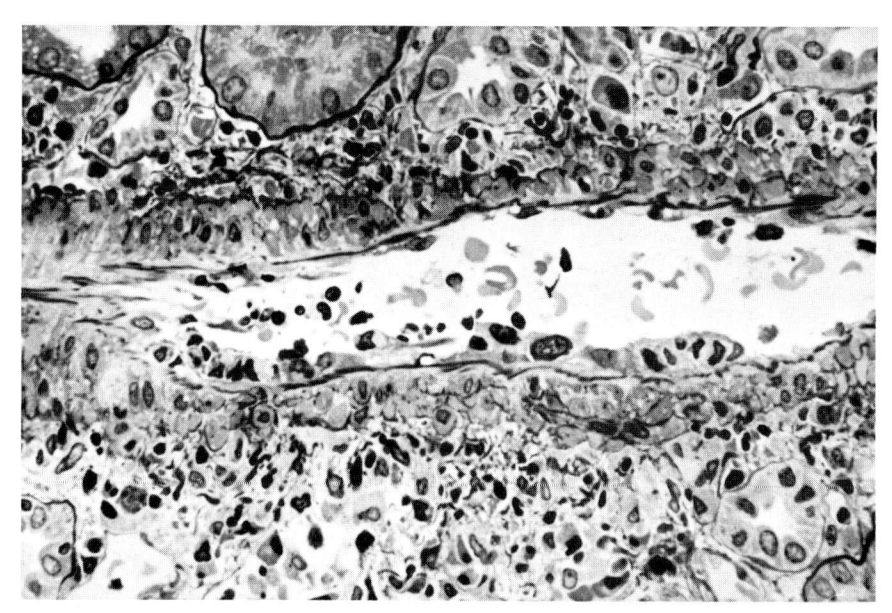

Figure 26-8. Specimen from a 35 year old woman who received a cadaveric renal transplant following a brief period of hemodialysis. Initially she had good renal function, but within 3 weeks had a progressively rising serum creatinine. Renal biopsy demonstrates marked endothelial injury in large vessels. Neutrophils are adherent to, and have infiltrated under, the endothelial cells. The endothelial cells in many zones are noted to be vacuolated as well as increased in number. Note the inflammatory cell infiltrate in the surrounding adventitial tissue and interstitial spaces. (Methenamine silver, ×300.)

in recipients of kidneys from living, related donors. Proliferation of endothelial cells, infiltration by neutrophils, and deposition of fibrin-fibrinogen and immunoglobulins in the walls of arteries and arterioles are very common in recipients of cadaveric organs, for example (Fig. 26-8), whereas acute vascular injuries are seen less frequently in renal biopsies from recipients of organs donated by a relative. Mild vascular lesions are associated with recovery of satisfactory renal function.

FLUORESCENCE MICROSCOPY. IgG and complement components in the walls of large and small arteries have been described in the vascular lesions, but their presence is variable. Fibrin also may be seen in severe vascular injuries.

Clinical Course and Prognosis

Early rejection is for the most part reversible with appropriate therapy. The outcome depends on the type and degree of injury, coupled with early diagnosis and appropriate therapy.

Occasionally an instance of the early rejection syndrome will prove particularly vigorous and respond poorly to therapy. Renal biopsy can be helpful in this situation; in addition to confirming the diagnosis, the biopsy can give important indications regarding the reversibility of the injury and the advisability of prolonging life-threatening medication. If interstitial infiltration, edema, and moderate amounts of tubular injury are the major lesions, response to treatment usually is good. The severe vascular lesions, on the other hand, may only be partially reversible, and treatment should be undertaken with great care, since kidney function may continue to decline despite aggressive therapy. In this case the patients have early irreversible rejection.

EARLY, IRREVERSIBLE REJECTION SYNDROME

Clinical Data

Occasionally a rejection reaction happens early in the posttransplant period, which proves to be extremely rigorous and does not respond to treatment. These patients often have fever, leukocytosis, and graft tenderness. Oliguria leads quickly to anuria, and the serum creatinine rises rapidly; thus, irreversible destruction of the transplant takes place virtually before appropriate therapy can be instituted. This syndrome is much more frequent in recipients of cadaveric kidneys than in those who received transplants from living, related donors.

Histology

The characteristics of early, irreversible rejection include hemorrhage, thrombosis, and diffuse tubular injury, but the major insult is vascular.

GLOMERULI. The vascular spaces in this syndrome often are indistinct because of swollen endothelial cell cytoplasm. In addition, the lumen frequently is occluded by fibrin-fibrinogen and other plasma proteins (Fig. 26–9).

INTERSTITIUM. Diffuse edema and foci of hemorrhage are the principal findings in the interstitium. Infiltration often is scanty or consists primarily of neutrophils (Fig. 26–10).

TUBULES. Diffuse swelling, vacuolation, and other evidences of injury, including obvious necrosis, frequently are found in the tubules (Fig. 26–11).

VESSELS. The most prominent lesion is marked endothelial cell proliferation and vessel wall disruption, with infiltration by inflammatory cells and deposits of fibrin-fibrinogen and other plasma components, including immunoglobulins (Fig. 26–12). These changes are prominent in arcuate and interlobular vessels, whereas thrombosis is common in smaller vessels (afferent arterioles, for instance).

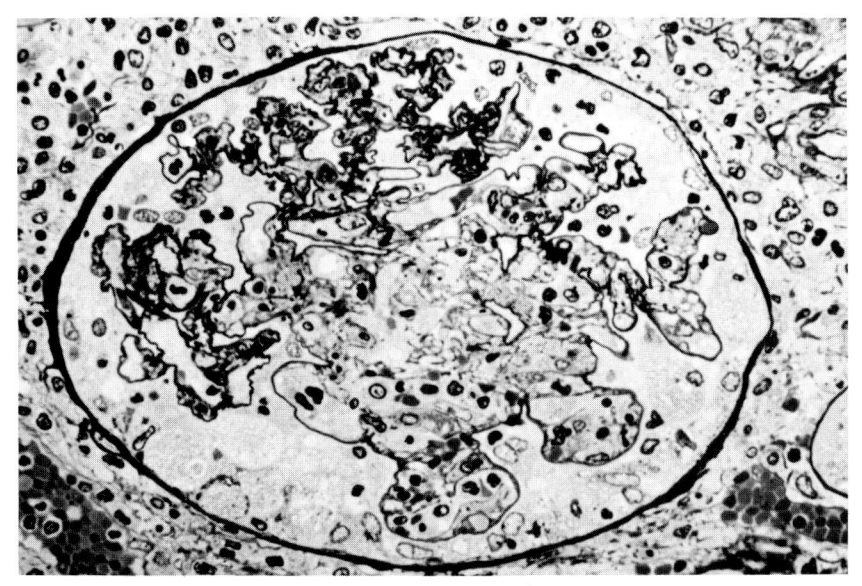

Figure 26-9 Specimen from a 37-year-old man who had received a cadaveric renal transplant which functioned well for approximately 1 week. Progressive deterioration led to nephrectomy at 6 weeks posttransplant. This biopsy was taken just prior to nephrectomy. There is diffuse endothelial-mesangial injury, with loss of the normal glomerular architecture. In the lower right hand portion of the illustration the mesangial regions are nearly completely effaced and capillary spaces are filled with cells. At the left, the capillary spaces are decreased and the peripheral basal lamina is wrinkled. (Methenamine silver, ×300.)

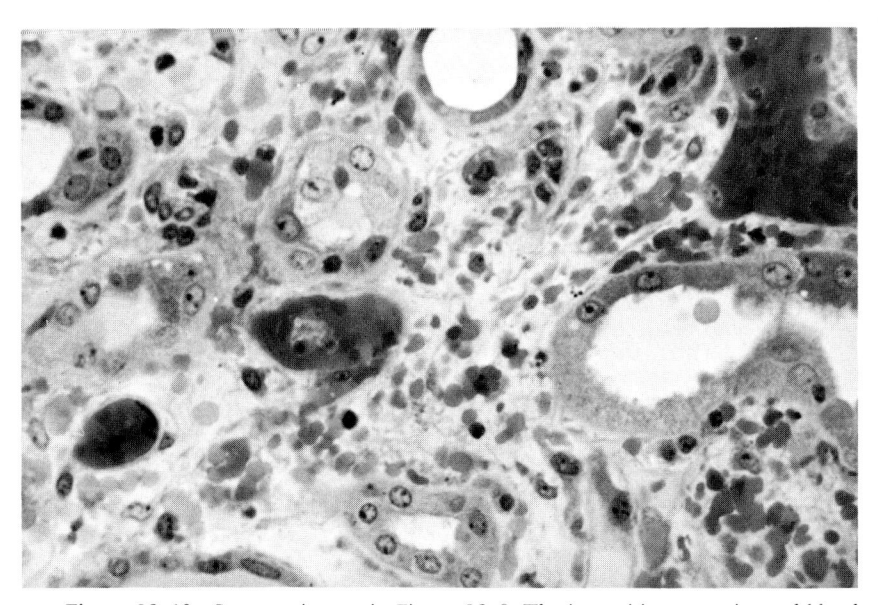

Figure 26-10 Same patient as in Figure 26-9. The interstitium contains red blood cells, edema fluid, and a small number of inflammatory cells. The tubules are widely spaced because of the interstitial lesion. (H&E, ×300.)

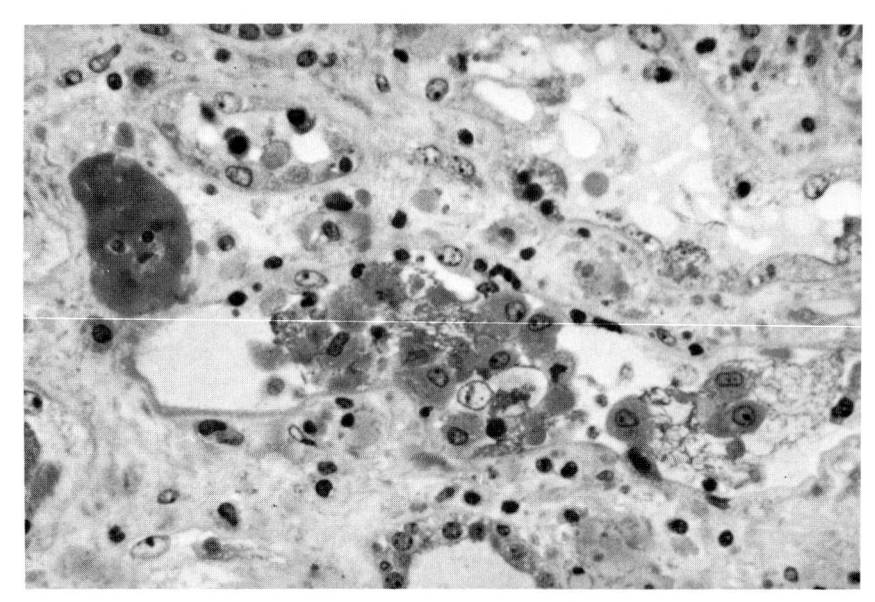

Figure 26-11 Same patient as in Figures 26-9 and 26-10. The tubular cells are diffusely affected. The lesion varies from mild vacuolation to complete necrosis. The interstitium is diffusely edematous and contains a small number of inflammatory cells. (H&E, ×300.)

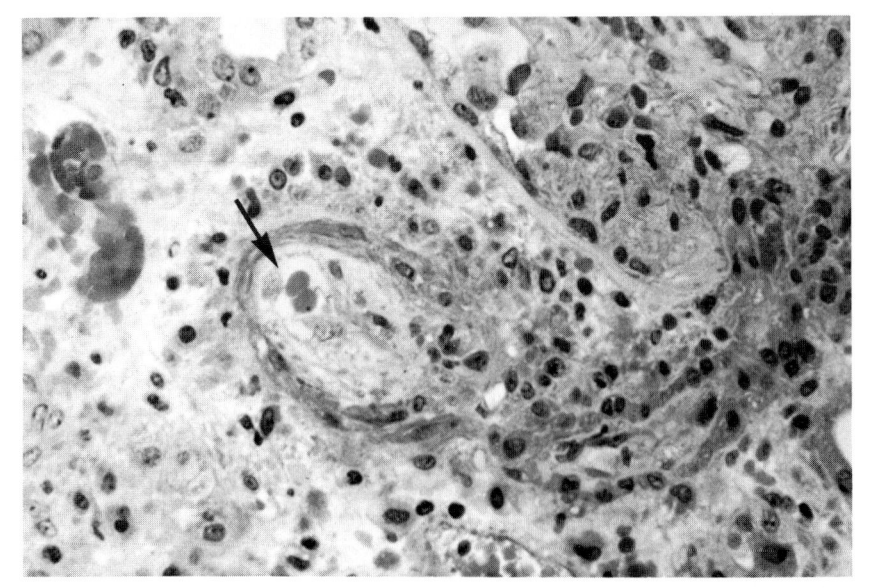

Figure 26-12 Same patient as in Figures 26-9 through 26-11. The afferent arteriole has a markedly compromised lumen due to swelling of endothelial cells. The lumen is eccentrically placed and contains two red blood cells (arrow). (H&E, ×300.)

Clinical Course and Prognosis

Even if vigorous anti-rejection therapy is employed, the kidney is rarely salvageable. Renal biopsy is particularly helpful in these cases, to determine the nature, extent, and potential reversibility. Based on the biopsy findings of vascular injury, an early decision on the continuation of immunosuppressive therapy may be made and a return to dialysis treatment considered.

LATE, IRREVERSIBLE REJECTION

The chances that rejection will occur decrease significantly following the first year, and the longer the graft remains, the greater is the likelihood of prolonged and possibly indefinite graft survival. A certain number of grafts undergo a slow, irreversible rejection process, however, clinically referred to as late or chronic rejection. The etiology of this syndrome is unclear, but it is thought to be immunologically mediated. Consequently, in the absence of clear evidence indicating the recurrence of the original lesion, the term "rejection" is applied to this situation also.

Clinical Data

The patients rarely are symptomatic in late, irreversible rejection unless the course has been particularly rapid. Minimally diminished renal function, however, is the first sign noted, usually becoming clinically apparent sometime after the first 6 months in the post-transplantation course. Hypertension and proteinuria, often in the nephrotic range, are common.

The main differential diagnoses in this syndrome are early rejection, recurrent renal disease, and vascular or obstructive abnormalities. The latter two can be detected by radiographic or radioisotopic techniques. Differentiation between early and late rejection is generally made by their clinical courses and responses to treatment. In this case, there would be no need for renal biopsy; however, the clinical picture may be unclear, and biopsy can be helpful in distinguishing these two syndromes and recurrence of the original disease in the transplanted kidney. The later syndrome will be discussed later in this chapter.

Histology

The general histologic picture indicates an increase in the amount of structural material (sclerosis) in all compartments. The result is slowly progressive atrophy of all components.

GLOMERULI. The overall cellularity appears to be decreased in the glomeruli. Conversely, the basal lamina and mesangial matrix are increased and have a "stiff" appearance. The capillary spaces, on the other hand, appear slightly decreased in area (Fig. 26-13).

Fluorescence microscopy is unrevealing, although granular basal lamina and mesangial (and occasionally linear) deposits of immunoglobulin, complement components, and fibrin-fibrinogen antigen have been described. Their significance, however, is unclear. Electron microscopy confirms the light microscopic impression of increased extracellular material, and the subendothelial space (lamina rara interna) often is widened by a sparsely staining, flocculent material. The endothelial cell cytoplasm usually is thickened.

INTERSTITIUM. The interstitial connective tissue is diffusely increased; thus, the tubules are separated from one another as well as from the capillaries. Chronic inflammatory cells are sparsely scattered throughout, but often are more concentrated around venules and small veins. Fluorescence and electron microscopy provide no additional information.

TUBULES. The most consistent change in the tubules is atrophy, with thickening of the basal lamina and low-lying epithelial cells.

VESSELS. Multilayering of myointimal cells, with a profuse increase in their adjacent basal lamina and elastic tissue, is the predomi-

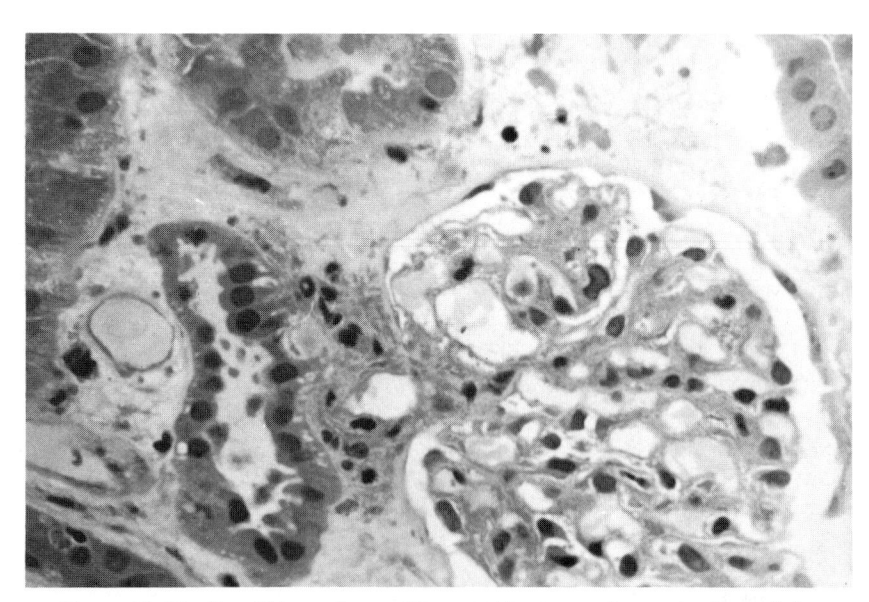

Figure 26-13 Renal biopsy from a 26 year old woman who received a graft from a living related donor 6 years ago. Serum creatinine has remained in the range of 1.2 to 1.4 mg/100 ml for the past 4 years. The major histologic changes are a decrease in the cellularity of glomeruli and moderate endothelial cell prominence throughout. The interstitium contains a slightly increased amount of connective tissue and sparsely scattered chronic inflammatory cells. (H & E, ×300.)

nant lesion in the vessels. There also is an increase in the basal lamina of the cells in the media, as well as an apparent reduction in their number, which may be pronounced in late lesions. The small blood vessels also are affected similarly, but the intimal changes are less pronounced. Recipients of cadaver grafts tend to have similar but markedly accentuated changes.

Clinical Course and Prognosis

Although this is a progressive lesion which will not respond to increased doses of immunosuppressive agents, the course is variable, and adequate function may continue for many months. It is common, for example, to have a sudden elevation of serum creatinine, which tends to stabilize or even slightly improve over time, but which can be followed by yet another elevation weeks or months later. This course continues until the degree of renal functional impairment requires reinstitution of dialysis therapy or placement of another graft.

The effects of therapy are difficult to evaluate because of the variable and occasionally remitting course. At best, however, therapy is of marginal help, and the possibility of a modest prolongation of function needs to be balanced against the possible adverse effects of increased immunosuppression. Renal biopsy can be helpful in this context to prevent overtreatment.

RECURRENCE OF RENAL DISEASE

Recurrence of the original renal disease in the transplanted kidney was first described in recipients of grafts from identical twins by Glassock and associates in 1968. It has subsequently been shown to occur with lesser frequency in allografts. Except for metabolic disorders (for instance, cystinosis and oxalosis) or systemic diseases, such as diabetes mellitus or systemic lupus erythematosus, primary glomerular diseases constitute the category which recurs most commonly. In general, these are the lesions associated with deposition of immunoglobulin or complement, leading to progressive sclerosis.

FOCAL AND SEGMENTAL SCLEROSIS. Patients with this lesion commonly have steroid-resistant nephrotic syndrome (Chapter 16). Although reports are limited, this lesion seems to have a very high incidence of recurrence (Hamburger et al., 1973). The lesion recurred in three of five transplant patients in the series of Mathew and associates (1975). The recurrence of nephrotic syndrome usually is evident in the first year following transplantation, but it can take place in a matter of hours. As in the original disease, the nephrotic syndrome is associated with progressive loss of renal function.

MEMBRANOPROLIFERATIVE GLOMERULONEPHRITIS. When the original disease was membranoproliferative glomerulonephritis, recurrence has been reported in about 20 per cent of patients. When the lesion is associated with dense intramembranous deposits (Chapter 16), the recurrence rate approaches 50 per cent. However, Mathew and associates (1975) have shown that membranoproliferative GN may be present in transplanted kidneys when the original lesion was another form of glomerulonephritis or nonglomerular disease. In such cases there was a higher incidence of membranoproliferative GN in those who developed anti-HLA antibodies or vesicoureteral reflux, suggesting that this histologic picture represents a nonspecific reaction to injury.

FOCAL AND SEGMENTAL PROLIFERATION. Although focal and segmental proliferation usually is associated with benign recurrent hematuria, occasionally a patient's condition may progress to renal failure. Mathew and associates (1975) reported that in two of 12 such patients, the lesion recurred in the graft.

GLOMERULAR DISEASE OF ACUTE ONSET AND RAPID PROGRESSION. This syndrome may be associated with antiglomerular basal lamina antibodies. Since these antibodies may persist in the circulation or are subject to recall, this disease theoretically should be likely to recur in the transplanted kidney. However, this has not proved to be the case. Transplantation has been undertaken successfully in many cases of proved antiglomerular basal lamina nephritis, and recurrence is rare.

Comment

Early in the renal transplantation experience there was considerable concern about recurrence of the original disease in the transplant. However, except for those noted above, this is fortunately a rare phenomenon. In addition, when recurrence becomes manifest, the course of the disease may parallel that of the original disease, affording the patient many years of adequate renal function.

References

1. Berthoux, F. C., Ducret, F., Colon, S., Blanc-Brunat, N., Zech, P. Y., and Traeger, J.: Renal transplantation in mesangioproliferative glomerulonephritis (MPGN): Relationship between the high frequency of recurrent glomerulonephritis and hypocomplementemia. Kidney Internat. 7:323, 1975.
2. Crosson, J. T., Wather, R. L., Raij, S., Anderson, R. C., and Anderson, W. R.: Recurrence of idiopathic membranous nephropathy in a renal allograft. Arch. Intern. Med. *135*:1101, 1975.

3. Glassock, R. J., Feldman, D., Reynolds, E. S., Dammin, G. J., and Merril, J. P.: Human renal isografts: a clinical and pathologic analysis. Medicine 47:411, 1968.
4. Gluckman, J. C., Beaufils, H., Berger, J., Hinglais, N., Legrain, M., and Küss, R.: Rapidly progressive glomerulonephritis with linear fluorescence in a kidney transplant. Clin. Nephrol. 1:40, 1973.
5. Hamburger, J., Berger, J., Hinglais, N., and Descamps, B.: Editorial: New insights into the pathogenesis of glomerulonephritis afforded by the study of renal allografts. Clin. Neph. 1:3, 1973.
6. Mathew, T. H., Mathews, D. C., Hobbs, J. B., and Kincaid-Smith, P.: Glomerular lesions after renal transplantation. Amer. J. Med. 59:177, 1975.
7. Raij, L., Hoyer, J. R., and Michael, A. F.: Steroid resistant nephrotic syndrome: Recurrence after transplantation. Ann. Int. Med. 77:81, 1972.

INDEX

Page numbers in *italics* refer to illustrations; (t) indicates tables.

Alport's syndrome. See *Nephritis, hereditary.*
Ammonium, excretion of, as index of renal damage, 74, *75*, 77
Amyloidosis, 301–307
  clinical features of, 302
  course of, 307
  histologic changes in, 303, *304–306*
Analgesic abuse, nephropathy from, 169–170
Arteriosclerosis, 141–143, *142, 143*
Artery, normal, structure of, *69*
  renal, acute occlusion of. See *Infarction, renal.*
Atrophy, of tubular epithelium, *50*, 66

Balkan nephropathy, 180–181
Basal lamina, glomerular, changes in, *37*, 64–65
  collapse of, *38*
  obsolescence of, *40*
  reduplication or splitting of, *39*
  of vessels, intimal and medial cell increases in, *60*, 70
  tubulo-interstitial, thickening of, *55*, 68
Biopsy, renal, blind, 4
  technique of, 16–18
  complications of, 15
  contraindications to, 14
  fixation of specimens, 21
  history of, 3–5
  in children, 19
  indications for, 13, 14(t)
  interpretation of specimens, 28–70
  methacrylate vs. paraffin embedding, 21–25, *22, 24, 26*
  of transplanted kidneys, 19–20
  percutaneous, 3
  technique of, 16–20

Biopsy (*Continued*)
  renal, blind, postbiopsy measures, 20
  processing of specimens for fluorescence microscopy, 25–27
  processing of specimens for light and electron microscopy, 20
  role of in diagnosis of renal disease, 11
  with television-monitored fluoroscopy, 18–19
Blood flow, renal, 74–75
  correlation of with renal disease, *73*, 74
  correlation of with tubulo-interstitial disease, *73*, 74
Bright's disease, 80

Capillaritis, 83
Cholesterol, crystals of, in atheromatous embolization, 141, *142, 143*
Clearance, creatinine, correlation of with glomerular disease, 71–74
  inulin, correlation of with glomerular disease, 71–74, *72*
  correlation of with interstitial disease, 71, *72*
  para-amino-hippuric acid, correlation of with vascular disease, *73*, 74
Complement, deposits of, in thickened glomerular basal lamina, *44*
  intramembranous, *46*
Concentrating ability. See *Kidney, concentrating ability of.*
Creatinine, clearance of. See *Clearance, creatinine.*
Cystic disease, of kidney, 176–179
  medullary, 178–179, *179*
Cystinosis, tubulo-interstitial nephropathy in, 175–176, *175, 176*

341

Deposits, amyloid, in amyloidosis, 303, 305, 306
  fibrin, in blood vessels of kidney, 62
  glomerular, intramembranous, 45, 46
    mesangial, 49
    of complement, 44
    subendothelial, of immunoglobulin, 42, 43
    subepithelial, 47, 48
  hyaline, in blood vessels of kidney, 61
  immunoglobulin, in blood vessels of kidney, 62
  in glomerular disease, 42–49, 65
  tubulo-interstitial, 55
Diabetes, glomerulosclerosis of, 284–293, 285–291. See also Glomerulosclerosis, diabetic.
Disease, Bright's, 80
  cystic, of kidney, 176–179
  glomerular, correlation of inulin clearance with, 71, 72
    interpretation of in biopsy specimens, 29, 31–49, 63–64
    of acute onset, 89–103, 90(t)
      classification of, 83(t)
      clinical features, 90–91
      course and prognosis of, 101–103
      glomerular changes, 91–95, 92–94, 96–99
      histologic features, 32(t), 91–101
      interstitial changes, 99–101, 102
      tubular changes, 98–99, 100
    of acute onset and rapid progression, 104–116
      changes in, by fluorescence microscopy, 108, 113, 114
        electron microscopic, 107, 111, 112, 113
        light microscopic, 106, 108–111, 109–112
      classification of, 83(t)
      clinical features, 105–107
      course and prognosis of, 114–116
      etiology of, 104, 105(t)
      histologic features, 31(t), 108–114
      recurrence of after transplantation, 338
    primary, classification of, 83(t)
    slowly progressive, 147–163. See also Hematuria, benign recurrent; and Nephritis, hereditary.
      classification of, 83(t)
      clinical features of, 148
      course and prognosis of, 156–157
      histologic changes in, 35(t), 39(t), 149–156, 150–156
    IgA. See Hematuria, benign recurrent.
  interstitial, correlation of inulin clearance with, 71, 72
  mesangial, primary, 195–200, 198, 199
  microcystic, 195–200

Disease (Continued)
  polycystic, of kidney, 177–178
  renal, associated with systemic syndromes, 235–320
    classification of, 80–84, 81(t), 83(t)
      by Volhard and Fahr, 81(t), 82
    clinical evaluation of, 6–12
    of acute onset, 87–143
    of pregnancy, 315–320
    recurrence of after transplantation, 337–338
    slowly progressive, 145–191
      glomerular, 147–163
      tubulo-interstitial, 165–181
      vascular, 38(t), 182–191
  tubulo-interstitial, acute diffuse interstitial nephritis. See Nephritis, acute diffuse interstitial.
    acute tubulo-interstitial injury, 118–123
      clinical features of, 119–120
      course and prognosis, 121–123
      histologic changes, 120–121, 120–122
    correlation of renal blood flow with, 73, 74
    in malignancy, 179–180
    interpretation of biopsy specimens, 50–55, 65–68
    of acute onset, 51(t)–53(t), 118–126. See also Renal failure, acute.
    slowly progressive, 165–181, 166. See also Nephropathy.
      conditions associated with, 165, 165(t)
    toxic nephropathy, 168–175
  vascular, and clearance of para-amino-hippuric acid, 73, 74
    interpretation of biopsy specimens in, 68–70
    of acute onset, 34(t), 62(t), 127–143
    slowly progressive, 182–191. See also Hypertension.
      clinical features of, 183
      course and prognosis, 187–191
      histologic changes in, 57(t), 183–187, 184–187, 188–191

Edema, as sign of renal disease, 8
  in tubulo-interstitial compartment, 53, 68
Elastic lamina, of vessels, thickening and reduplication of, 59, 70
Ellis Type 1 glomerulonephritis, acute, 83(t). See also Disease, glomerular, of acute onset.
  rapidly progressive, 83(t). See also Disease, glomerular, of acute onset and rapid progression.

Ellis Type 2 glomerulonephritis, 83(t).
  See also *Disease, glomerular, slowly progressive.*
Embedding, of biopsy specimens, 20. See also *Methacrylate embedding; Paraffin embedding.*
Embolization, atheromatous, 141–143, *142, 143*
  cholesterol crystals in, 141, *142, 143*
Endothelial cells, hypercellularity and swelling of, in glomerular disease, *34*
Epithelial cells, diffuse hypercellularity of, in glomerular disease, *31*
  fusion of foot processes of, in glomerular disease, *33*
  segmental hypercellularity of, in glomerular disease, *32*
Epithelium, tubular, atrophy of, *50, 66*
  cytoplasmic swelling and/or frank necrosis, *51, 66*
Extracellular material, of tubulo-interstitial compartment, changes in, *53, 55, 68*
  vascular, changes in, *59–62, 70*

Fibrin, deposits of, in renal blood vessels, *62*
Fibrosis, interstitial, *54, 68*
Filtration rate. See *Glomerular filtration rate.*
Fixation, of biopsy specimens, 21
Fluorescence microscopy, processing of biopsy specimens for, 25–27
Fluoroscopy, television-monitored, in renal biopsy, 18–19

GBL. See *Basal lamina, glomerular.*
GFR. See *Glomerular filtration rate.*
Glomerular basal lamina. See *Basal lamina, glomerular.*
Glomerular disease. See *Disease, glomerular.*
Glomerular filtration rate, 71–74. See also *Clearance.*
  relationship of to tubulo-interstitial disease, 71–74, *72, 73*
Glomerulonephritis, 80. See also *Disease, glomerular; Nephrotic syndrome.*
  acute, characteristics of, 81(t)
  chronic, 83(t). See also *Glomerulonephritis, slowly progressive.*
    characteristics of, 81(t)
  Ellis Type 1, acute, 83(t). See also *Disease, glomerular, of acute onset.*
    rapidly progressive, 83(t). See also *Disease glomerular, of acute onset and rapid progression.*

Glomerulonephritis (*Continued*)
  Ellis Type 2, 83(t). See also *Disease, glomerular, slowly progressive.*
  evolution of, 82–84, *84*
  extracapillary, with crescents, 83(t)
  exudative, 83(t)
  focal, in systemic lupus erythematosus, 239, *240, 241,* 251(t)
  focal necrotizing, 83(t)
  lesions associated with, 82–83, 83(t)
  lobular, *215,* 216, *216, 217*
  membranoproliferative, 204(t), 205–218, 211(t)
    recurrence of after transplantation, 338
    with dense intramembranous deposits, 46(t), 205, 211(t), *214–215*
    with subendothelial deposits, 44(t), 205, 211(t), *212–213*
  minimal lesion, 203–205, 204(t)
  poststreptococcal, acute, 83(t), 89. See also *Disease, glomerular, of acute onset.*
  proliferative, 83(t), 204(t), 205–218
  rapidly progressive, 83(t). See also *Disease, glomerular, of acute onset and rapid progression.*
  sclerosing, 83(t), 204(t), 218–231
  subacute, 83(t). See also *Disease, glomerular, of acute onset and rapid progression.*
    characteristics of, 81(t)
  subchronic, 83(t). See also *Disease, glomerular, slowly progressive.*
Glomerulosclerosis, diabetic, 37(t), 284–293
  course and prognosis of, 292
  diffuse sclerotic lesion of, 286, *287*
  insudative lesion of, *287, 288, 288*
  nodular lesion of, 285–286, *285, 286*
Glomerulus(i), appearance of in methacrylate- vs. paraffin-embedded specimens, 21–23, *22*
  changes in, in amyloidosis, 303, *304, 305*
    in diabetic glomerulosclerosis, 285–288
    in early irreversible transplant rejection, *332, 333*
    in early reversible transplant rejection, *328, 330*
    in hemolytic uremic syndrome, 272, *274–275*
    in late irreversible transplant rejection, 336, *336*
    in scleroderma, 295, *296*
    in systemic lupus erythematosus, 239, *240*
    in thrombotic thrombocytopenic purpura, *280, 282*
  collapse of glomerular basal lamina, *38*
  disease of. See *Disease, glomerular.*

Glomerulus(i) (Continued)
  disease of, cellular changes in, 31–36, 63–64
    deposits in, 42–49, 65
    extracellular changes in, 37–41, 64–65
    interpretation of in biopsy specimens, 29, 63–64
  endothelial cell changes in, hypercellularity and swelling, 34
  epithelial cell changes in, diffuse hypercellularity, 31
    fusion of foot processes, 33
    segmental hypercellularity, 32
  glomerular basal lamina changes, 37, 64–65
  inflammatory cells in, 36
  intramembranous deposits, complement, 46
    immunoglobulin, 45
  mesangial cell changes in, hypercellularity, 35
  mesangial deposits, immunoglobulin, 49
  mesangial matrix of, increase in, 41
  normal, 30
  obsolescence of glomerular basal lamina, 40
  reduplication or splitting of glomerular basal lamina, 39
  subendothelial deposits, complement, in GBL, 44
    immunoglobulin, diffuse and irregular, 42
    diffuse and linear, 43
  subepithelial deposits, 47, 48
Goodpasture's syndrome, 83(t). See also Disease, glomerular, of acute onset and rapid progression.
Gout, 174
Granulomatosis, Wegener's. See Wegener's granulomatosis.
Glycosuria, as sign of renal disease, 10

Heavy metal nephropathy, 171, 172
Hematuria, as sign of renal disease, 8
  benign recurrent, 157–160
    clinical features of, 157–158
    course and prognosis of, 158–160
    histologic features of, 32(t), 157, 158, 159
Hemolytic uremic syndrome, 271–279
  characteristics of, 271(t)
  course and prognosis of, 279
  histologic changes in, 272, 274–278
Henoch-Schönlein purpura, 265–269
  histologic changes in, 266–267, 268
Hyalin, deposits of, in renal blood vessels, 61

Hypercellularity, vascular, intimal cell, 56, 70
  medial cell, 57, 70
Hypertension, and slowly progressive renal vascular disease, 182–191
Hyperuricemia, tubulo-interstitial nephropathy in, 174

IgA disease. See Hematuria, benign recurrent.
Immune complex disease, 90, 90(t)
Immunoglobulin, deposits of, in glomeruli, intramembranous, 45
    mesangial, 49
    subendothelial, 42, 43
    subepithelial, 47, 48
  in renal blood vessels, 62
Infarction, renal, 133–137
  clinical features of, 134–135
  course and prognosis of, 136–137
  histologic changes in, 134, 135, 135, 136
Infiltrate, inflammatory, in vascular compartment, 58, 70
Inflammatory cells, in glomerular disease, 36
  in interstitium, 53, 66–68
Inflammatory infiltrate, in tubulo-interstitial compartment, 52, 66–67
  in vascular compartment, 58
Interstitium. See also Tubulo-interstitial compartment.
  appearance of in methacrylate- vs. paraffin-embedded specimens, 23
  histologic changes in, in systemic lupus erythematosus, 247, 250
  inflammatory cells in, 52, 66–68
Intimal cells, hypercellularity of, 56, 60, 70
Inulin, clearance of. See Clearance, inulin.

Kidney, acidifying ability of, correlation of with renal damage, 75, 76, 77
  biopsy of. See Biopsy.
  blood flow of. See Blood flow, renal; Vessels, blood, of kidney.
  concentrating ability of, as indicator of tubulo-interstitial disease, 74, 75, 77
  correlation of structure and function in, 71–78. See also Clearance; Glomerular filtration rate.
  cystic diseases of, 176–179
  diseases of. See Disease and names of specific disorders, such as Glomerulonephritis.
  clinical evaluation of, 6–12
  function of, 71–78. See also Glomerular filtration rate.

Kidney (*Continued*)
  function studies of, 9
  in systemic lupus erythematosus, 237–252
  transplantation of, 321–338
    and recurrence of original disease, 337–338
    rejection of, 323–338. See also *Rejection syndromes.*
  transplanted, biopsy of, 19–20
  tubulo-interstitial compartment of. See *Tubulo-interstitial compartment.*
  vascular compartment of. See *Vessel(s), blood, of kidney.*
Kimmelstiel-Wilson syndrome, 284

Lamina, basal. See *Basal lamina.*

Matrix, mesangial, of glomeruli, increase in, *41*
Medial cell hypercellularity, *57, 60,* 70
Medullary cystic disease, of kidney, 178–179, *179*
Membranoproliferative glomerulonephritis. See *Glomerulonephritis, membranoproliferative.*
Mesangial cells, hypercellularity of, in glomerular disease, 35
Mesangial disease, primary, 195–200
Methacrylate embedding, appearance of glomeruli in, 21, *22*
  appearance of interstitium in, 23
  appearance of tubules in, 23, *24*
  appearance of vessels in, 23, *26*
  comparison of with paraffin embedding, 25
Microcystic disease, 195–200
Micturition, changes in, as sign of renal disease, 7
Myeloma, multiple, 309–313
  clinical features of, 309–310, *312, 313*
  course and prognosis of, 311–313
  histologic changes in, 310–311, *312, 313*

Necrosis, and cytoplasmic swelling, of tubular epithelium, 51, *66*
  renal cortical, 137–139
    clinical features of, 137–138
    course and prognosis of, 138
    histologic changes in, 137, *137, 138*
Nephritic syndrome, acute, 83(t). See also *Disease, glomerular, of acute onset.*

Nephritis, acute diffuse interstitial, 124–126
  clinical features of, 124
  course and prognosis of, 125–126
  histologic changes in, 55(t), *124,* 125, *125*
  immunofluorescence of, 125, *125*
  hereditary, 160–163
    clinical features of, 160–161
    course and prognosis of, 163
    histologic changes in, 161–163, *162, 163*
  nephrosis with, 202
Nephropathy, Balkan, 180–181
  tubulo-interstitial, 165–181. See also *Disease, tubulo-interstitial.*
    analgesic abuse, 169–170, *170*
    conditions associated with, 165, 165(t)
    developmental, 176–179
    endemic, of Balkans, 180–181
    heavy metal, 171, *172*
    hereditary, 176–179, *179*
    in cystinosis, 175–176, *175, 176*
    in hyperuricemia, 174
    metabolic, 174–176
    radiation, 173
    toxic, 168–174
Nephrosclerosis, malignant, 127–133
  clinical features of, 128
  course and prognosis of, 132–133
  histologic changes in, 56(t), *128,* 129–131, *129–133*
Nephrosis, 83(t), 202. See also *Nephrotic syndrome, primary.*
Nephrotic syndrome, infantile, 195–200
  clinical features, 195–196
  course and prognosis of, 197–200
  histologic changes in, 39(t), 197, *198–199*
  primary, 201–232, 202(t)
    associated with systemic disease, 202, 202(t)
    classification of, 83(t)
    distinguishing features of, 204(t)
    membranoproliferative, 204(t), 205–208, 211–218, *212–215, 216, 217*
    characteristics of, 204(t), 211(t)
    minimal lesion, 203–205, 204(t), *206, 207*
    sclerosing, 204(t), 218–232, *220–222, 224–230.* See also *Sclerosis.*
    pure proliferative, 204(t), 205, *209, 210,* 217

Oliguria, as sign of renal disease, 7
Output, urinary, changes in, as sign of renal disease, 7

PAH. See *Clearance, para-amino-hippuric acid*.
Pain, as sign of renal disease, 8
Para-amino-hippuric acid, clearance of. See *Clearance, para-amino-hippuric acid*.
Paraffin embedding, appearance of glomeruli in, 22, 23
  appearance of interstitium in, 23
  appearance of tubules in, 23, *24*
  appearance of vessels in, 25, *26*
  comparison of with methacrylate embedding, 25
Polyarteritis nodosa, 253, 253(t), 258–264
  clinical features of, 258
  course and prognosis of, 263–264
  large vessel type, histologic changes in, 258–261, *259–261*
  microvascular form, histologic changes in, 258, 261–263, *262–263*
Polycystic disease, of kidney, 177–178
Poststreptococcal glomerulonephritis, acute, 83(t), 89. See also *Disease, glomerular, of acute onset*.
Pregnancy, renal disease of, 315–320. See also *Toxemia, of pregnancy*.
Progressive systemic sclerosis. See *Scleroderma*.
Proteinuria, as indicator of glomerular change, 78
  as sign of renal disease, 10
Purpura, Henoch-Schönlein, 265–269, *266–267*
  thrombotic thrombotocytopenic, 271(t), 280–283, *280, 281*
Pyelonephritis, chronic infectious, 167–168
Pyuria, as sign of renal disease, 10

Radiation nephropathy, 173
Radiography, in diagnosing renal disease, 10
Rejection syndromes, transplant, characteristics of, 325(t)
  early irreversible, 332–335, *333–334*
  early reversible, 325(t), 327–332, *328–331*
  immediate irreversible, 324–327, 325(t), *326, 327*
  late irreversible, 335–337, *336*
Renal failure, acute, 118–126
  major causes of, 118, 119(t)
Renal function studies, 9
Renal function tests, as indicators of renal damage, 71–78

Scleroderma, 294–300
  clinical features of, 294
  course and prognosis of, 298–300

Scleroderma (*Continued*)
  histologic changes in, 56(t), 295–298, *296–299*
Sclerosis, focal, 204(t), 218–219, *220–222*, 231
  focal and segmental, recurrence of after transplantation, 337
  membranous, 204(t), 218, 219–232, *224–230*
  progressive systemic. See *Scleroderma*.
Swan-neck lesion, 175, *175*
Systemic lupus erythematosus, 237–252
  clinical course and prognosis of, 247–252, 251(t)
  diffuse proliferative lesion of, 239–246, *242–246*, 251(t)
  focal proliferative lesion of, 239, *240, 241*, 251(t)
  histologic changes in, 36(t), 42(t), 238–247
  organs involved in, 238(t)
  sclerosing lesions of, 246–247, *248–249*, 251(t)

Thrombosis, renal vein, 134, *136*, 139–140. See also *Infarction, renal*.
Thrombotic thrombocytopenic purpura, 271(t), 280–283
  histologic changes in, *280–281*, 282
Toxemia, of pregnancy, 315–320
  clinical features of, 315–316
  course and prognosis of, 320
  histologic changes in, 34(t), 316–320, *316–319*
Transplantation, of kidney, 323–338
  and recurrence of original disease, 337–338
  transplant rejection and. See *Rejection syndromes*.
Tubules. See also *Tubulo-interstitial compartment*.
  appearance of in methacrylate- vs. paraffin-embedded specimens, 23, *24*
Tubulo-interstitial compartment, basal laminar thickening, 55, 68
  cellular changes in, 50–52, 66–68
  changes in, in amyloidosis, 303, *306*
  in diabetic glomerulosclerosis, 288, *289, 291*
  in early irreversible transplant rejection, 332, *333, 334*
  in early reversible transplant rejection, *329, 330*, 330
  in hemolytic uremic syndrome, 273, *276*
  in multiple myeloma, 311, *312, 313*
  in scleroderma, 295, *297*
  deposits in, 55

Tubulo-interstitial compartment (*Continued*)
  disease of, interpretation of biopsy specimens in, *50–55*, 65–68
  edema in, 53, 68
  extracellular material changes in, 53–55, 68
  interstitial fibrosis of, *54*, 68
  interstitial inflammatory changes in, *52*, 66–68
  normal structure, *67*
  tubular epithelium atrophy, *50*, *66*

Urination, frequency of, changes in, as sign of renal disease, 7
Urine, color of, change in, as sign of renal disease, 8
  osmolarity of, maximal, relationship of to interstitial disease, 74, 75, 77
  output of, changes in, as sign of renal disease, 7

Vascular compartment. See *Vessel(s), blood, of kidney.*
Vasculitis, clinical syndromes associated with, 253, 253(t)
Vein, renal, thrombosis of. See *Infarction, renal; Thrombosis, renal vein.*
Vessels, blood, appearance of, in methacrylate- vs. paraffin-embedded specimens, 23, *26*
  of kidney, basal lamina increase in intimal and medial cells, *60*, *70*
    cellular changes in, 56–58, 68–70
    changes in in diabetic glomerulosclerosis, 289, *290*, *291*

Vessels (*Continued*)
  blood, changes in in early irreversible transplant rejection, *332*, *334*
    changes in in early reversible transplant rejection, *330*, *331*
    changes in in hemolytic uremic syndrome, 273–279, *276–278*
    changes in in scleroderma, 295–298, *298*, *299*
    changes in in systemic lupus erythematosus, *247*, *250*
    diseases of. See *Diseases, vascular.*
    elastic laminar thickening and reduplication, *59*, *70*
    extracellular material changes, 59–62, *70*
    fibrin deposits in, *62*
    hyaline deposits in, *61*
    immunoglobulin deposits in, *62*
    in amyloidosis, 303, *306*
    in malignant nephrosclerosis, *132*, *133*
    in slowly progressive renal vascular disease, *188–191*
    in thrombotic thrombocytopenic purpura, *281*, *282*
    inflammatory infiltrate in, *58*, *70*
    intimal hypercellularity, *56*, *70*
    medial hypercellularity, *57*, *70*
    structure of, normal artery, *69*

Wegener's granulomatosis, 253–257
  clinical features of, 254
  course and prognosis of, 255
  histologic changes in, 254–255, *256–257*